HEALTH & WELLNESS SERIES

DIABETES
MEALS FOR GOOD HEALTH
COOKBOOK

THIRD EDITION

Complete Meal Plans & 100 Recipes

KAREN GRAHAM, RD, CDE
Registered Dietitian &
Certified Diabetes Educator

MANSUR SHOMALI, MD, CM
Endocrinologist & Diabetes Expert

Robert
ROSE

Diabetes Meals for Good Health Cookbook, Third Edition

Text copyright © 2020, 2012, 2008 Karen Graham, RD, CDE
Photographs and illustrations copyright © 2020, 2012, 2008 Durand & Graham, Ltd. *(except as listed below)*
Cover and text design copyright © 2020, 2012, 2008 Robert Rose Inc.

Some of the content of this book was previously published as *Meals for Good Health* (Paper Birch Publishing, 1998–2007).

Disclaimer

The suggestions and information contained in this publication are based on a thorough assessment of the latest research and information. Reasonable steps have been taken to ensure the accuracy of the information presented. However, we cannot ensure the safety or efficacy of any product or service described in this publication. Individuals are advised to consult a physician or other appropriate health care professional before undertaking any diet, exercise, activity or treatment program or taking any herb or medication referred to in this publication. Professionals must use and apply their own professional judgment, experience, and training and should not rely solely on the information contained in this publication before prescribing any diet, exercise, treatment or medication. While we thank the professional expertise of the reviewers of this publication, neither they nor the authors or publisher assumes any responsibility or liability for personal or other injury, loss or damage that may result from the suggestions or information in this publication.

The recipes in this book have been carefully tested by our kitchen and our tasters. To the best of our knowledge, they are safe and nutritious for ordinary use and users. For those people with food or other allergies, or who have special food requirements or health issues, please read the suggested contents of each recipe carefully and determine whether or not they may create a problem for you. All recipes are used at the risk of the consumer. For those with special needs, allergies, requirements or health problems, in the event of any doubt, please contact your medical adviser prior to the use of any recipe.

This book is not intended as a substitute for professional medical care. Only your doctor can diagnose and treat a medical problem.

Use of brand names is for educational purposes only and does not imply endorsement.

Library and Archives Canada Cataloguing in Publication

Title: Diabetes meals for good health cookbook : complete meal plans & 100 recipes / Karen Graham, RD, CDE,
  Registered Dietitian & Certified Diabetes Educator, Mansur Shomali, MD, CM, endocrinologist & diabetes expert.
Other titles: Diabetes meals for good health
Names: Graham, Karen, author. | Shomali, Mansur, author.
Description: Third edition. | Series statement: Health & wellness series | Includes index. | Originally published under the title:
  Diabetes meals for good health. Toronto : R. Rose, 2008. | Companion to Karen Graham's The complete diabetes guide.
Identifiers: Canadiana 20190234512 | ISBN 9780778806547 (softcover)
Subjects: LCSH: Diabetes—Diet therapy—Recipes. | LCGFT: Cookbooks.
Classification: LCC RC662 .G72 2020 | DDC 641.5/6314—dc23

Editor: Janice Madill, Easy English; and reviews on pages 1-42 by Joanne Seiff and Cathy Richards
Robert Rose Proof Editor: Kathleen Fraser
Indexer: Gillian Watts
Food Photographer (except as noted below): Brian Gould, Brian Gould Photography Inc.
Food Stylists: Judy Fowler and Katie Fowler
Production & Design Updates: Daniella Zanchetta & Joseph Gisini/PageWave Graphics Inc.
Cover Design: Kevin Cockburn/PageWave Graphics Inc.
Hand Illustrations (page 12): Sandi Storen
Nutrient Analysis: Barb Selley and Cathie Martin of Food Intelligence (2nd edition); and Karen Graham calculated the
  net carbs and any recipe and nutrient revisions in this 3rd edition. Canadian Nutrient File and USDA FoodData Central
  were primary sources of nutrient information.
Recipe Contributor Third Edition: Sally McKenney, Crabcakes (adapted with permission, page 108)

Additional Image Credits: Front cover: top photo © Andrew Lipsett; other images © Getty Images. Back cover: photo of Karen Graham © David McIlvride; photo of Dr. Shomali © Juliette Bogus. Breakfast photo on page 8 © Andrew Lipsett. Photos on pages: 4, 5, 6, 12, 14, 16, 17, 19, 21, 22, 24, 28, 33, 34, 41, 46, 58, 68, 78, 80, 82, 90, 92, 102, 117, 120, 125, 129, 132, 133, 136, 137, 140, 141, 144, 145, 149, 152, 153, 156, 157, 161, 164, 165, 168, 169, 176, 177, 180, 181, 184, 185, 188, 189, 192, 193, 197, 200, 201, 204, 205, 208, 212, 213, 216, 220, 221, 224, 225, 228, 229, 232, 233 (cardamom pods), 236, 237, 240, 244, 249, 252, 256, 257, 260, 261, 264, 265, 269, 271, 276, and 277 © Getty Images. Salt icon (pages 277–285) © Getty Images.

The publisher gratefully acknowledges the financial support of our publishing program by the Government of Canada through the Canada Book Fund.

Canada

Published by Robert Rose Inc.
120 Eglinton Avenue East, Suite 800, Toronto, Ontario, Canada M4P 1E2
Tel: (416) 322-6552 Fax: (416) 322-6936
www.robertrose.ca

Printed and bound in China

2 3 4 5 6 7 8 9 LEO 28 27 26 25 24 23 22 21

Contents

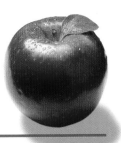

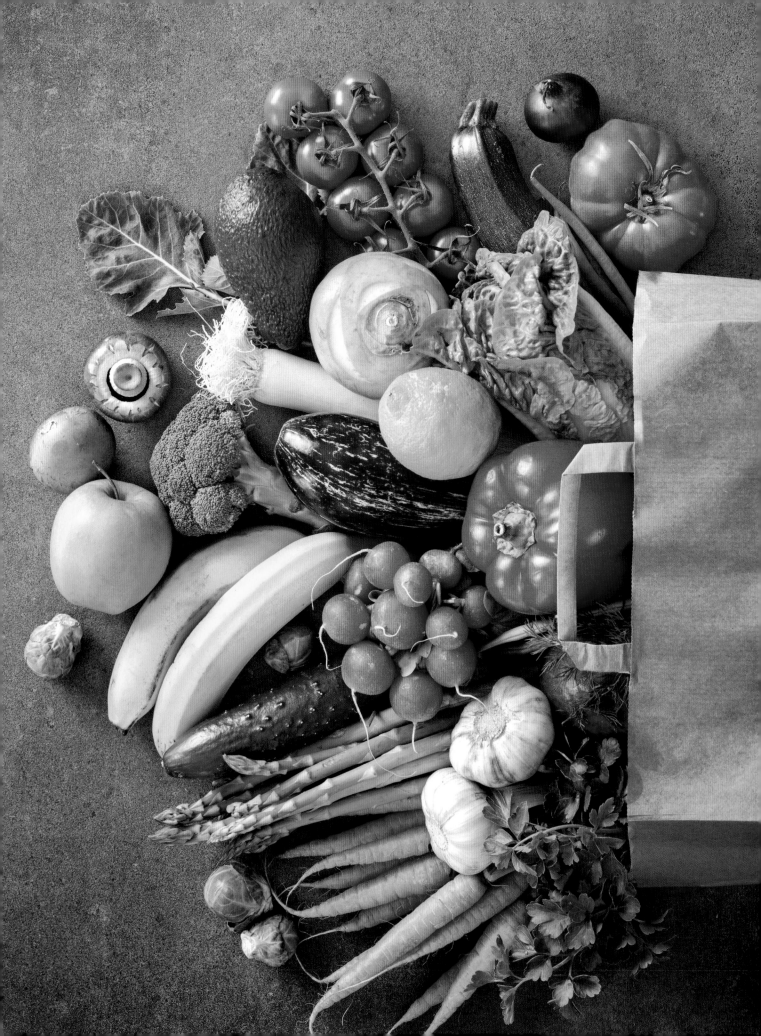

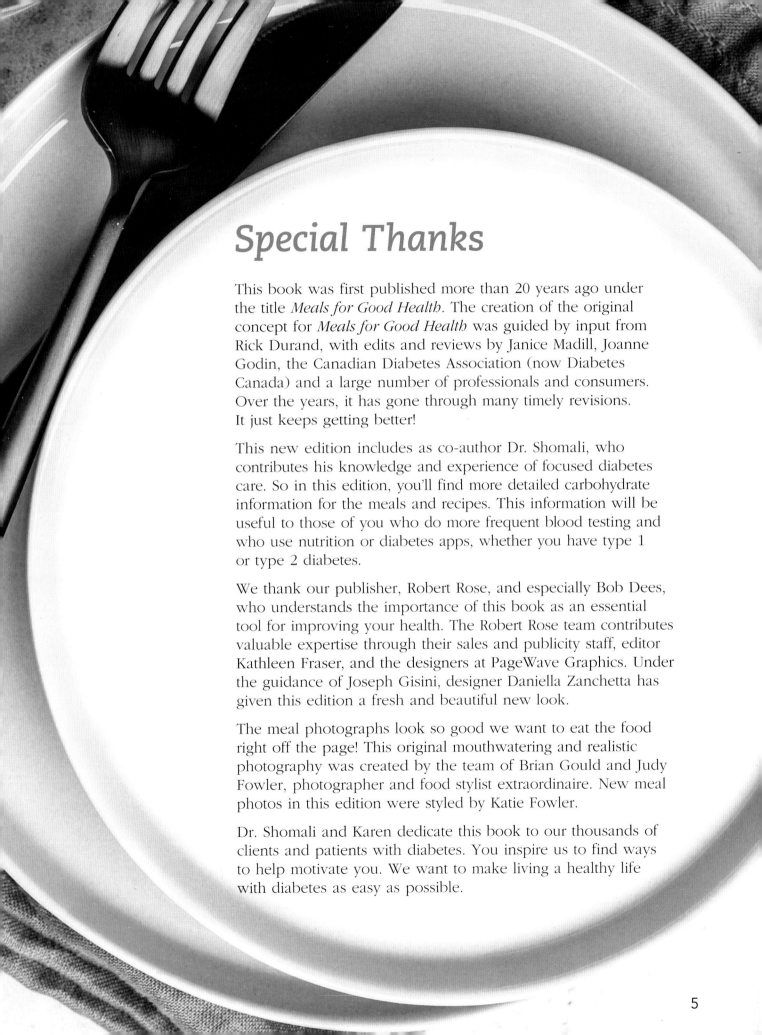

Special Thanks

This book was first published more than 20 years ago under the title *Meals for Good Health*. The creation of the original concept for *Meals for Good Health* was guided by input from Rick Durand, with edits and reviews by Janice Madill, Joanne Godin, the Canadian Diabetes Association (now Diabetes Canada) and a large number of professionals and consumers. Over the years, it has gone through many timely revisions. It just keeps getting better!

This new edition includes as co-author Dr. Shomali, who contributes his knowledge and experience of focused diabetes care. So in this edition, you'll find more detailed carbohydrate information for the meals and recipes. This information will be useful to those of you who do more frequent blood testing and who use nutrition or diabetes apps, whether you have type 1 or type 2 diabetes.

We thank our publisher, Robert Rose, and especially Bob Dees, who understands the importance of this book as an essential tool for improving your health. The Robert Rose team contributes valuable expertise through their sales and publicity staff, editor Kathleen Fraser, and the designers at PageWave Graphics. Under the guidance of Joseph Gisini, designer Daniella Zanchetta has given this edition a fresh and beautiful new look.

The meal photographs look so good we want to eat the food right off the page! This original mouthwatering and realistic photography was created by the team of Brian Gould and Judy Fowler, photographer and food stylist extraordinaire. New meal photos in this edition were styled by Katie Fowler.

Dr. Shomali and Karen dedicate this book to our thousands of clients and patients with diabetes. You inspire us to find ways to help motivate you. We want to make living a healthy life with diabetes as easy as possible.

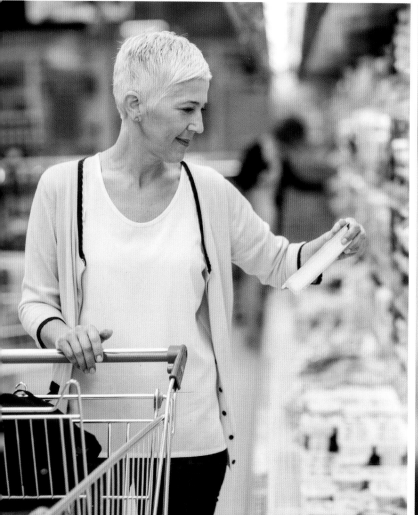
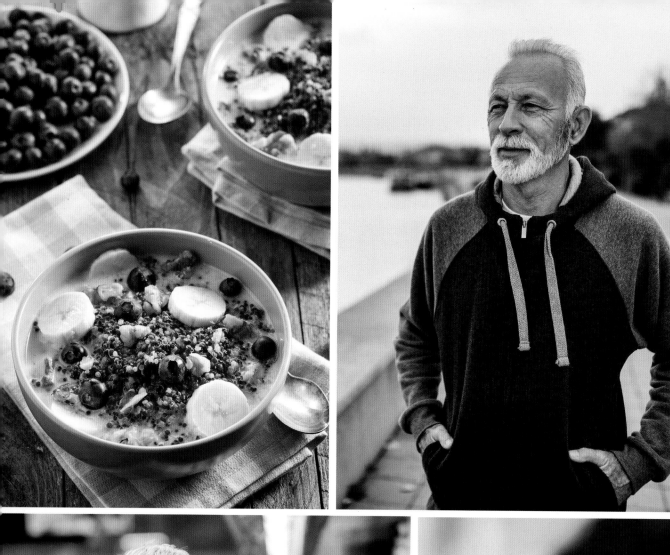
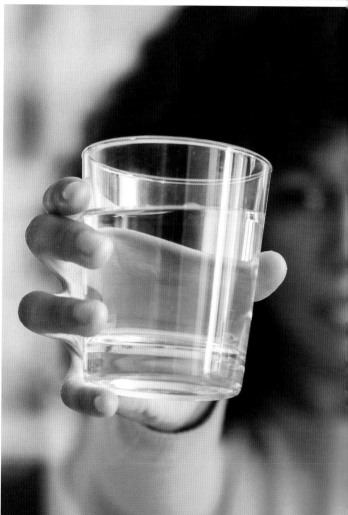

Ten Changes for Good Health

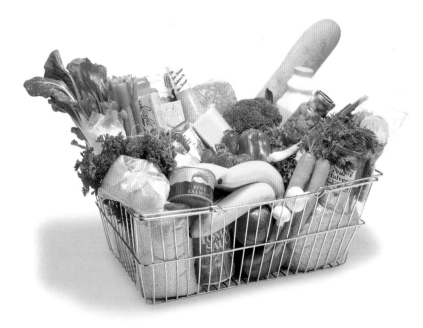

1. Eat Breakfast

People who eat breakfast find it easier to lose weight and keep it off. They are also more likely to get all of the nutrients they need each day for good health.

TAKE ACTION
- Start eating a small breakfast.
- Next, eat less in the evening.

Breakfast is the best way to start your day.

When you eat breakfast, you have more energy. Your body will "switch on" and start using up your fat. If you overeat in the evening, when you are less active, your body will store fat.

If you have a family at home, then gather and eat together. Research shows that eating meals together helps us connect with each other. This builds bonds and friendships and makes families stronger.

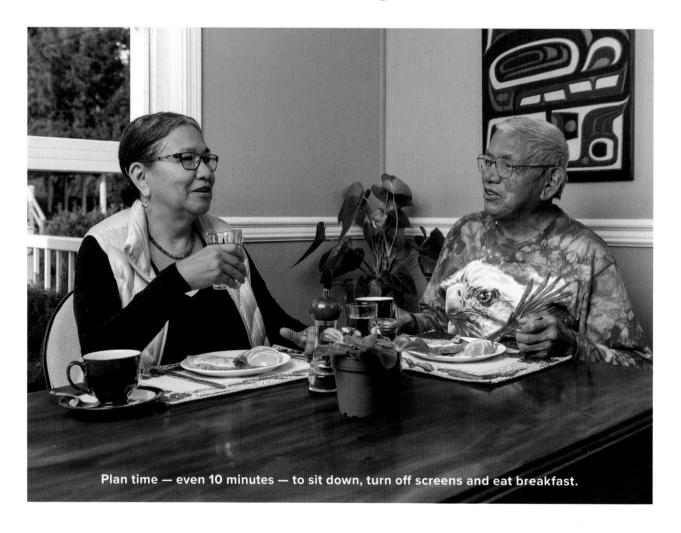

Plan time — even 10 minutes — to sit down, turn off screens and eat breakfast.

2. Eat Proper Portions

TAKE ACTION

- Choose either the small or large meal plans in this book. See *How to Use the Meal Plans* on pages 35–42.
- Divide your plate, and eat more vegetables!
- Choose meal portions the size of your hand.

Eat slowly to avoid overeating. Put down your fork, knife and spoon between bites. Drink water with your meals. Turn off the TV and other screens, and focus on what you are eating. Save leftovers for the next meal.

Use a smaller plate or bowl for meals

Your smaller portions of food will look like more on a smaller plate or bowl, and will feel more satisfying.

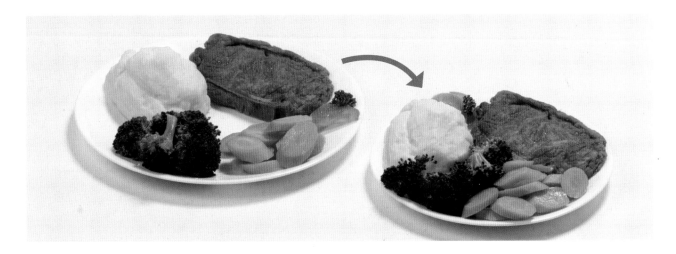

Divide Your Plate

Fill Up on Vegetables and Fruits

Vegetables and fruits are naturally low in fat and are full of fiber, vitamins and minerals. Eat more low-calorie vegetables, as listed on page 149. If you fill up on vegetables and fruits, you will find it easier to cut back on meats, fats, desserts and high-fat snack foods.

vegetables

starch | **protein**

This healthy balance of foods will fill you up but not load you down with calories.

Divide Your Plate

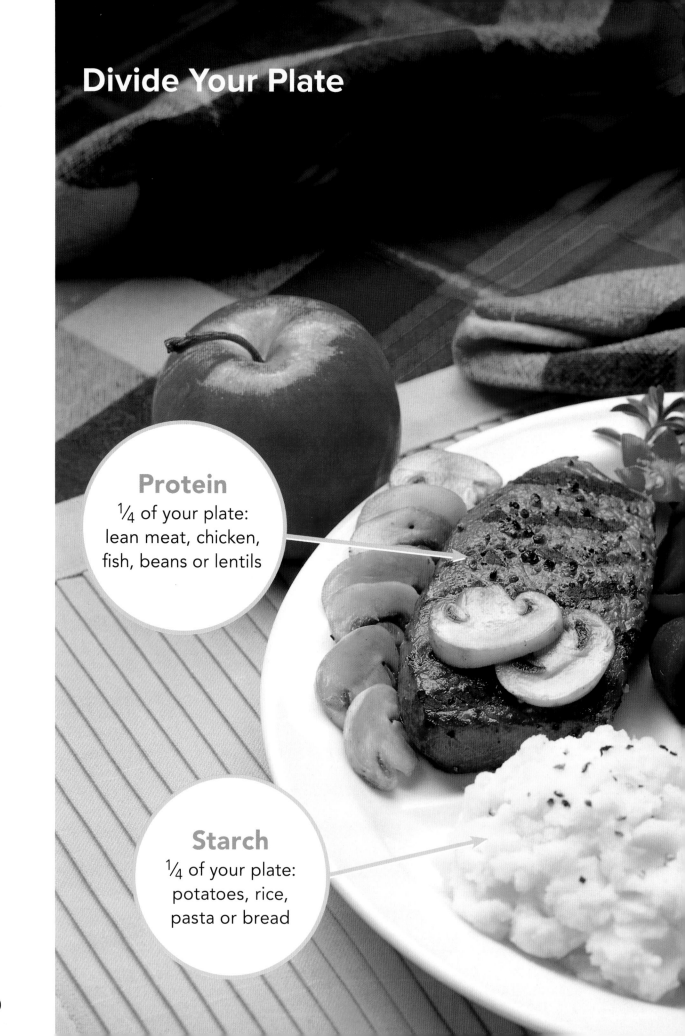

Protein
¼ of your plate:
lean meat, chicken,
fish, beans or lentils

Starch
¼ of your plate:
potatoes, rice,
pasta or bread

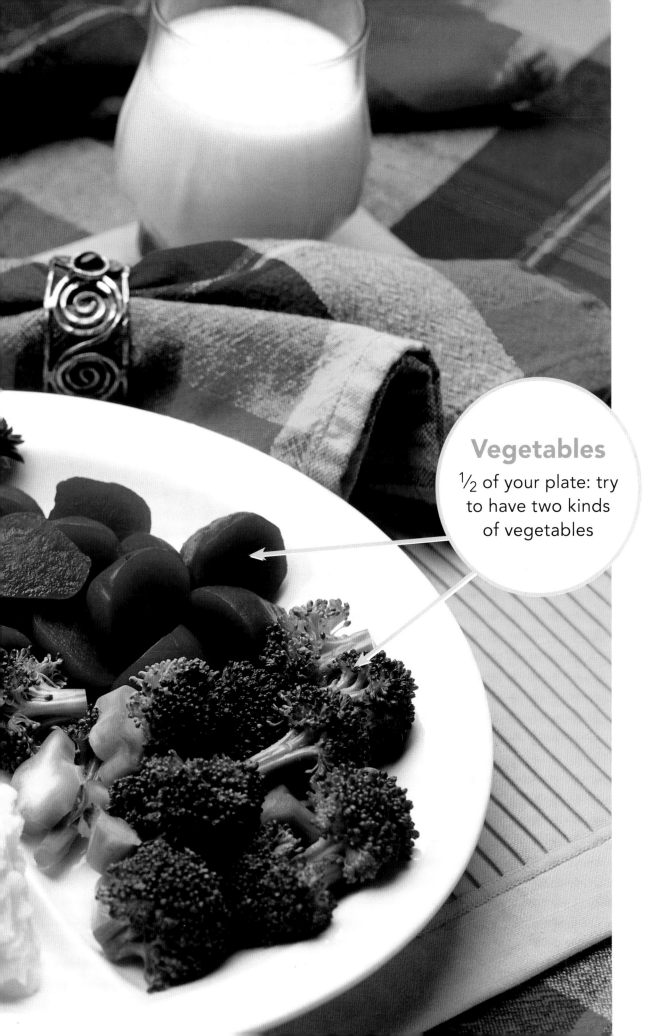

Vegetables

½ of your plate: try to have two kinds of vegetables

Choose Meal Portions the Size of Your Hand

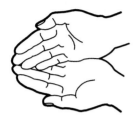

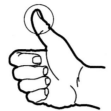

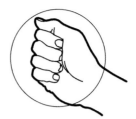

Vegetables and fruits: Fill your hands with these.

Fats and sugars: Use an end-of-thumb portion of oil, fat, butter or margarine and of sugar.

Grains and starches: Choose 1 to 2 fist-size portions of rice and other grains, bread and potatoes.

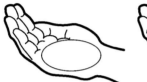

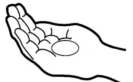

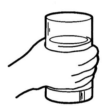

Protein: Choose one palm-size portion of chicken, meat, eggs, beans or lentils, *or* half a palm-size portion of nuts, seeds or cheese.

Drink water with every meal.

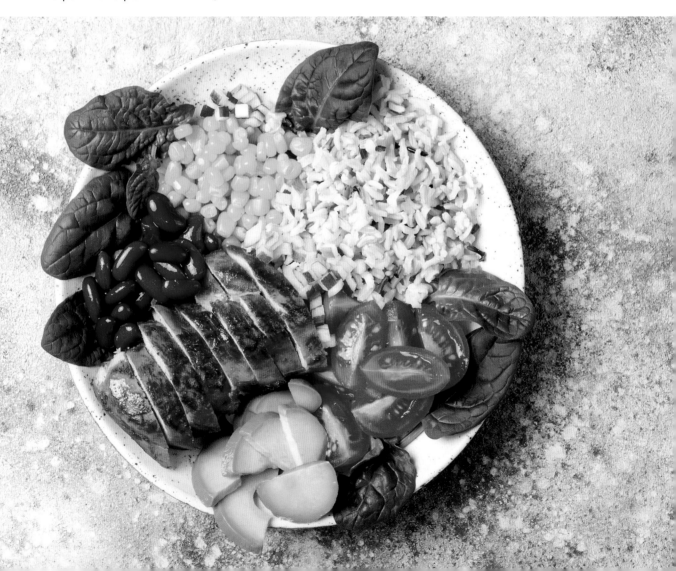

3. Eat a Variety of Foods

TAKE ACTION

- At each meal choose a variety of foods as shown in each of the meals in this book.
- Eat vegetables and fruits of different colors to get a variety of important nutrients.

Vegetables and Fruits

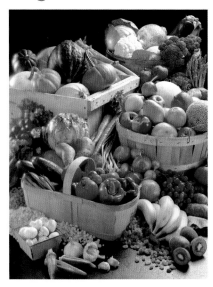

Grains and Starches

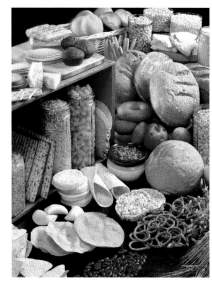

High-Fiber Foods

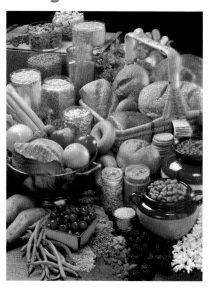

Calcium-Rich Foods

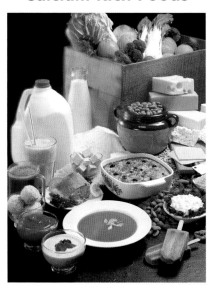

Proteins

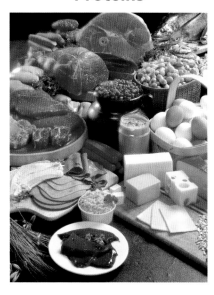

Healthy Fats

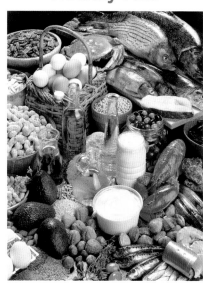

The North American diet has changed over the past century. We now eat fewer grains and starches and we eat more meat and processed foods. Processed foods add extra fat, sugar and salt to our diets. These additives are listed on food labels, so it's important to read the labels. We suffer from diseases such as diabetes, heart disease and cancer that are linked to these changes in our food choices.

Vegetables and Fruits

Fresh vegetables and fruits. These have no label. This means they have no added sugar, salt or fat.

Frozen vegetables and fruits. Check the label and choose frozen vegetables and fruits without added sugar, salt or fat.

Canned vegetables and fruits. Fruits canned in water or juice are a better choice than fruits canned in syrup. Vegetables canned in salt can be rinsed in water to remove about a third of the salt.

Limit your dried fruit portions. Dried fruit has more sugar than fresh fruit because the water has been taken out. For example, 2 tbsp (30 mL) of raisins have 4 tsp (16 g) of sugar, the same as ½ cup (125 mL) of grapes.

When you are hungry between meals, eating a vegetable or a fruit is better than eating a high-fat snack food or a rich dessert. You will find a variety of snack choices on pages 278–285.

FOOD FACT

Vegetables and fruits give you energy. They are low in fat. They add vitamins, minerals and extra fiber to your diet. They help reduce your risk for cancer.

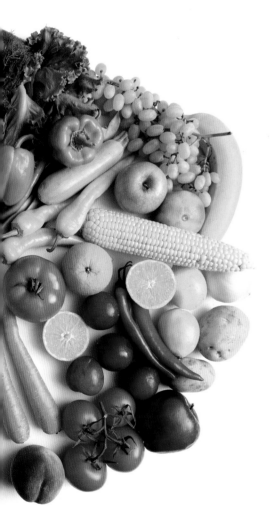

HEALTH TIP

Eat the whole fruit or vegetable — don't juice it.
Juice raises your blood sugar faster than whole fruit or vegetables. It is also not as filling, so it's easier to have too much. One cup (250 mL) of apple juice is equivalent to 2 apples and 1 cup of carrot juice is equal to 2 carrots.

1 cup of apple juice = 28 grams of carbohydrate
1 cup of beet juice = 24 grams of carbohydrate
1 cup of carrot juice = 14 grams of carbohydrate

Limit Juice

- You may be surprised to learn that "unsweetened" fruit juices have sugar.
- One cup (250 mL) of unsweetened apple, orange or grapefruit juice has 6 to 7 teaspoons of natural sugar, which is equal to 24 to 28 grams of carbs.
- One cup (250 mL) of grape and prune juice have almost 10 teaspoons of sugar, which is equal to 40 grams of carbs.
- Since juice has less fiber and is not as filling as fresh fruit, it is easy to drink too much.
- Vegetable juices, such as tomato juice, have less sugar than fruit juices but often contain more salt.

Check how much your drinking glasses hold. Unless you are drinking water, use the smaller glasses. The glasses of apple juice seen below don't really look that different, but the glass on the right holds *three times as much*. That means an extra 7 teaspoons (or 28 grams) of sugar! A 16 oz (about 500 mL) bottle of juice from a vending machine can have 15 teaspoons of sugar.

FOOD FACT

If you drink a lot of juice, it will be harder for you to lose weight and your blood sugar will go up.

Eating fresh fruit instead of drinking juice should be your everyday choice. Fresh fruit has more fiber than juice and is more filling.

Portion sizes of unsweetened apple juice

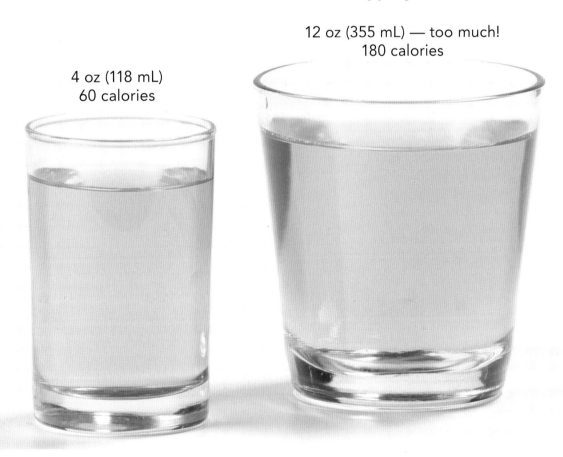

12 oz (355 mL) — too much!
180 calories

4 oz (118 mL)
60 calories

FOOD FACT

Good for the environment
When you fill up more of your plate with grains, starches, vegetables and fruits, you eat lower on the food chain. This means these foods are less damaging to the environment than a low-carb diet, which typically includes lots of meat.

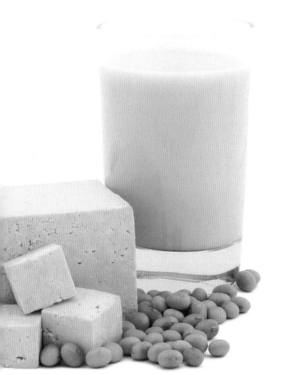

Choose Whole Grains

Whole grains such as whole wheat or rye, oats, barley, brown rice, bulgur, quinoa, couscous and corn contain fiber. Fiber is a natural laxative. It may help reduce your risk for colon cancer and help lower your blood cholesterol and blood sugar. It's good food for your healthy gut bacteria. Fiber helps you feel full and can help you lose weight.

Calcium-Rich Foods

Calcium is a mineral that makes your bones and teeth strong. It is found in milk and foods made from milk, such as yogurt and cheese, as well as in dried beans and soft fish bones. Vitamin D helps calcium work. This vitamin is found in fatty fish. It is also added to milks and some milk products.

Infants and growing children need extra calcium as their bones and teeth grow. Many people believe that milk and other calcium foods are just for kids. The truth is, we need calcium and vitamin D all our adult life to keep our bones strong.

Skim or 1% milk and yogurt are lower-fat choices.

You can get your daily calcium from other foods too. Try:

- tofu made with added calcium
- fortified soy drinks. These have the same protein and calcium as cow's milk; buy unsweetened.
- cashew, almond, rice or coconut beverages. They don't have very much protein, so if choosing these, read labels carefully to make sure they have added calcium and vitamin D and are unsweetened (no added sugar).
- beans, such as baked beans
- seeds and nuts, such as almonds and sesame seeds
- fish bones, such as those in canned salmon
- dark green, leafy vegetables, such as broccoli, Brussels sprouts, okra, kale and Chinese cabbage
- a few fruits, such as dried figs and oranges

Proteins

Vegetable proteins

- Tofu, made from soy beans, is a good meat replacement.
- Fortified soy drinks contain protein.
- Nuts, including peanuts and peanut butter, and seeds, such as sunflower seeds, are a good source of healthy fats.
- Kidney beans, brown beans, chickpeas and dried peas are low in fat and high in fiber.
- There are smaller amounts of vegetable protein in whole-grain breads and oatmeal than in the foods listed above.

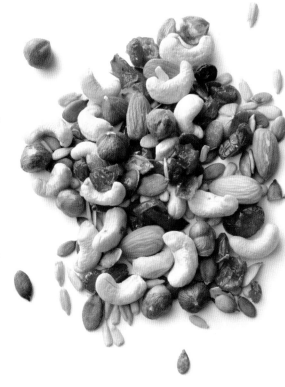

Animal proteins

Lean meats are a good protein choice. Remember to remove the skin from chicken and turkey. Lean hamburger, round roast or steak, lamb, goat, pork, deer, rabbit, bison and caribou are also good choices. Take care to trim off the fat and avoid eating it.

Eggs are an excellent source of protein to choose instead of meat. (See page 20, *Cholesterol in food*.)

Fish: Try to eat fish at least twice a week. Ocean perch, red snapper, cod, haddock, sole, shrimp and lobster are low-fat fish. Light tuna, pink salmon and sardines canned in water are good choices too. Bluefish is a medium-fat fish. The fattier fishes are lake trout or red (sockeye) salmon. The fattier fishes offer the best source for healthy omega-3 fat.

Dairy: Milk and milk products, especially cheese and Greek yogurt, are a good source of protein. Cheese has more salt than lean meats, eggs or fish but usually less salt than processed meats.

DOCTOR'S TIP

Fish is an important part of a healthy diet. However, if you are pregnant, check with your doctor or health care provider about how much fish you can eat. High levels of pollution in fresh and salt water habitats can contaminate fish and may harm a growing infant.

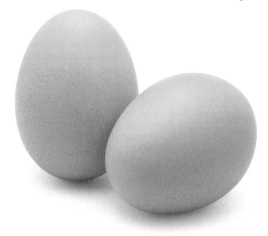

Healthy Fats

Good Choices

Polyunsaturated and monounsaturated fats are found in:

Vegetable oils

- Common vegetable oils include canola, olive, peanut, corn, soybean, safflower and sunflower seed oil.
- Specialty oils are made from avocado, pumpkin seeds, walnuts, macadamia nuts, grape seeds, sesame seeds, hemp seeds, flax seeds and wheat germ.
- Some oils such as virgin olive oil, will say "cold pressed" on the label. These are often the most expensive, but the healthier fats are better preserved in these oils.
- Choose soft tub non-hydrogenated margarines or salad dressings that are made from these oils.

Whole foods

- Avocados, olives and olive oil are rich in monounsaturated fats; these fats can help reduce blood cholesterol.
- Nuts such as walnuts, almonds, hazelnuts, pecans, peanuts and pistachios contain both kinds of fat.
- Seeds such as sunflower, sesame and flax seeds are sources of healthy fats.

Best Choices

Omega-3 fat is a type of polyunsaturated fat that is healthy for your brain and eyes. Research shows it may lower your risk for heart attacks and stroke because it lowers triglycerides (blood fat) and helps keep blood from clotting.

Fish, especially cold water ocean fish, is the best source of omega-3 fats. Fish can also contain some omega-6 fat, monounsaturated fat or smaller amounts of saturated fat. Fish is rich in selenium, B vitamins and vitamin D.

Omega-3 fat is found in:
- sardines, salmon, trout, bass, mackerel, herring, anchovies, sturgeon, halibut and tuna
- shellfish such as shrimp, lobster, clams, oysters, mussels and snow crab
- ground flax seed (flaxseed meal) or flaxseed oil and pumpkin seeds
- non-hydrogenated canola oil or soybean oil, or the margarines or salad dressings made from these oils
- walnuts
- omega-3 fortified products such as eggs, yogurt, milk and cheese (check for omega-3 on labels)
- soy nuts, soybeans, soy flour or wheat germ

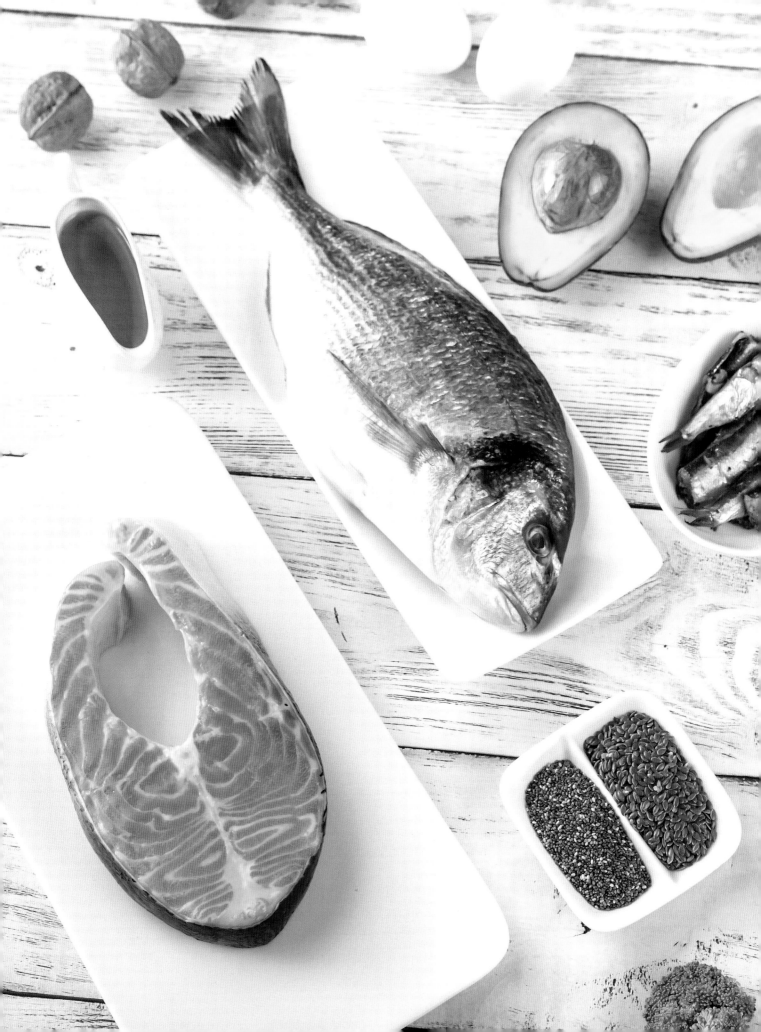

4. Eat Less Saturated Fat

FOOD FACT

Banned Trans Fats

Trans fats are man-made from vegetable oils. Because they have a long shelf life, they were used in many food products. But they are bad for our blood vessels and heart. In 2018, they were banned in most commercial foods.

This ban is good. But, keep in mind that today's food products can still be high in saturated fats. Unhealthy palm oil is now frequently being added to food products.

HEALTH TIP

All fats (saturated fats and healthy fats) are high in calories. So regardless of the type of fat you eat, if you eat too much and then put on weight, this will make your blood sugar and cholesterol go higher. Practice moderation: a teaspoon or two of olive oil to a salad or potato, not several tablespoons.

TAKE ACTION

- Eat less meat, butter, cream, bacon and fried foods.
- Eat fewer processed foods.

Eating less saturated fat helps to reduce cholesterol and keep your heart and blood vessels healthy, and lowers your risk for some kinds of cancer.

Saturated fat is found in:

- lard, butter, and meat gravy
- meats such as beef, pork, lamb, skin-on chicken and turkey
- processed meats such as bacon, bologna, wieners, salami, sausages, liverwurst and canned meats
- eggs, high-fat hard cheese and cottage cheese, cream cheese, cream, high-fat sour cream, high-fat yogurts and whole milk
- ice cream, chocolate, cookies and baked goods
- deep-fried foods and fast foods such as french fries, fried chicken, hamburgers and hot dogs
- coconut, coconut oil, palm oil and ghee (clarified butter)

Some early evidence suggests that coconut oil or ghee may help raise good cholesterol, but we lack studies to help us understand the risks or benefits to the heart when they are eaten over many years. We do know that evidence shows that unsaturated oils are healthful. See page 18.

The meals in this book lower saturated fat by limiting portions of meats and added fats. Lean meats are mostly offered rather than fried and deep-fried meats. Rich desserts and high-fat snacks are limited, and lighter choices are suggested.

Cholesterol in food

If your blood cholesterol is high, don't eat liver and other organ meats more than once a month. People used to be told they couldn't eat eggs if their cholesterol was high. Yet eggs are a great source of protein and other nutrients, and are a lower-cost protein food. So, if you choose a lean meat or reduced meat diet, then, if you want, go ahead and have an egg breakfast a few times a week. You can also include eggs as part of a lunch and dinner meal during the week.

5. Drink More Water

TAKE ACTION
- Aim for six to eight glasses of water a day.
- Keep your water glass or water bottle handy.

Water is the best calorie-free drink. Dietitians suggest getting about eight glasses of water a day. Eight glasses equals a 2 qt. (2 L) plastic soft drink bottle. Many of us get most of our water in our coffee, tea, juice or soft drinks each day. Our bodies don't need all the caffeine or sugar in these drinks. Drink less coffee, tea and diet soft drinks, and skip the juice and regular pop.

Your body needs water to work properly. Water helps the body break down stored fat. Water helps keep you regular. It helps clear your urine and reduce your risk of urinary tract infections. Drinking water helps replace fluids when you exercise.

Some tips to help you start drinking more water
Remind yourself
Often we simply forget to drink water. If you like water cold, keep a bottle or jug of water in the fridge. Keep a water glass on your table or desk. When you see the jug or glass, you will remember to drink water.

Drink water in the morning
We are naturally thirsty when we first wake up. Drink water first thing in the morning.

Drink water with meals
Get into the habit of drinking water with all your meals and snacks. Add a slice of lemon to your water for a fresh taste.

Drink water whenever you feel hungry
Water fills your stomach so you feel full and eat less.

HEALTH TIP

If you are a smaller body size, you may need only six glasses daily, whereas if you are a larger size, you may need more than eight glasses. Your need for water and other fluids increases in warm weather, with exercise and when your blood sugar is up.

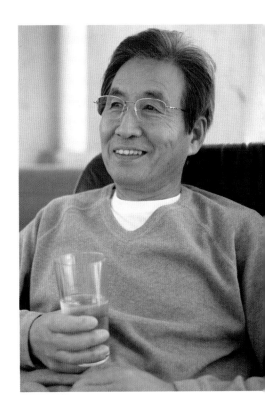

6. Limit Sweet Drinks and Sugars

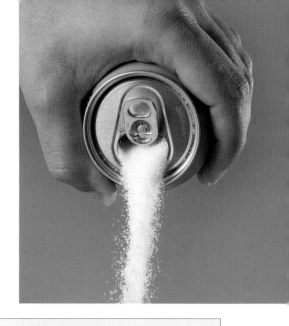

TAKE ACTION

- Drink fewer soft drinks, fruit juices and other sweetened beverages.
- Read labels and choose less sugary processed foods.
- Enjoy fresh fruit and small, light desserts.

Teaspoons of sugar in a 16-ounce (2 cups/500 mL) serving of a beverage

Different brands have different amounts of sugar or carbohydrate in them. Check labels and the serving size. One teaspoon (5 mL) of sugar (or other carbohydrate) is equal to 4 grams.

21 to 34 teaspoons (84 to 136 grams carbs)	• Vitamin Water Essential • Gatorade energy drink • Triple Thick Shake or Fruit Smoothie Supreme • Frappuccino malt coffee • Prune juice, unsweetened
16 to 20 teaspoons (64 to 80 grams carbs)	• Boost Original or Ensure • Commercial shakes or fruit smoothies • Cranberry juice cocktail • Pineapple juice or grape juice, both unsweetened • Eggnog, non-alcoholic • Instant Breakfast, regular, made with sugar
11 to 15 teaspoons (44 to 60 grams carbs)	• Colas (Coke and Pepsi), cream soda, fruit drinks or Tang • Many energy drinks • Iced specialty coffees • Orange juice or apple juice, both unsweetened • Slushes or Slurpees • Chocolate milk • Rice or soy beverage (sugar varies), both sweetened
7 to 10 teaspoons (28 to 40 grams carbs)	• Grapefruit juice, unsweetened • Iced tea, made from instant powder with sugar • Instant Breakfast, made with milk, no sugar added • Powerade sports drink • Kool-Aid made with sugar • Mountain Dew, Sprite, ginger ale or tonic water • Boost Diabetic, Ensure Diabetes or Glucerna
3 to 6 teaspoons (12 to 24 grams carbs)	• White milk • Tomato juice or V8 • Sweetened (flavored) instant coffee powders; caffe latte
No Sugar	• Tap water, plain bottled water, mineral water or soda water • Diet and "zero" soft drinks, Sugar Free Kool-Aid, Sugar Free Tang, Crystal Light, Vitamin Water Zero or Gatorade Zero • Tea, herbal tea, perked or instant coffee, no sugar added

Limit Sweet Drinks

We drink a lot of sugar every day. High-sugar drinks include fruit drinks, fruit juice, sweetened coffees, regular soft drinks, sweetened crushed ice drinks, chocolate milk and milk shakes. One cup (250 mL) of unsweetened fruit juice or 1 cup of regular soft drink has about 7 tsp (35 mL) of sugar, which adds 28 g of carbohydrate and 110 calories. Instead, choose water or diet drinks.

Limit pure sugars

We need to limit pure sugars — white sugar, brown sugar, icing sugar, corn syrup, maple syrup, molasses and honey. One type of pure sugar is not better or worse than another. These pure sugars give us calories we don't need and very little nutrition. Such sugars are called "empty calories."

Desserts

Sugars, and often fats, are packed into all our favorite desserts: cakes, cookies, pies, tarts, donuts, muffins, chocolates and candies. This is what makes them so tasty and why it is often so hard to stop at one. Grocery stores sell these goodies in supersize servings. How to resist? Don't linger in the parts of the grocery store when they sell these products. Plan to skip dessert if you eat out. Buy these less often and then you won't eat them.

Processed foods

Most processed foods contain sugar. In fact, it is hard to find a food label without sugar on the ingredient list. If sugar is the first ingredient, it means the food has more sugar than anything else. Try to limit these sugary foods.

Other types of sugar

You may see words such as sucrose, fructose, sorbitol and mannitol on food labels. Sucrose and fructose are pure sugars and they are not low-calorie. Sorbitol and mannitol are types of sugars, called sugar alcohols. These have fewer calories than table sugar, but they aren't sugar-free. They raise the blood sugar more slowly, but may cause gas and bloating.

Cookies, candies and chocolates made with sorbitol may be higher in fat and calories than regular kinds. Check the labels.

HEALTH TIP

Sugar is found naturally in fruits, some vegetables and even milk. Starches found in breads and cereals change into sugar after you eat them. The sugar in these foods gives you energy. These foods also have many other nutrients. These foods are good for you in the amounts shown in the meals and snacks.

Enjoy the lighter dessert choices and recipes in this book. You'll find more light desserts in our other books in this *Health & Wellness* series (see back cover).

FOOD CHARTS

See the charts on page 292 for information on sugar in cereals.

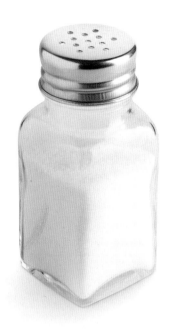

7. Limit Salt and Alcohol

TAKE ACTION

- Eat out less often in restaurants and eat less of processed foods. These foods are often loaded in salt.
- Drink less alcohol.

Limit salt

Cutting back on salt is a good healthy change for everyone. The benefits of cutting back on salt are many and can include:
- reduced high blood pressure
- reduced swelling in your legs and feet
- less work for your kidneys (which is so important if you have chronic kidney disease)

To cut back on salt

Eat less of:
- take-out and restaurant meals
- frozen ready-to-eat meals
- ham, bacon and deli meats
- ready-made scones, biscuits and muffins
- canned foods with salt added
- canned and packaged soups and broths
- table salt added to your food or recipes

Eat more of:
- homemade meals made with whole foods and less salt
- low-sodium or unsalted foods, such as unsalted soda crackers
- fresh or frozen vegetables
- brands with less sodium — check the amount of sodium per serving on the Nutrition Facts label
- seasonings other than salt during cooking and at the table: try black pepper, spices and herbs, garlic powder, lemon juice, lime juice or vinegar. (Try the Spice Mix on page 140.)

DOCTOR'S TIP

Other changes that can reduce high blood pressure:

- Drink less alcohol.
- Find ways to better manage your stress.
- Choose more potassium-rich foods, such as vegetables and fruits.
- Eat less saturated fat — choose low fat dairy and lean meats — and include fish and nuts as a source of healthy fat
- Walk or do other exercise regularly.
- Lose weight (if you are overweight); even a few pounds can help.

- Quit smoking or smoke less.
- Take your blood pressure medications as advised by your doctor and have your blood pressure checked regularly.

There are many things on this list. Look for just one thing that you could focus on first. Maybe the time is right to go for a daily walk. Or schedule 10 minutes during each day for quiet relaxation to help manage stress.

Salt in the recipes in this book

Salt enhances flavors and is needed for rising of baked goods. Some of our recipes include salt, baking powder, baking soda, bouillon, soy sauce or seasoning salt, but used in lesser amounts than standard recipes.

The meals also include some salty foods, such as dill pickles, sauerkraut, sausages, ham and wieners. In the portions shown, these foods can be part of a healthy diet if eaten occasionally (once or twice a month).

If you need to cut out more salt, choose:
- sliced cucumber instead of a dill pickle
- plain cabbage instead of sauerkraut
- unsalted beef or pork instead of sausages or wieners
- leftover cooked meat or chicken, or an egg instead of processed meat on sandwiches
- reduced or no-salt broths
- salt-free seasoning mixes

FOOD CHARTS

The charts on pages 291–317 show you how much salt is added to processed and restaurant foods.

HEALTH TIP

Once you start to cut back on salt, you will notice that many processed and restaurant foods begin to taste too salty.

Limit alcohol

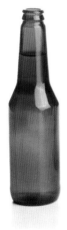
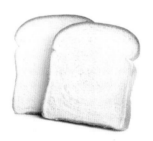

One beer or 2 ounces (60 mL) of hard liquor, such as whisky or rum, has about the same number of calories as two slices of bread.

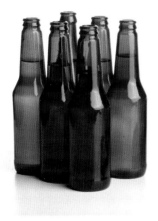
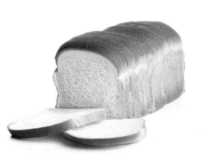

Six beers have 900 calories, equal in calories to about a loaf of bread. That's a lot. Six diet soft drinks have only 20 calories.

CAUTION!

- Alcohol is not recommended for children and teenagers, and women who are pregnant or breastfeeding.
- Always talk to your doctor or pharmacist about how your medications react with alcohol.
- If you take insulin or diabetes pills, drinking alcohol can cause a low blood sugar episode. To avoid this problem, don't drink; or limit yourself to one or two drinks and have something to eat with your drink.
- Alcohol increases your risk of getting cancer, especially liver and breast cancer.
- Even one drink a day increases a woman's risk for breast cancer. The more you drink, the more likely you are to get breast cancer.

Alcohol is high in calories. If you want to lose weight, you must look at everything you eat and drink, including alcohol. Like sugar, alcohol is full of "empty calories". Mostly we don't include alcohol with the meals or snacks in this book, but it can be an occasional choice. You might enjoy a glass of wine or bottle of beer with a meal, or perhaps a drink before a meal or in the evening. Any of these choices have similar calories. Drink alcohol on a daily basis only if your doctor advises it.

The calories in hard liquor, such as whisky, come from the alcohol alone. Three-quarters of the calories in beer comes from the alcohol with the rest coming mostly from sugar. In liqueurs, just over half the calories come from alcohol and the rest come from sugar.

To reduce calories from alcoholic drinks:

- Drink less beer, wine, liqueurs, coolers, ciders and hard liquor. Instead drink water, diet beverages, no-alcohol low-calorie beer, or coffee or tea.
- Choose a light or extra-light beer, which has less sugar and less alcohol than regular beer.
- Instead of drinking a whole beer, have just half a beer and mix it with diet ginger ale.
- Read the labels on no-alcohol beers and no-alcohol wines; most have sugar (though usually less sugar than soft drinks) but are still a better choice than regular beer that has alcohol.
- If you want to have a glass of wine, choose dry wine. This has less sugar than sweet wine.
- Avoid liqueurs, which are heavy on alcohol and sugar.
- If you choose to have a drink of hard liquor, mix it with a diet soft drink or water, instead of juice or regular soft drink.
- Drink water before and with your meals, instead of alcohol. Alcohol often makes you feel hungrier.

Alcohol is more than just a source of calories; it is an addictive drug. If you drink too much alcohol, it will affect more than your weight. Alcohol will make it hard to make other changes in your life.

Drinking less alcohol or quitting drinking can be a difficult choice, but help is available.

8. Read Labels for Home Cooking

TAKE ACTION

- Choose foods with less added sugar;
  1 tsp of sugar = 1 tsp of carbohydrate = 4 grams
- Choose foods with less fat: 1 tsp of fat = 5 grams

Read Nutrition Facts labels so you know what you are eating. Plan your shopping trip carefully. Use a list so you buy healthy foods. If you are hungry when you go grocery shopping, you will be easily tempted to buy the high-fat and high-sugar snacks. Try to go shopping after you've had something to eat. Remember, whatever you buy, you or your family will eat. You don't need to buy more cookies, ice cream and chips just because you've eaten them all up.

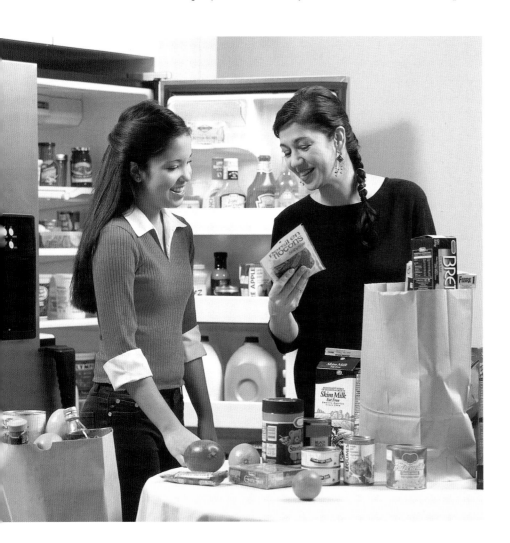

FOOD CHARTS

You'll find lots of shopping tips in the charts on pages 291–317.

HEALTH TIP

Limit Restaurant Meals

When you cook meals at home, *you* control the ingredients and portion size.

When you eat in a restaurant, you lose some of that control. Portions are most often large and high in fat, sugar and salt. It is hard for anyone to refuse these big servings. One good solution is to eat less often in restaurants and more often at home. When you do eat out, go online and check the calories of the menu items. Compare the restaurant calories and nutrients to those of the meals in this book (see page 37).

READING FOOD LABELS

Food labels list the amount of carbohydrates and sugar in grams

Four grams (4 g) of carbohydrate will break down into about 1 tsp (5 mL) of sugar, whether it comes from grains and starches or pure sugar. For example, 20 grams of carbs divided by 4 equals 5 teaspoons of sugar.

The "sugars" listing on a label separates the pure sugar from the grains and starches part of the carbohydrate. Both starch and sugar will end up as sugar in your blood stream. Sugars on the food label also includes natural sugars such as those from fruits, vegetables or milk. Rather than focusing on sugar alone, look at the total carbohydrate. From this number, subtract the fiber to get the net carbs (see page 39).

- A 355 ml can of cola has 39 g of total carbohydrate; of those, 39 g are sugars (10 tsp/50 mL) and 0 g fiber. The net carbs are therefore 39 g.
- A granola bar with 21 grams of carbohydrate, 8 g of sugars and 1 g fiber has 20 g net carbs, because 21 minus 1 equals 20.

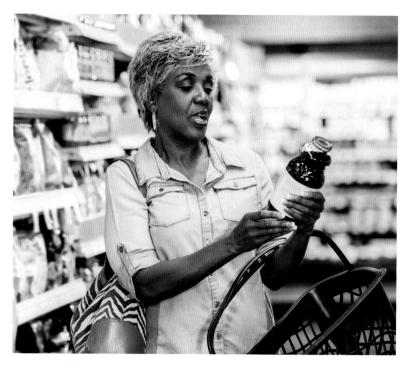

"My goodness, this juice has a lot of natural sugar!"

CAUTION

- When fat is reduced, the food loses flavor so more sugar may be added.
- When a food contains less sugar, more fat may be added.
- Extra salt may be added in low-sugar or low-fat products.

These are sneaky changes. You won't know unless you look at the nutrient label.

HEALTH TIPS

When grocery shopping, try to avoid the aisles most tempting for you, especially the bakeshop, potato chips, cookie or ice cream aisles. Spend more time in the fruits and vegetable aisles.

A food that has fewer than 20 calories in a serving is so low in calories that it will not have an effect on your weight.

READING FOOD LABELS

Food labels list the amount of fat in grams

Five grams (5 g) of fat is the same as 1 tsp (5 mL) of fat. On labels, serving sizes will vary. If one serving of three crackers has 5 g of fat, you will eat a whole teaspoon of fat when you eat those three crackers. That is a lot of hidden fat. A serving of three to five crackers with 2 g of fat or less would be a better choice.

Milks

Today there are so many kinds of milk sold. Cow's milk and fortified soy beverage have calcium and vitamin D. They also contain a good combination of protein and other nutrients essential for healthy bones and teeth. Skim and 1% milk have less saturated fat than 2% or whole milk and are healthy choices. Choose unsweetened soy beverage.

Almond, cashew or rice beverages have little protein and may not have the same amount of vitamins and minerals as milk or soy beverage. If you are buying these, make sure they are fortified with calcium and vitamin D, and are unsweetened.

Yogurts

Yogurt varieties have different amounts of fat and sugar. If available, choose 0%, 1% or 2%. If flavored, sugar will be added unless a low-calorie sweetener like sucralose or aspartame replaces some or all of the added sugar. "Plain" means no sugar has been added, making this a good choice. You can add your own fruit or mix one container of plain yogurt with a flavored variety. Greek yogurt has fewer carbohydrates (and more protein) than regular yogurt, but it has a bit less calcium than regular yogurt.

Ice cream

Ice cream has little calcium, so it does not count as a milk serving. Calories vary from 120 to 250 calories per $\frac{1}{2}$ cup (125 mL); choose the lighter one. Now the trick is to keep your portion to that smaller size (see page 253).

The Food Charts on pages 291–317 have lots of tips on comparing food products from less healthy to healthy.

FOOD FACT

When a label says cholesterol-free or no trans fat, the food may still be high in vegetable fat and calories. Remember, all types of animal fat and vegetable fat have the same high number of calories per ounce (gram).

HEALTH TIP

You may find a smaller portion of the thicker Greek Yogurt is as satisfying as a larger portion of regular yogurt. Try plain yogurt as an alternative to sour cream or whipped topping.

9. Walk for Health

DOCTOR'S TIP

Sore knees or hips? A physiotherapist can help you find the best way to move for your health. Walking poles are often helpful.

HEALTH TIPS

Walking has many benefits. It can:

- help prevent you from gaining unwanted weight, and may help you lose weight
- help regulate your blood sugar
- help you look and feel better
- keep your bones and muscles strong
- help you breathe deeper and easier
- often reduce back pain and other joint pain
- improve circulation, which is important for brain health and can reduce swelling in your legs and feet
- help you reduce your stress and help you sleep better at night

TAKE ACTION

- Build short walks into your everyday life.
- Work toward a goal: walk 25 minutes or more every day.

Experts recommend about 30 minutes of exercise a day. For people with diabetes, a minimum of 150 minutes per week is recommended. If half an hour is too long for you, instead go for three 10-minute walks a day.

Walking is the best exercise for most of us. You can walk when you want and where you want. Start off slowly and try walking a little faster and further each week.

There is a difference between being active or busy, and exercising. Compare the way we live today with how people lived a hundred years ago. People used to walk to work, to the store, to the post office, to school, to church and to the dance hall. Working in the home and on the land was hard exercise. Today, we sit for hours a day, whether at home or at work. Television, computers and cell phones too often replace active play and work. Long periods of inactivity makes us unhealthy.

Are you simply too tired to go for a walk? When your muscles are weak, you will feel tired. It may seem strange, but the only way to have the energy for walking is to go for a walk. Start with one block, or up and down the hallway. Once you become more fit, you will find that walking gives you energy.

Are you so busy you can't find the time to go for a walk? Finding the time for a walk means making a few changes. Think about how often you go outside to do something — such as go to your car or the bus stop, or to get the mail. Once you are outside, take an extra 20 minutes to go for a walk. Walking is an important part of keeping healthy. We usually can find the time to do things we think are important.

If you have diabetes, walking helps you lower your blood sugar. If you have high blood cholesterol, walking helps you lower your blood cholesterol. If you have high blood pressure, walking will help bring it down.

It may take several months to get into a walking routine. Once you start walking regularly, you will feel better. You may have lost weight and, with more energy, you may now be ready to do more exercise, as it gets easier with each passing day.

DOCTOR'S TIP

Walking for just 15 minutes half an hour after you eat a meal brings down your blood sugar.

Put this book down and go for a walk.

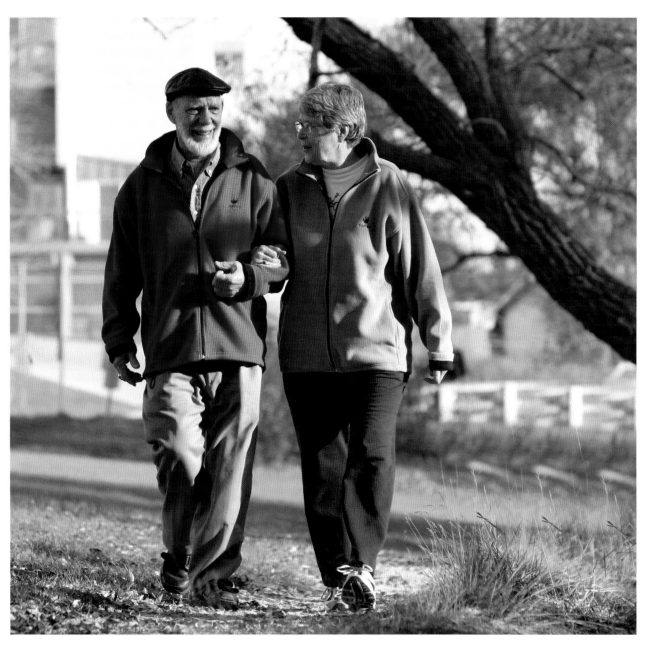

Here are some helpful walking tips

First, start walking more each day.

When you go shopping, park at the far end of the lot and walk. When you take the bus, get off one stop early and walk that extra block.

Walking up and down stairs is great exercise. Start by walking down stairs or getting off the elevator one floor early.

Wear comfortable shoes or boots that fit well. It's important to give your feet good support.

Then, start walking as a regular exercise.

Try to go for a walk twice a week. It may help to walk at the same time each day so it becomes a habit — a good habit. Screen time wastes good walking time.

Boldly mark your calendar after each walk. Feel proud of yourself.

Next, walk further. Walk more often. Walk faster and swing your arms.

Walk faster and further. Over time you will likely see your blood sugar, blood cholesterol and blood pressure improve.

Now that you are walking, you may decide to also do some swimming, biking or dancing. Using an exercise bike or a treadmill are also excellent ways to exercise. Lifting weights or using stretch bands keeps your muscles strong and helps lower high blood sugar too.

Walking takes time but it gives you a lifetime of better health.

DOCTOR'S TIPS

Recommended exercise for adults and seniors

When you are ready, try 150 minutes of walking or aerobic exercise each week. This can be split into three 10-minute sessions a day.

Children and teens should get 60 minutes each day.

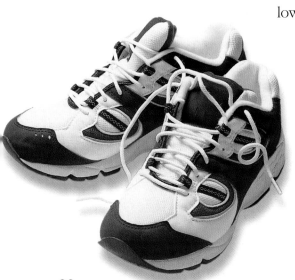

10. Take Care of Yourself

TAKE ACTION

- Get a good night's sleep.
- Take one step at a time — changes take time.
- Regularly, step back and look at the good changes you've made.

Treat yourself the way you would a good friend

When you feel sad or upset, ask yourself, What can I do right now to care for myself in a positive way? What would you do for a friend in the same situation as yourself? Do more of these things for yourself.

Try to get better sleep and go for a regular walk

A sound sleep helps to renew your body and spirits each day. When you don't sleep well, your body makes hormones that can make you hungry and stressed and overeat. A night of sleep rests you, and a walk during the day keeps you going. A walk improves your blood circulation and mood.

Take one step at a time

Important work and change takes time and effort. Set reasonable goals, but give yourself time to get used to changes in how you are eating or exercising. Don't expect big changes overnight. Write down what you are doing right, even the small things.

Do make an effort, but give yourself a break when you need it

Remember, it's what you do 90% of the time that counts most. Now and again you will fall off the healthy pattern you are trying to set. This is normal. Don't put yourself down. We all make mistakes; this is how we learn and move forward.

Be mindful

Try to notice what is happening in the present. What are you thinking and feeling? Are there voices in your mind that aren't being kind to you? Search for the kinder voice from within.

Ask yourself, what triggers make you eat? Practice eating slowly and enjoy the flavors of each bite of food.

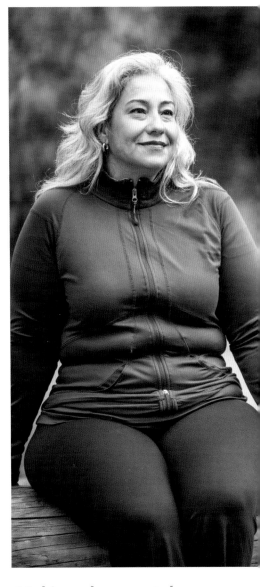

Making changes takes time and effort — but you are worth it!

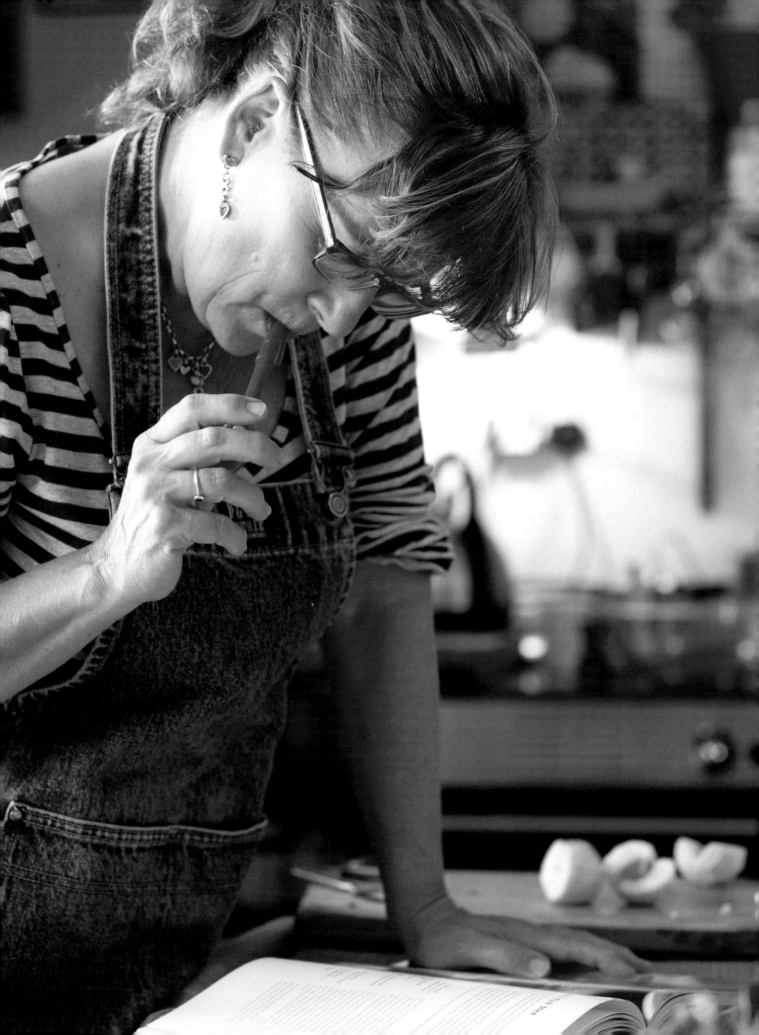

How to Use the Meal Plans

Our philosophy is that all foods fit, in the right amounts. It's what you do 90% of the time that counts.

HEALTH TIP

If you have special dietary needs, talk to your dietitian, diabetes educator or doctor for individual diet recommendations.

DOCTOR'S TIP

Read this if you are on diabetes pills, insulin, heart pills or blood pressure pills:

When you make changes such as eating less or exercising more you may not need as many pills or as much insulin. If you feel weak, shaky or dizzy when exercising, before meals or when getting out of bed, your medications may need to be adjusted. Check your blood sugar with your meter, and share the results with your health care provider. They may make adjustments to your diabetes medications.

All Foods Fit!

You are more likely to have long-term success in establishing a healthy weight and blood sugar if you don't feel you are on a diet. We wanted a cookbook that doesn't use trendy foods with ingredients that you've never heard of. Our cookbook has family favorites adapted to be as healthy as possible. We know life is busy. Our book has recipes that are fast and easy to make. Our book teaches moderation and a balanced way to eat well. The goal is always to enjoy foods.

These real meals and snacks are for everyday people, and are dietitian and doctor approved!

Read through the next five pages to learn how to use this book as a complete diabetes meal planner to achieve your goal to maintain or lose weight, and to manage your blood sugar levels.

Calories of the Meals

The beautiful life-size photographs on the following pages show you how to organize your daily calorie needs (from 1,200 to 2,200 calories) into delicious meals and snacks. All the calories and carbs are counted for you, making it an easy-to-use daily meal planer. For each meal there are two photographs. The life-size photograph is the large meal and the small photograph is the small meal. All large meals have the same calories and all small meals have the same calories (see next page). The large dinners each have 730 calories, and no matter which one you choose you always get the same calories.

This book shows large and small meals and different-sized snacks. This section will help you decide what meal size and how many snacks you will need.

Portions will be different for each member of your family. The small meals would be enough for most small children and older adults who are less active. Growing children and teenagers and physically active adults may need portions larger than even the large meals and large snacks. To meet their calcium needs, children and teenagers, and pregnant and breastfeeding mothers, should include a serving of milk (or milk substitute), yogurt or cheese with each meal.

Should I Choose the Large or Small Meals?

There are two ways to help you quickly choose either the large or small meals:

1. Use the general rule.
2. Use your hand size.

1. General Rule

If you are trying to lose weight, here is a general rule:

- Women choose 1,200 to 1,800 calories daily.
- Men choose 1,500 to 2,200 calories daily.

Use the Daily Meal Plan Chart below to choose your meal plan.

A. Daily Meal Plan Chart

Small meals with no snacks	1,200 calories
Small meals with two small snacks	1,300 calories
Small meals with one small and two medium snacks	1,450 calories
Small meals with one small, one medium and one large snack	1,550 calories
Large meals with no snacks	1,620 calories
Large meals with two small snacks	1,720 calories
Large meals with one small and two medium snacks	1,870 calories
Large meals with one small, one medium and one large snack	1,970 calories
Large meals with three large snacks	2,220 calories

B. Make Your Own Meal Plan

You can create your own meal plan for your calorie level. You can mix and match different-size meals and snacks, depending on your schedule and calorie needs.

SAMPLE MEAL PLAN

Large breakfast	370
Small snack	50
Small lunch	400
Large snack	200
Large dinner	730
Medium snack	100
Total calories	**1,850**

NOTE: There is a plus or minus 5 to 10 percent range in calories for the meals and snacks.

Calories for the small meals:
- Breakfast has 250 calories.
- Lunch has 400 calories.
- Dinner has 550 calories.

Calories for the large meals:
- Breakfast has 370 calories.
- Lunch has 520 calories.
- Dinner has 730 calories.

Calories for the snacks:
- Low-calorie snack has 20 calories or less.
- Small snack has 50 calories.
- Medium snack has 100 calories.
- Large snack has 200 calories.

2. Hand Size

Hand size is the second way to decide whether to start with the large or small meals.

- Go to page 114–115, to the life-size photograph of Dinner 1.
- If the palm of your hand is about the size of the 1½ chicken breasts and your fist is about the size of the 1½ potatoes, then choose the large meals.
- If the palm of your hand is closer in size to the one piece of chicken and your fist is about the size of the one potato, then the small meals are for you (shown in the small inset photograph).
- You may want to add several snacks to your daily meal plan. But if you are trying to lose weight, start with the small snacks or the low-calorie snacks.
- Over time, based on your weight loss or gain, adjust the meal size and the number and size of snacks.

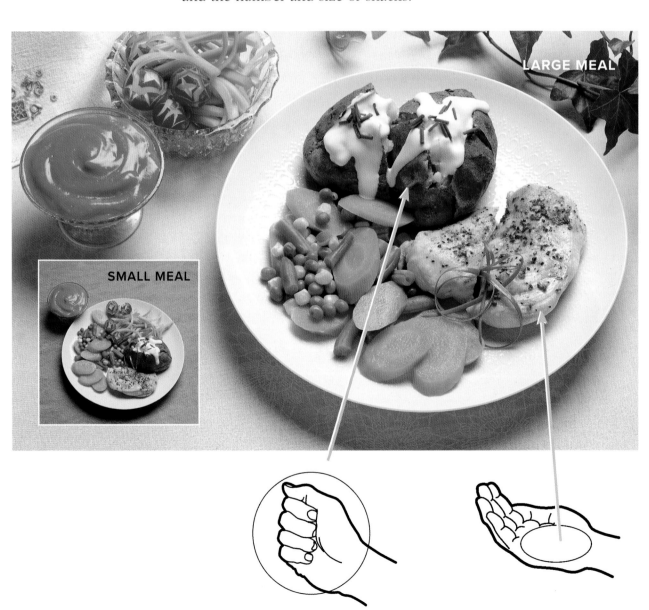

LARGE MEAL

SMALL MEAL

Carbohydrates of Meals

Listed for all meals in this book are Diabetes Food Choices and carbohydrates (carbs). Some diabetes apps and diabetes educators use total carbs, others use net carbs, so we list both. See sidebar for definition of net carbs.

Diabetes Food Choices

The American Diabetes Association and Diabetes Canada have developed diabetes food groups (Food Choices) as a way to help meal planning. For those using this system, we've listed Food Choices for every meal. A Carbohydrate Choice has 15 grams of total or net carbs, and depending on the type of carbohydrate food, 1 to 8 grams of protein. A Protein Choice has 7 grams of protein and 3 to 5 grams of fat. And a Fat Choice has 5 grams of fat.

	NUTRIENTS PER CHOICE		
Food Choices	**Carbs**	**Protein**	**Fat**
Carbohydrates			
Grains and Starches	15 g	3 g	0 g
Fruits	15 g	1 g	0 g
Milk & Alternatives	15 g	8 g	variable
Other Choices	15 g	variable	variable
Vegetables	< 5 g	2 g	0 g
Fat	0 g	0 g	5 g
Protein	0 g	7 g	3–5 g

In this book, net carbs are used to calculate Food Choices, according to Diabetes Canada recommendations.

Comparing Carbohydrate Choices with Total Carbs or Net Carbs

You may notice that the Carbohydrate Choices for a meal are sometimes not exactly equivalent to the total or net carbs. There are a couple of reasons for this.

1. Food Choices generally do not include carbohydrate from vegetables and miscellaneous sources such as nuts, seeds and condiments. As a result, Carbohydrate Choices assigned to meals containing these foods (especially vegetables) will not account for all the carbs.

2. On the other hand, the Carbohydrate Choices may account for slightly more carbs. This happens because not all food choices in a group have exactly the same nutrients and because food choice counts are rounded.

What is a net carb?

- Net carb and available carb are the same thing. We use the term net carbs.

- Total carbohydrate minus fiber equals net carbs. Fiber is a carbohydrate, which in its whole (unprocessed) form is not digested, so does not affect your blood sugar.

- For example, 30 grams total carbohydrate minus 5 grams of fiber equals 25 grams net carbs.

- Half of the carbs from sugar alcohols are subtracted when calculating net carbs. Sugar alcohol are ingredients that end in "ol" such as xylitol or sorbitol.

- For example, 30 grams of total carbohydrate minus 10 grams of sorbitol equals 25 grams of net carbs.

HEALTH TIP

When you focus *only* on carbs, you might forget about the importance of the vitamins and minerals that come from a variety of foods. Remember, carbohydrate foods balance with other foods to form a healthy diet. This variety helps your body be healthy and heal, and helps you to reduce infections.

DOCTOR'S TIPS

Use our meal plans to learn how to eat less while still enjoying your food. Eating less can lead to weight loss and better blood sugar levels.

If you check your blood sugar before a meal, you can use the carb information listed to adjust what you eat. If your blood sugar is high, try to eat less of the higher carb foods at that meal. After your meal, go for a walk — this also helps bring down blood sugar.

Carb Counting

Carb counting is when you add up the total amount of carbohydrates in your meal or snack. You can use the carb numbers listed with the meal menus and snacks in this book. For other meals and snacks, search FoodData Central (USDA) or Canadian Nutrient File, or use a nutrition app. For foods with labels, you will need to start reading those labels.

The good news is that most people do not need to count carbs when using this book! With this book, if you choose the large or small meals with a consistent number of snacks, then every day you will get a similar number of calories and portions (see page 37 and 42). The maximum carbs for each meal group (breakfast, lunch and dinner and large and small meal) is listed on page 42. To allow for favorite meals which might be higher in carbs, such as pasta or pizza, there is some variation between the carb content of meals in each group.

Beyond Carbohydrates: Other Factors that Affect Your Blood Sugar

While carbs have the greatest effect on your blood sugar, there are other factors that also have an effect. This explains why your blood sugar levels can vary after meals that have similar amounts of carbohydrate. Also, unless you always do a blood sugar test before and after a meal, it is hard to monitor the effect of a particular meal. Here are a few examples of things that might alter your blood sugar after a meal:

Diabetes medications and insulin
- What you are taking, how much and when you last took it can alter blood sugar.
- Certain diabetes medications, such as Acarbose, can affect how sugars are digested.

Exercise
- When you last walked can affect how quickly you digest foods.

Stress
- When you are under stress, your blood sugar can swing up or down.

Food
- Different types of fiber affect how quickly we absorb blood sugar. For example, soluble fiber found in oatmeal and lentils slows the absorption of carbohydrates more than fiber in whole wheat does.
- A larger meal will enter your blood stream faster.
- Carbohydrates from table sugar and refined grains (such as white flour) can raise your blood sugar a bit faster than whole grains.
- When a food also has protein and fat, this can slow down the rise of your blood sugar. Yet, if you've eaten a big portion of protein and/or fat, some will convert to blood sugar. For example, you may notice that after you eat pizza, which has both protein and fat as well as carbs, the pizza can raise your blood sugar more than expected hours later.
- The digestion and release of sugar can be slowed down by foods like lemon juice or vinegar, or the tannins in a cup of tea.

Carb counting can be useful in these two situations:

1. **If you check your blood sugar before meals:** You can change what you eat in order to keep your blood sugar in range. Total carbs and net carbs are listed for every single meal item and snack. If your blood sugar is high, try to eat less of the higher carb foods at that meal.

2. **If you take fast-acting insulin with your meals:** You can match the dose of insulin you take to the carbs in your meals and snacks. If you eat more or less of a food item included in a meal, you can also work out a new carb total and insulin amount for your meal. Your diabetes educator can teach you how to adjust your insulin dose. This will depend on the carbs of your meal, and how much insulin your body needs to digest the carbs. For example, a typical dosing would be one unit of insulin for every 10 to 15 grams of carbohydrate.

DOCTOR'S TIP

If your blood sugar is high before a meal, try to eat less of the higher carb foods at that meal. If you go for a walk after you've finished your meal, this also helps bring down blood sugar.

About the Recipes

Check the recipes for the number of servings. Some recipes will serve up to six people. If you live on your own, you may want to cut the recipes in half. If you are cooking for a large family, the recipes can be doubled. Leftovers can be safely kept in your fridge for three days, or frozen to be eaten later.

This book's 100 tested recipes are:

- easy to make
- low-cost and use mostly common ingredients
- reduced in fat, sugar and salt
- family favorites
- easy to freeze

Ingredients Used in Nutrient Calculations

We used the following standard ingredients unless otherwise specified. Remember these ingredients when you are shopping for and creating meals at home:

- Skim milk
- Cheddar, Swiss and mozzarella cheese (25 to 35% fat)
- Sour cream (4%)
- Yogurt (0 to 2%) if fruit flavored, sweetened in part with a low-calorie sweetener
- Light salad dressings (30 calories or less per 1 tbsp/15 mL)
- Lean ground beef/hamburger (less than 17% fat)
- Rice and pasta are made without added salt
- 3 medium boiling potatoes and 2 medium baking potatoes (1 lb/500 g)
- Granulated white sugar, when sugar is listed
- Large eggs

If there is a choice of ingredients or amount in a recipe, the first listed was calculated for the nutrition information.

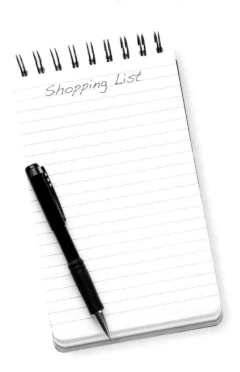

Shopping List

Calories and Carbs of Meals and Snacks

The meals in this book are color-coded as follows:

15 Breakfast Meals

LARGE MEALS have 370 calories
• total carbs 60 grams or less
• net carbs 50 grams or less

SMALL MEALS have 250 calories
• total carbs 50 grams or less
• net carbs 40 grams or less

15 Lunch Meals

LARGE MEALS have 520 calories
• total carbs 90 grams or less
• net carbs 80 grams or less

SMALL MEALS have 400 calories
• total carbs 70 grams or less
• net carbs 60 grams or less

40 Dinner Meals

LARGE MEALS have 730 calories
• total carbs 110 grams or less
• net carbs 100 grams or less

SMALL MEALS have 550 calories
• total carbs 90 grams or less
• net carbs 80 grams or less

4 Snack Groups

• **Low-calorie** snacks (20 calories or less)*
• **Small** snacks (50 calories)*
• **Medium** snacks (100 calories)*
• **Large** snacks (200 calories)*

* Carbs vary between the snacks.

No matter which meal you choose, every dinner has either 730 calories (for large meals) or 550 calories (for small meals). The same goes for Breakfasts, Lunches and Snacks, only with fewer calories. Calories are consistent across each group — so you can pick and choose meals and snacks without having to count calories yourself!

Meals, Recipes and Snacks

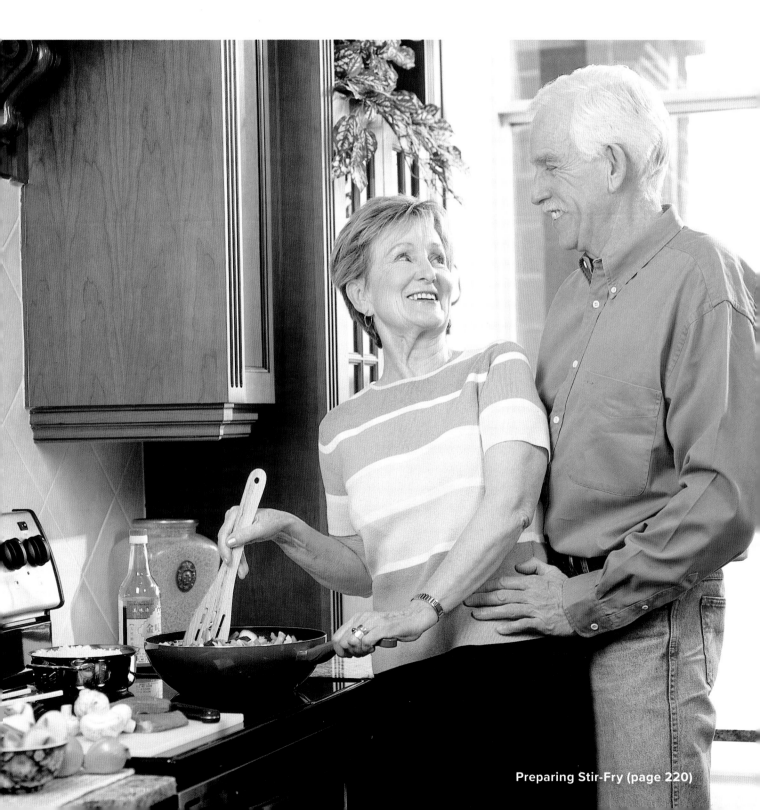

Preparing Stir-Fry (page 220)

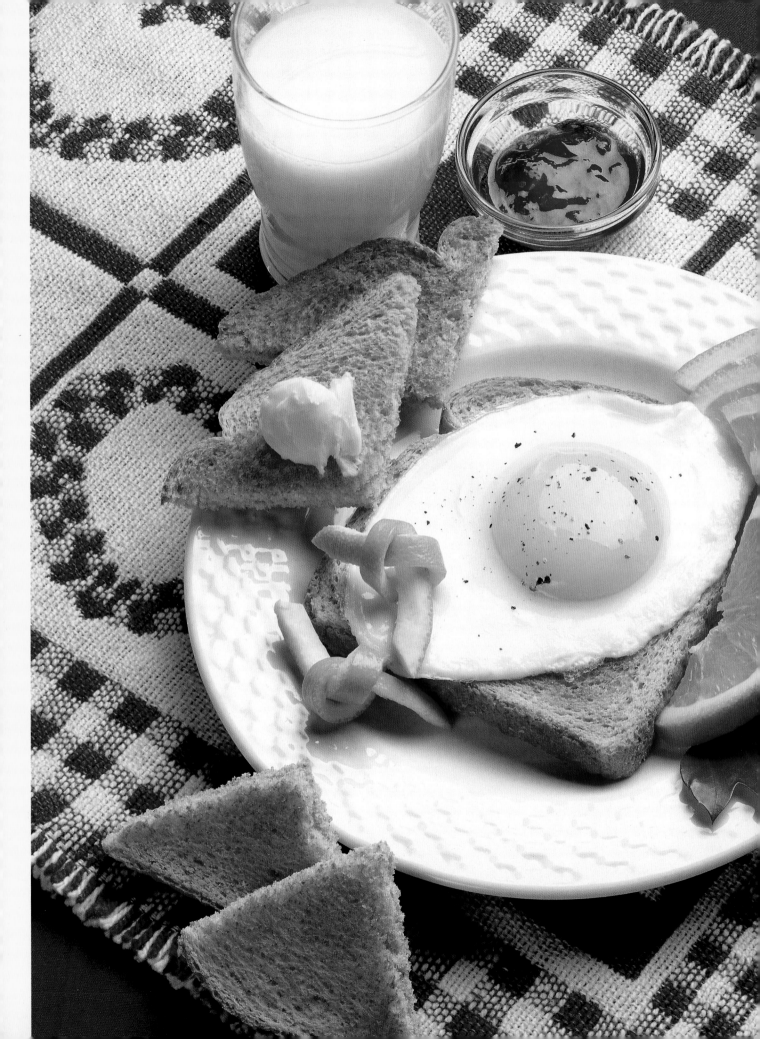

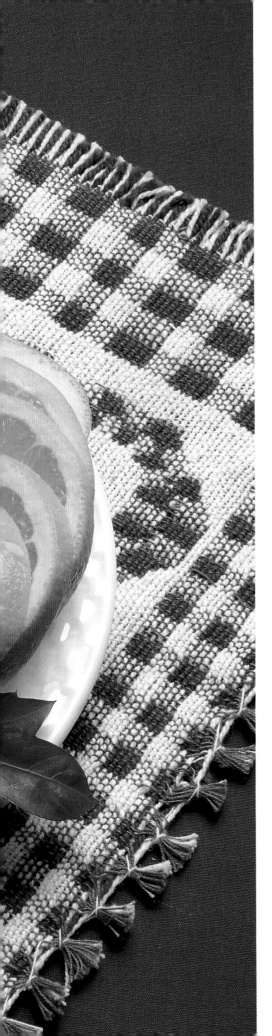

Breakfast Meals

- Each large breakfast has **370 calories**
  Total carbs: 60 g or less | Net carbs: 50 g or less

- Each small breakfast has **250 calories**
  Total carbs: 50 g or less | Net carbs: 40 g or less

BREAKFAST 1

Cold or Hot Cereal

FOOD FACTS

The nuts topping your cereal add a source of protein to help slow down the rise in blood sugar after breakfast.

FOOD CHARTS

See page 291: Oatmeal.

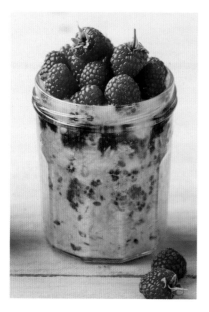

Cold Cereal

Look at the cereal labels before you buy. Choose cereals that have little or no added sugar. One serving should have less than 5 grams of sugar and less than 2 grams of fat.

Another thing to look for when you buy cereals is fiber. Cereals with a lot of fiber are a good choice. These would include bran cereals and whole wheat or whole-grain cereals. Check the label for the amount of fiber per serving.

Hot Cereal

Hot cereals such as porridge (oatmeal), oat bran, whole grain cereals and cornmeal cereal are high in fiber. If you add 1 to 2 tsp (5 to 10 mL) of ground flax seeds (flaxseed meal) or chia seeds, or 1 tbsp (15 mL) of nuts to your cereal, you will have a source of omega-3 fats.

Overnight oats

This can be a change to cooked oatmeal. Use the portions shown in the menu box below. In a bowl combine the raw oats, chopped fruit and milk (or use plain yogurt). For extra flavor you can add a sprinkle of cinnamon or ginger, and for extra fiber you can add flax seeds or chia seeds. Cover and let sit overnight and enjoy cold the next morning.

DOCTOR'S TIP

Research shows that people who eat breakfast find it easier to lose weight and keep it off and are more likely to get all the nutrients the body needs to be healthy.

Food Choices	Large Meal	Small Meal
Carbohydrate	3½	3
Fat	2½	1

Your Breakfast Menu	Large Meal (370 calories)	Total Carbs	Net Carbs	Small Meal (250 calories)	Total Carbs	Net Carbs
Cereal – All-Bran Flakes	1 cup (250 mL)	27	22	¾ cup (175 mL)	20	17
Skim or 1% milk	1 cup (250 mL)	12	12	¾ cup (175 mL)	9	9
½ medium banana	3-inch (7.5 cm) piece	12	11	3-inch (7.5 cm) piece	12	11
Sliced almonds or other nuts	¼ cup (60 mL)	4	1	2 tbsp (30 mL)	2	1
		55 g	46 g		43 g	38 g

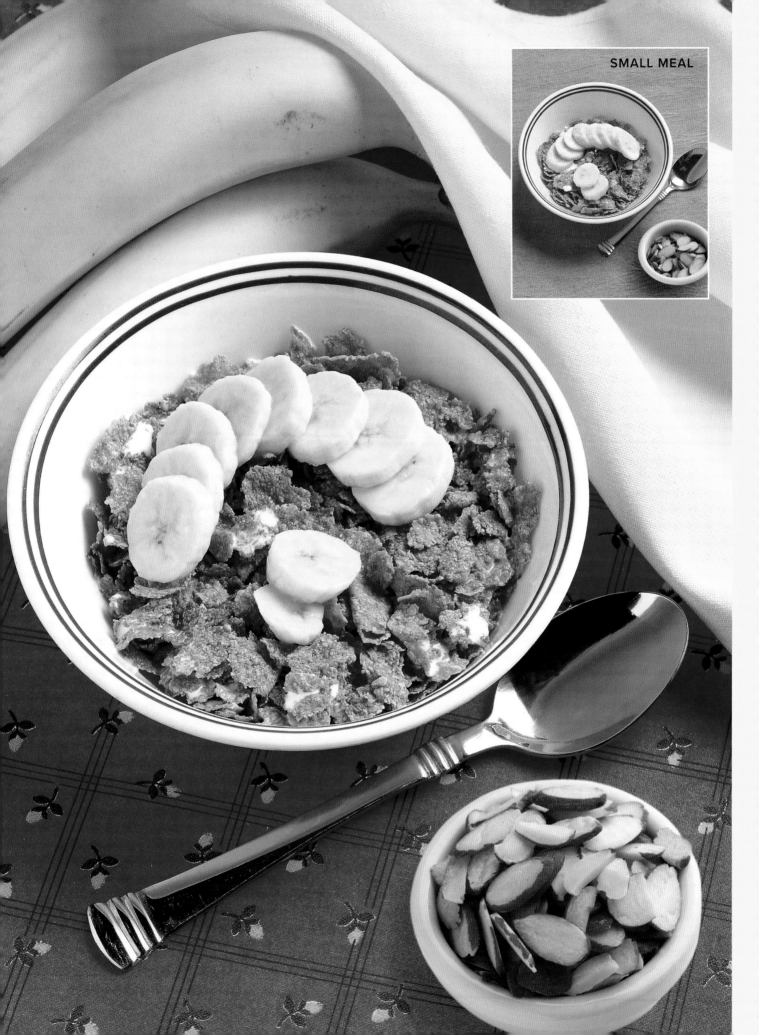

SMALL MEAL

Egg & Toast

In the morning, we all need good food to get our brains going!

Boil an egg, or poach or fry it in a nonstick pan with no added fat. To boost your heart health, choose eggs that have been enriched with omega-3 fats.

Large eggs have almost the same yolk size as small eggs. Large eggs are larger because they have more egg white. This means that a small egg has about the same cholesterol as a large egg.

Bread slices vary from brand to brand. We recommend thinner-sliced bread with 70 calories and 16 grams of carbohydrate or less per slice. Whole-grain is the best choice; whole wheat or rye bread are good choices.

This breakfast includes a half fruit choice: half an orange, or several slices of tomato.

FOOD FACT

Sugar, honey and jam have fewer calories than butter or margarine. This is because a gram of sugar has fewer calories than a gram of fat.

- 1 tsp (5 mL) of sugar, honey or regular jam or jelly has 20 calories.
- 1 tsp (5 mL) of butter or margarine has about 45 calories.

FOOD CHARTS

See page 294: Restaurant Egg Breakfast.

HEALTH TIP

Eat your fruit rather than drink it

Fresh fruit is a better choice than fruit juice. This is because fresh fruit has more fiber and is more filling. So most of the time, choose fresh fruit, and have juice only occasionally.

- One fruit choice such as an orange or apple or half a banana equals 1/2 cup (125 mL) of unsweetened juice.
- Tomato juice or vegetable juice is lower in sugar than fruit juice, so the fruit choice would equal 1 cup (250 mL) of unsweetened vegetable juice.

Food Choices	Large Meal	Small Meal
Carbohydrate	3	2
Protein	1	1
Fat	1	1

Your Breakfast Menu	Large Meal (370 calories)	Total Carbs	Net Carbs	Small Meal (250 calories)	Total Carbs	Net Carbs
Egg (cooked without fat)	1 egg	0	0	1 egg	0	0
Whole-grain or whole wheat toast	2 slices	32	27	1 slice	16	13
Margarine	1 tsp (5 mL)	0	0	–	0	0
Jam or jelly	1 tsp (5 mL)	5	5	1 tsp (5 mL)	5	5
Skim or 1% milk	1/2 cup (125 mL)	6	6	1/2 cup (125 mL)	6	6
Orange slices	1/2 medium orange	8	7	1/2 medium orange	8	7
		51 g	**45 g**		**35 g**	**31 g**

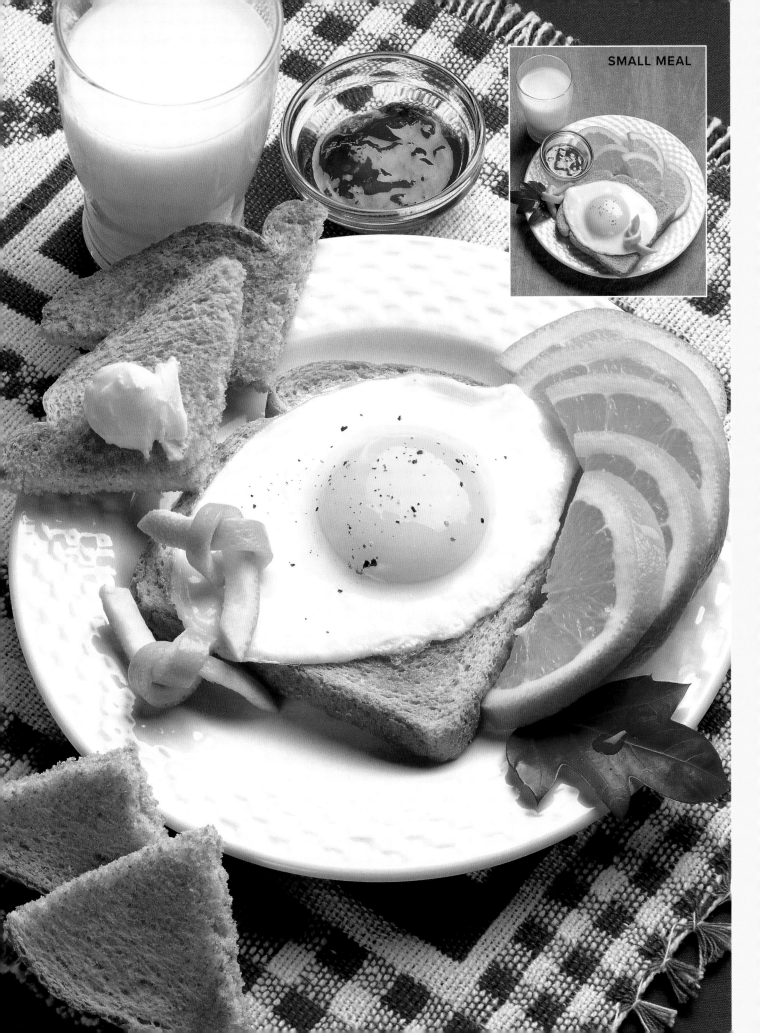

SMALL MEAL

BREAKFAST 3

Pancakes & Bacon

Protein-Powered Pancakes

Makes sixteen 4-inch (10 cm) pancakes

1 cup (250 mL) flour
$\frac{1}{2}$ tsp (2 mL) salt
1 tsp (5 mL) baking powder
1 tbsp (15 mL) sugar
3 eggs
1 tbsp (15 mL) oil, margarine
  or butter, melted
1$\frac{1}{4}$ cups (300 mL) skim milk

PER PANCAKE	
Calories	61
Carbohydrate	8 g
Fiber	0 g
Net Carbs	8 g
Protein	3 g
Fat, total	2 g
Fat, saturated	0 g
Cholesterol	35 g
Sodium	99 mg

1. In a large bowl, mix together flour, salt, baking powder and sugar.
2. In a medium bowl, beat egg with a fork. Add the fat and milk to egg, and mix well.
3. Add egg mixture to the flour mixture. Stir until smooth. It helps to stir with a wire whisk. If it is too thick, add a little more milk.
4. In a greased nonstick pan, cook on medium heat. Use just under $\frac{1}{4}$ cup (60 mL) of batter for each pancake. Once the pancakes have small bubbles, turn them over.

OPTIONS

Look at the labels on light syrup. Two tablespoons (30 mL) should have fewer than 60 calories. Two tablespoons (30 mL) of this light syrup are the same as 1 tbsp (15 mL) of most regular syrups.

Instead of syrup, you may prefer to have some berries or sliced fruit on your pancakes.

HEALTH TIP

For extra fiber, add 1 tbsp (15 mL) of bran to your batter.

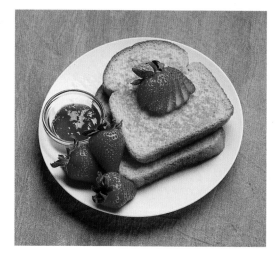

French toast instead of pancakes

Protein power your French toast too. Use three eggs and $\frac{1}{4}$ cup (60 mL) of milk for three slices of bread. (Have two slices of French toast for large meal and one slice for small meal.)

Food Choices	Large Meal	Small Meal
Carbohydrate	3	2
Protein	1	$\frac{1}{2}$
Fat	1$\frac{1}{2}$	1

Your Breakfast Menu	Large Meal (370 calories)	Total Carbs	Net Carbs	Small Meal (250 calories)	Total Carbs	Net Carbs
Protein-Powered Pancakes	3 pancakes	24	23	2 pancakes	16	15
Syrup	1$\frac{1}{2}$ tbsp (22 mL), or 3 tbsp (45 mL) light syrup	24	24	1 tbsp (15 mL), or 2 tbsp (30 mL) light syrup	16	16
Bacon, crisp strips	2 strips	0	0	1$\frac{1}{2}$ strips	0	0
		48 g	**47 g**		**32 g**	**31 g**

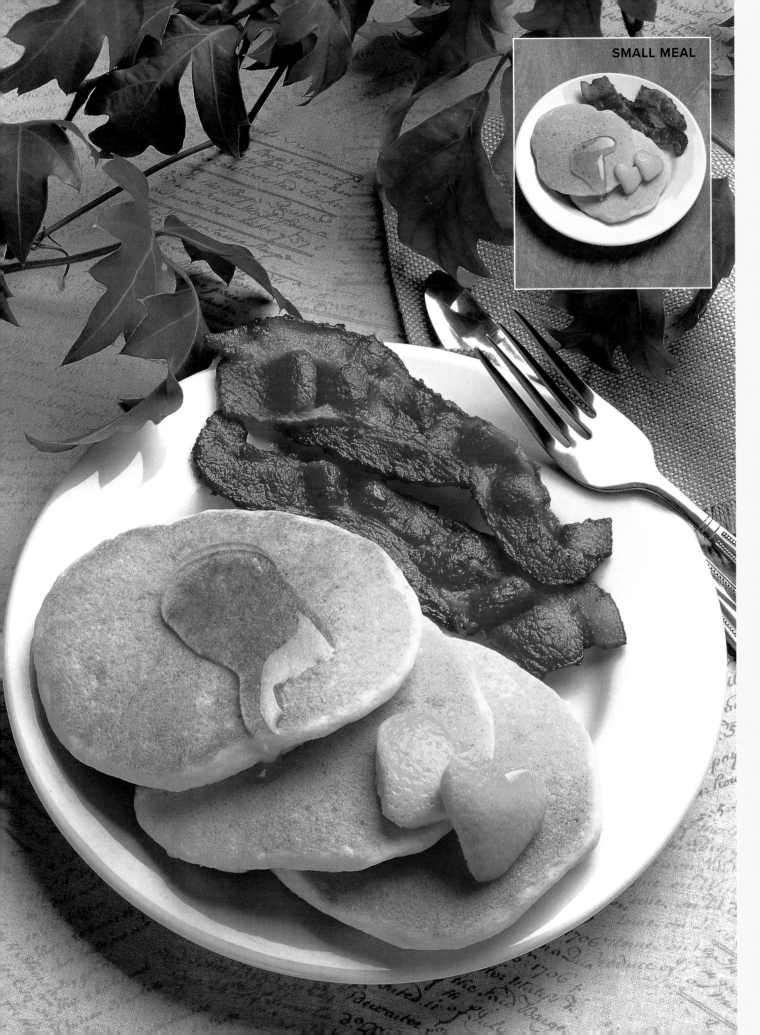

SMALL MEAL

BREAKFAST 4

Toast & Peanut Butter

This simple breakfast has protein to start your day. One tablespoon (15 mL) of peanut butter is a good source of protein. But peanut butter has a lot of fat, so put it on a dry piece of toast — you don't need to add extra fat.

Half an apple is served with this breakfast.

Here are a few examples of other fruit servings:

- ½ cup (125 mL) of unsweetened applesauce
- 2 medium kiwis
- ¼ of a small melon
- 1 small banana
- 1 orange
- ½ grapefruit. See Breakfast 8 for a new way to enjoy grapefruit.

For the large meal, try the peanut butter on your first piece of toast and 1 tsp (5 mL) of jam or jelly on your second piece of toast.

Regular or Diet Jams

A light (or "diet") jam or jelly should have fewer than 10 calories in 1 tsp (5 mL) and 30 calories in 1 tbsp (15 mL). Two teaspoons (10 mL) of this light jam are about the same as 1 tsp (5 mL) of regular jam or jelly.

Jams marked "no sugar added" may in fact have added sugar in the form of concentrated fruit juice. These jams often have almost the same amount of carbohydrate as regular jam.

OPTIONS

In place of the ½ cup (125 mL) of milk, you could have 1 cup (250 mL) of hot cocoa marked "light."

FOOD CHARTS

See page 295: Jam.

Food Choices	Large Meal	Small Meal
Carbohydrate	3½	2
Protein	½	½

Your Breakfast Menu	Large Meal (370 calories)	Total Carbs	Net Carbs	Small Meal (250 calories)	Total Carbs	Net Carbs
Whole-grain or whole wheat toast	2 slices	32	27	1 slice	16	13
Peanut butter	1 tbsp (15 mL)	3	2	1 tbsp (15 mL)	3	2
Jam or jelly	1 tsp (5 mL) regular jam, or 2 tsp (10 mL) diet jam	5	5	–	0	0
Skim or 1% milk	½ cup (125 mL)	6	6	½ cup (125 mL)	6	6
Apple slices	½ medium apple	11	10	½ medium apple	11	10
		57 g	**50 g**		**36 g**	**31 g**

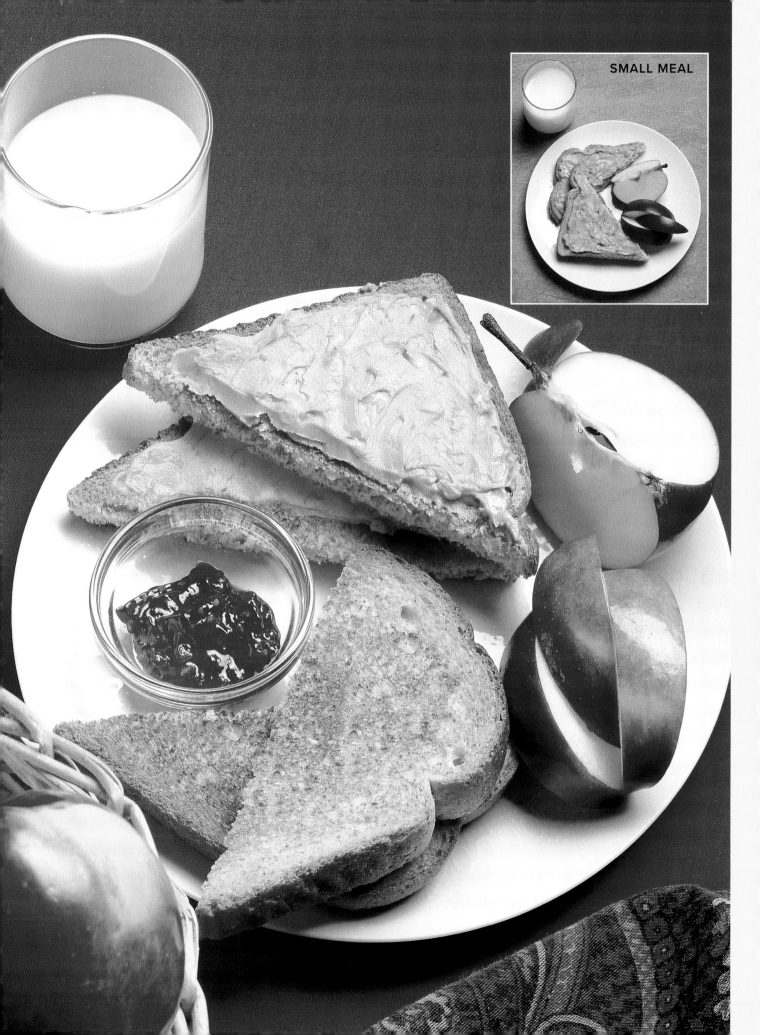

SMALL MEAL

BREAKFAST 5

Spinach & Eggs

This is an easy, lower-carb breakfast. Eggs cooked on a bed of spinach or your favorite greens, served with a slice of whole-grain toast. Include a serving of fresh homemade salsa, also known as *pico de gallo* in Spanish.

OPTIONS

Choose your greens!

Instead of spinach, try arugula, beet tops or kale. If using kale, first cut out the stems. A 1½-cup (375 mL) portion of kale should be enough, as it is a rougher green than spinach.

With scrambled eggs

If you don't like your egg yolks runny, you can mix the eggs in a bowl before pouring them on top of the bed of spinach, and cook with the lid on.

Food Choices	Large Meal	Small Meal
Carbohydrate	1	1
Protein	2	2
Fat	2½	0

Spinach & Eggs

Serves 1

¼ cup (60 mL) water
2 cups (500 mL) lightly packed
  fresh spinach leaves
2 eggs

1. Pour the water into a small nonstick frying pan. Place spinach on top. At medium heat, simmer for 1 to 2 minutes, until spinach is wilted. Add a bit more water if needed to keep the spinach moist.
2. Break eggs on top and cover with a lid. Continue to simmer for another 2 to 3 minutes, until the egg whites are cooked; the yolks will be runny.

PER SERVING	
Calories	157
Carbohydrate	3 g
Fiber	1 g
Net Carbs	2 g
Protein	14 g
Fat, total	10 g
Fat, saturated	3 g
Cholesterol	372 mg
Sodium	189 mg

Fresh Salsa (Pico de Gallo)

Makes 1 cup (250 mL)

1 large tomato, finely chopped
2 tbsp (30 mL) finely chopped
  fresh cilantro
1 tbsp (15 mL) finely chopped
  white or red onion
⅛ tsp (0.5 mL) salt
¼ tsp (1 mL) black pepper
Juice of 1 lime (or 2 tbsp/30 mL bottled)
Few dashes of hot pepper sauce or
  ¼ jalapeño pepper, finely chopped (optional)

PER ¼ CUP SALSA	
Calories	11
Carbohydrate	3 g
Fiber	1 g
Net Carbs	2
Protein	0
Fat, total	0
Fat, saturated	0
Cholesterol	0
Sodium	75 mg

1. In a bowl, combine all ingredients; let stand for 10 minutes before eating. Cover and refrigerate leftovers for up to 3 days.

Your Breakfast Menu	Large Meal (370 calories)	Total Carbs	Net Carbs	Small Meal (250 calories)	Total Carbs	Net Carbs
Spinach & Eggs	1 serving	3	2	1 serving	3	2
Whole-grain toast (38 g slice)	1 slice	14	12	1 slice	14	12
Margarine or butter	1 tsp (5 mL)	0	0	–	–	–
Fresh Salsa (or store-bought salsa)	¼ cup (60 mL) (2 tbsp/30 mL if store-bought)	3	2	¼ cup (60 mL) (2 tbsp/30 mL if store-bought)	3	2
Avocado	⅓ medium	4	1	–	–	–
		24 g	17 g		20 g	16 g

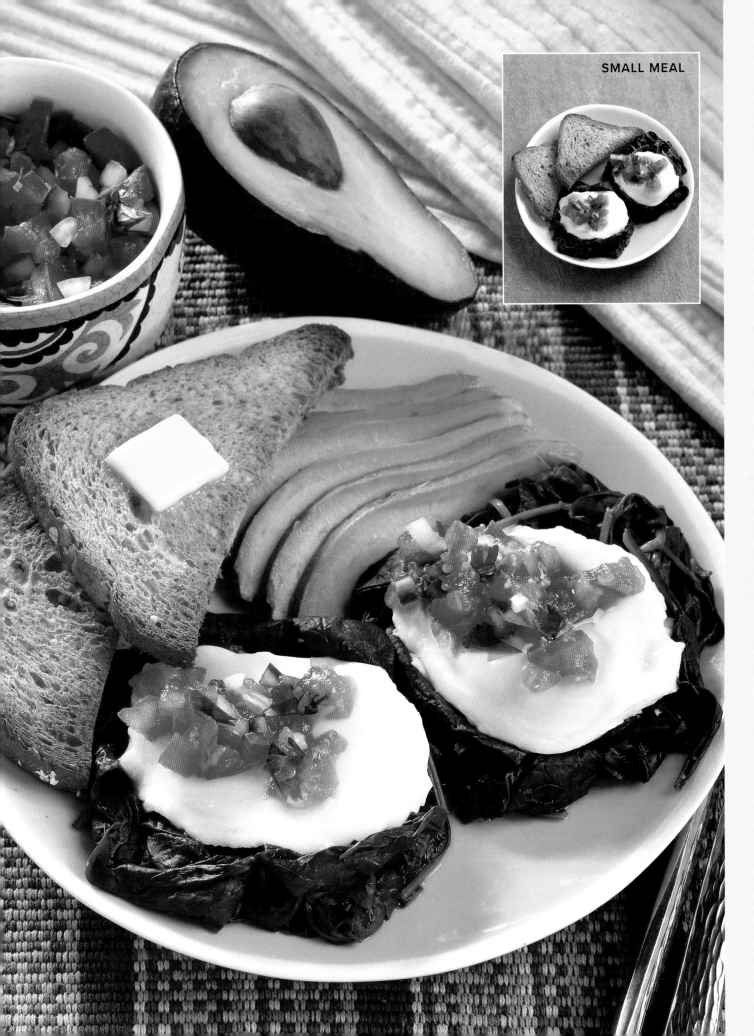

SMALL MEAL

Muffin & Yogurt

Bran Muffins

Makes 12 medium muffins

1 cup (250 mL) flour
1½ tsp (7 mL) baking powder
½ tsp (2 mL) baking soda
½ tsp (2 mL) salt
¼ cup (60 mL) unsweetened applesauce
¼ cup (60 mL) vegetable oil
¼ cup (60 mL) packed brown sugar
¼ cup (60 mL) molasses (or honey)
1 egg
1 cup (250 mL) skim milk
1 cup (250 mL) wheat bran
½ cup (125 mL) raisins

PER MUFFIN	
Calories	156
Carbohydrate	27 g
Fiber	3 g
Net Carbs	24 g
Protein	4 g
Fat, total	5 g
Fat, saturated	0 g
Cholesterol	16 mg
Sodium	259 mg

FOOD CHARTS

See page 310: Muffin or Donut.

OPTIONS

For the small meal, you could have a ½-oz (15 g) slice of cheese instead of yogurt.

HEALTH TIP

These homemade muffins have a lot less sugar and fat than larger store-bought or coffee shop muffins.

1. In a medium bowl, mix flour, baking powder, soda and salt together.
2. In a large bowl, combine applesauce, oil, brown sugar, molasses and egg. Stir with a wooden spoon until well mixed.
3. Add the milk, then add wheat bran to the large bowl.
4. Add flour mixture to the large bowl. Then add raisins. The mixture will be wet.
5. Spoon into a greased nonstick muffin tin. Bake in a 400°F (200°C) oven for 20 to 25 minutes. They are ready when a toothpick put into the center of a muffin comes out clean.

Food Choices	Large Meal	Small Meal
Carbohydrate	3	3
Protein	1	0

Your Breakfast Menu	Large Meal (370 calories)	Total Carbs	Net Carbs	Small Meal (250 calories)	Total Carbs	Net Carbs
Bran Muffin	1	27	24	1	27	24
Greek yogurt (0 to 2%), flavored, less sugar	½ cup (125 mL)	6	5	½ cup (125 mL)	6	5
Orange	½ medium	8	7	½ medium	8	7
Piece of cheese	1 oz (30 g)	0	0	–	0	0
		41 g	**36 g**		**41 g**	**36 g**

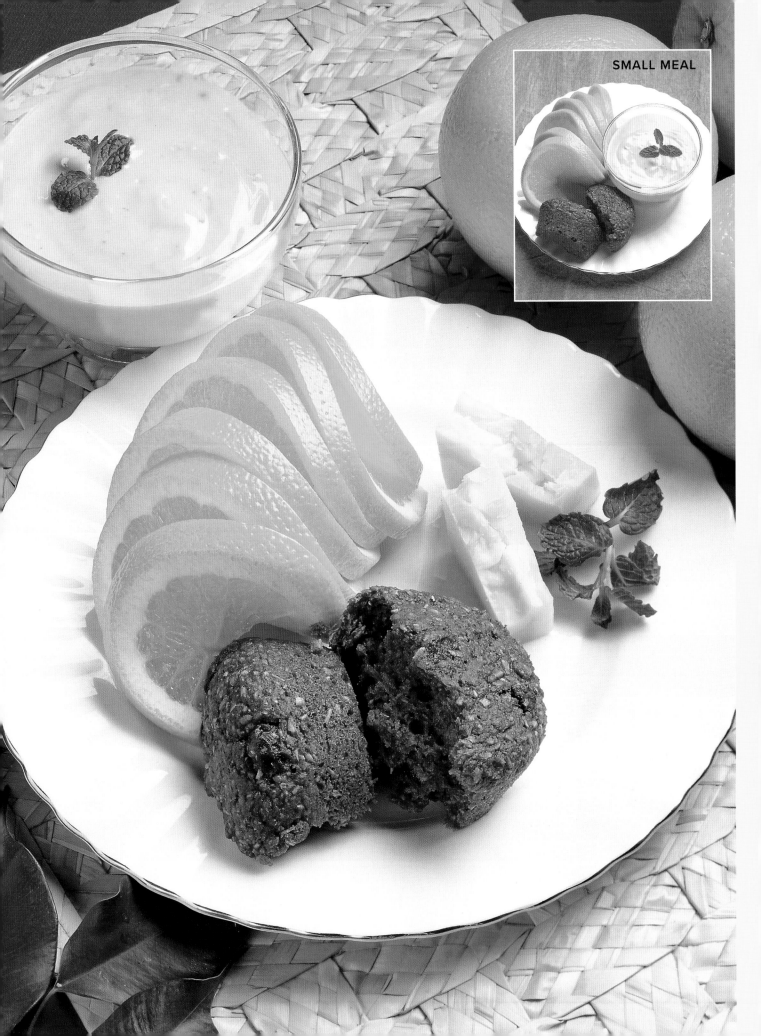

SMALL MEAL

BREAKFAST 7

Raisin Toast & Cheese

Raisin toast makes a nice change. As with all types of bread, make sure it is in the 70 calorie range (thin slice), or else adjust your portion to match the carbs in the thin sliced bread.

Grapefruit treat

A nice way to have grapefruit is to sprinkle it with a bit of cinnamon and sugar (or low-calorie sweetener). Then, microwave it for 30 seconds or broil it until warm.

Grapefruit and Statins

Grapefruit can interact with some medications. For example, grapefruit can increase the side effects of some statin cholesterol medications. If you see a warning on your medication bottle, check with your pharmacist. You might be advised to replace the grapefruit with a different fruit.

OPTIONS

Instead of two slices of raisin toast, you could have one raisin scone or one hot cross bun.

DOCTOR'S TIP

When you eat breakfast, even the small one, you will wake up your body and have more energy. In this way, eating breakfast will help you control your blood sugar throughout the day.

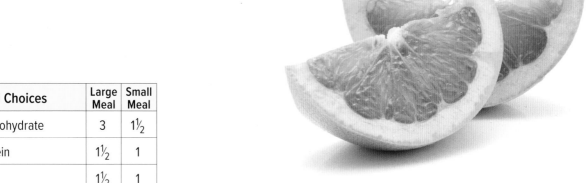

Food Choices	Large Meal	Small Meal
Carbohydrate	3	1½
Protein	1½	1
Fat	1½	1

Your Breakfast Menu	Large Meal (370 calories)	Total Carbs	Net Carbs	Small Meal (250 calories)	Total Carbs	Net Carbs
Raisin toast	2 slices	27	25	1 slice	13	12
Margarine or butter	1½ tsp (7 mL)	0	0	1 tsp (5 mL)	0	0
Jam or jelly	1 tsp (5 mL)	5	5	–	0	0
Gouda cheese (light or original)	1½ oz (40 g)	1	1	1 oz (30 g)	1	1
Grapefruit	½ small	10	8	½ small	10	8
		43 g	**39 g**		**24 g**	**21 g**

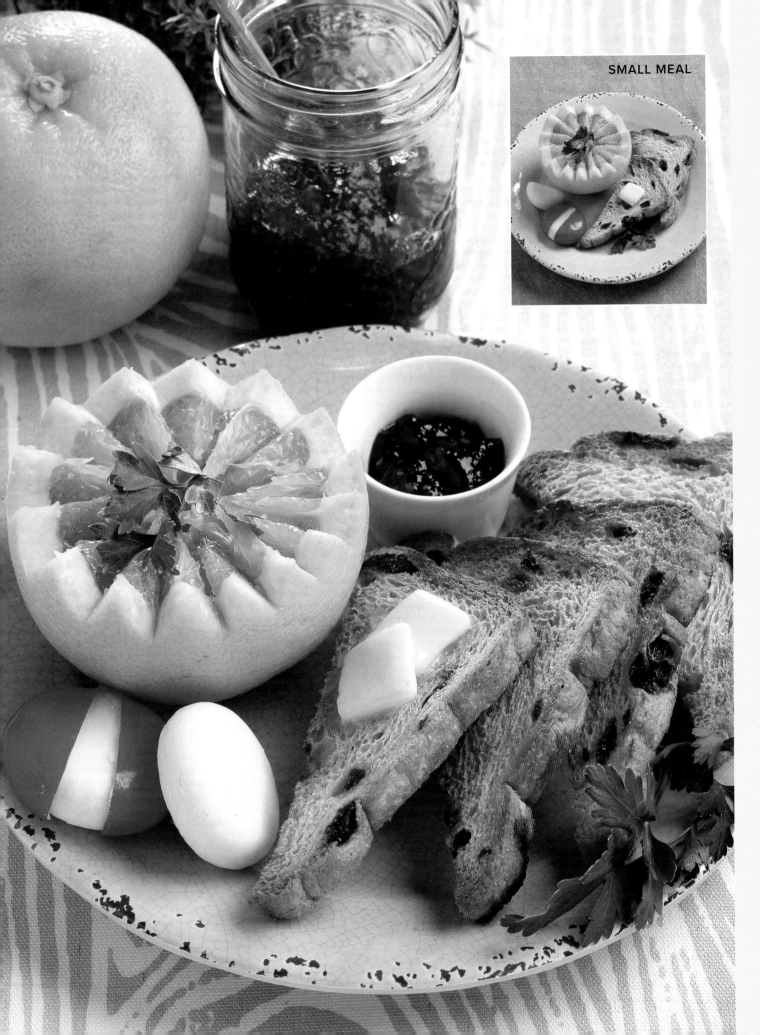

SMALL MEAL

BREAKFAST 8

Tuna Scramble

If you love fish any time of the day, try this tasty one-skillet breakfast made with either canned tuna or salmon. Serve with arugula salad and cherry tomatoes.

Tuna Scramble

2 large or 3 small servings

1 tbsp (15 mL) butter, margarine or oil

4 green onions, chopped

2 tbsp (30 mL) sweet pepper, finely chopped

1 medium 3-inch (7.5 cm) precooked potato, chopped

2 eggs

1 can of tuna (5 oz/213 g) or
½ can of salmon, drained

¼ cup (60 mL) of shredded regular fat Cheddar cheese, lightly packed

Salt and pepper to taste

PER LARGE SERVING	
Calories	345
Carbohydrate	18 g
Fiber	2 g
Net Carbs	16 g
Protein	30 g
Fat, total	16 g
Fat, saturated	8 g
Cholesterol	276 mg
Sodium	360 mg

1. In a nonstick frying pan, melt fat at medium heat.
2. Add potato, onions and pepper and cook until potatoes are lightly browned.
3. In a small bowl, beat eggs with a fork. Mix in tuna and cheese.
4. Add egg mixture to the pan with the vegetables and stir until cooked.

Arugula Salad

2 servings

Over ½ cup (125 mL) of arugula, drizzle 1 tsp (5 mL) of vinegar and ½ tsp (2 mL) of oil.

RECIPE TIP

Quick and easy cooked potatoes

Poke a potato with a fork and microwave for a couple of minutes.

OPTIONS

Scrambled eggs without the fish

Follow the Tuna Scramble recipe, but omit the fish and use four eggs. Remember this recipe is enough for two large servings.

HEALTH TIP

Drink water with all your meals, including breakfast.

Food Choices	Large Meal	Small Meal
Carbohydrate	1	1
Protein	4	2½
Fat	1	½

Your Breakfast Menu	Large Meal (370 calories)	Total Carbs	Net Carbs	Small Meal (250 calories)	Total Carbs	Net Carbs
Tuna Scramble	½ of recipe	18	16	⅓ of recipe	12	10
Arugula Salad	¼ cup to ⅓ cup (60 to 75 mL)	1	1	¼ cup to ⅓ cup (60 to 75 mL)	1	1
3 cherry tomatoes (or a couple of tomato slices)	3	2	1	3	2	1
		21 g	**18 g**		**15 g**	**12 g**

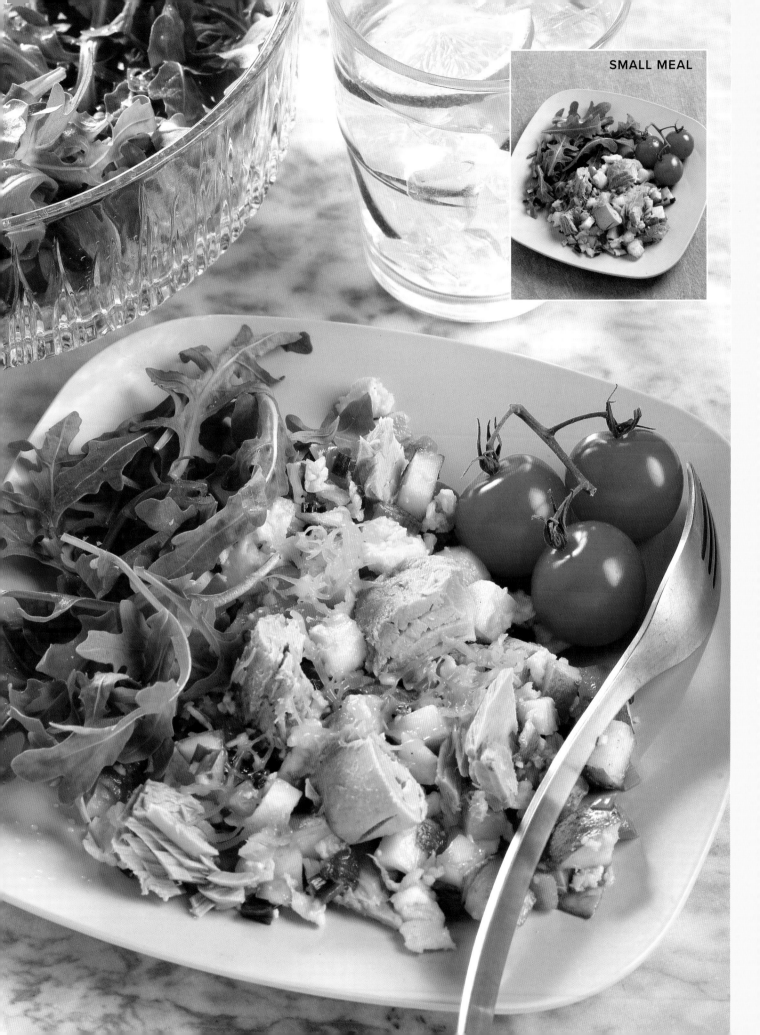

SMALL MEAL

Homemade Waffle

This waffle is so fast and easy to make using a waffle iron. Top your waffle with fresh fruit, nuts, and a touch of syrup for a delectable start to your morning.

The number of waffles this recipe makes will depend on the size and shape of your waffle iron. One cup (250 mL) of batter will make four 4-inch (10 cm) waffles or, if you have a 7-inch (18 cm) round waffle iron, two larger waffles.

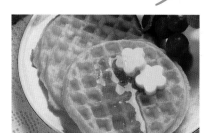

Store-bought frozen ready-to-eat 4-inch (10 cm) waffles

Standard store-bought waffles have more carbohydrate and less protein than this home-made waffle. Compare the portions for one or two store-bought waffles:

	One 4-inch	Two 4-inch
Calories. .	88	176
Carbs . . .	14 g	27 g
Net carbs	13 g	25 g
Protein. . .	2 g	4 g
Fat.	3 g	5 g
Sodium . .	262 mg	524 mg

Homemade Waffle

Makes 1 cup (250 mL) of batter, enough for four 4-inch (10 cm) square waffles

2 tbsp (30 mL) flour
¼ cup (60 mL) skim milk powder
   (fat free instant skim milk powder)
1 tsp (5 mL) baking powder
Pinch of salt
⅛ tsp (0.5 mL) nutmeg
2 eggs
3 tbsp (45 mL) 0 to 2% plain Greek yogurt

1. In a medium bowl, whisk together all ingredients until smooth.
2. Using an oiled hot waffle iron, pour half the batter (½ cup/125 mL) in iron and cook until lightly browned.

PER ½ CUP (125 ML) BATTER	
Calories	162
Carbohydrate	15 g
Fiber	0
Net Carbs	15 g
Protein	14 g
Fat, total	5
Fat, saturated	2 g
Cholesterol	191 mg
Sodium	232 mg

Food Choices	Large Meal	Small Meal
Carbohydrate	3	2½
Fat	3	1

Your Breakfast Menu	Large Meal (370 calories)	Total Carbs	Net Carbs	Small Meal (250 calories)	Total Carbs	Net Carbs
Homemade Waffle	two 4-inch (10 cm)	15	15	two 4-inch (10 cm)	15	15
Margarine or butter	1 tsp (5 mL)	0	0	–	–	–
Syrup	1 tbsp (15 mL) regular, or 2 tbsp (30 mL) light	16	16	½ tbsp (7 mL), regular or 1 tbsp (15 mL) light	8	8
Fruit, grapes and berries	½ cup (125 mL)	11	8	⅓ cup (75 mL)	7	5
Chopped nuts, raw or toasted	2 tbsp (30 mL)	4	4	1 tbsp (15 mL)	2	2
Coffee or tea with single milk, low-calorie sweetener	1 cup (250 mL)	1	1	1 cup (250 mL)	1	1
		47 g	**44 g**		**33 g**	**31 g**

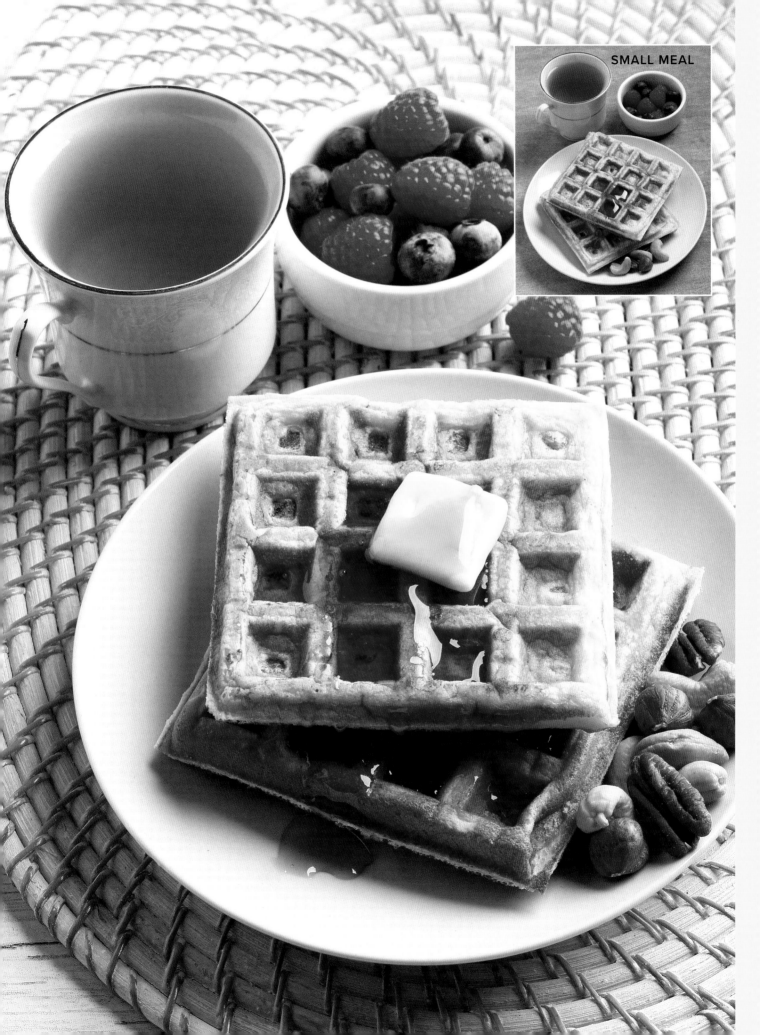

SMALL MEAL

Smoothie & Protein Bar

Two recipes with similar calories for protein smoothies follow. The Soy Fruit Smoothie is the one shown in the photograph.

Choose a high-protein bar with no more than 150 calories. They come in different flavors like oats and nuts (shown in photo) or chocolate. These are lower in carbs than standard granola bars. The diabetic bars such as Glucerna bars are high in fiber and may contain sugar alcohols which, like fiber, are poorly absorbed and reduce the net carbs.

Soy Fruit Smoothie

Makes 2 cups (500 mL)

5¼ oz (150 g) flavored dessert tofu (such as peach, mango, berry or lime)
¼ cup (60 mL) 0 to 2% plain Greek yogurt
½ cup (125 mL) almond milk, unsweetened
2 peach halves (fresh or canned, juice-packed) or ½ small banana

1. Place all ingredients in a blender and blend until smooth.

PER 1 CUP (250 ML)	
Calories	107
Carbohydrate	14 g
Fiber	1 g
Net Carbs	13 g
Protein	7 g
Fat, total	1 g
Fat, saturated	0 g
Cholesterol	3 mg
Sodium	78 mg

Spinach Fruit Smoothie

Makes 2 cups (500 mL)

½ cup (125 mL) 0 to 2% flavored Greek yogurt, less sugar, or plain
½ cup (125 mL) almond milk, unsweetened
3 tbsp (45 mL) skim milk powder
½ cup (125 mL) raw spinach or other greens, packed
2 peach halves (fresh or canned, juice-packed) or ½ small banana
1 tsp (5 mL) honey
Pinch cinnamon (optional)

1. Place all ingredients in a blender and blend until smooth.

PER 1 CUP (250 ML)	
Calories	97
Carbohydrate	16 g
Fiber	1 g
Net Carbs	15 g
Protein	6 g
Fat, total	2 g
Fat, saturated	0 g
Cholesterol	5 mg
Sodium	85 mg

Food Choices	Large Meal	Small Meal
Carbohydrate	3	2
Protein	2	1½

Your Breakfast Menu	Large Meal (370 calories)	Total Carbs	Net Carbs	Small Meal (250 calories)	Total Carbs	Net Carbs
Soy Fruit Smoothie or Spinach Fruit Smoothie	2 cups (500 mL)	28	26	1 cup (250 mL)	14	13
High-protein bar	1 (about 150 calories)	18	14	1 (about 150 calories)	18	14
		46 g	**40 g**		**32 g**	**27 g**

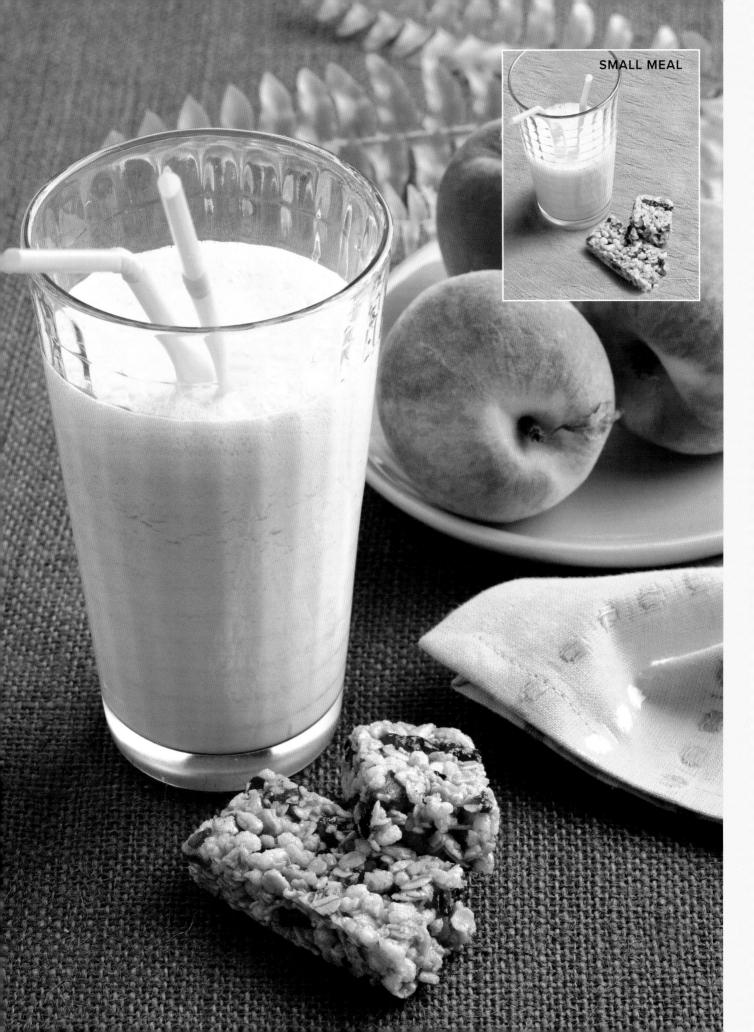

SMALL MEAL

Fiesta Breakfast

Mexican Rice & Beans

Makes just over 2 cups (500 mL)

2 tsp (10 mL) olive oil or vegetable oil

1 small or ½ medium onion,
  finely chopped

3 cloves garlic, minced

½ tsp (2 mL) ground cumin

½ tsp (2 mL) dried oregano

1 tbsp (15 mL) fresh cilantro
  or parsley, chopped

¼ tsp (1 mL) hot pepper flakes (optional)

1 cup (250 mL) canned black beans (½ of a 19-oz/540 mL can)

1 cup (250 mL) cooked rice

PER ¾ CUP (175 ML)	
Calories	196
Carbohydrate	34 g
Fiber	5 g
Net carbs	29 g
Protein	7 g
Fat, total	4 g
Fat, saturated	1 g
Cholesterol	0 mg
Sodium	204 mg

1. To a frying pan, add oil, onions, garlic, cumin, oregano, cilantro and hot pepper flakes. Cook, stirring, over medium heat until onions are soft.
2. While onions are cooking, empty beans into a sieve, rinse them with cold water and drain.
3. Stir cooked rice and rinsed beans into the pan with the cooked onions. Place in a covered casserole dish in a warm oven while you scramble the eggs. Or refrigerate, to reheat the next morning.

Café Almondo

Makes 1 cup (250 mL)

1 cup (250 mL) almond beverage,
  unsweetened

1 tsp (5 mL) instant coffee or
  ¼ cup (60 mL) strong coffee

Sweetener, to taste

PER 1 CUP (250 ML)	
Calories	34
Carbohydrate	2 g
Fiber	1 g
Net carbs	1 g
Protein	8 g
Fat, total	3 g
Fat, saturated	0 g
Cholesterol	0 mg
Sodium	131 mg

1. In a microwave, heat almond beverage until boiling, for 2 to 3 minutes, then add instant (or hot) coffee and low-calorie sweetener. (If you use regular sugar, limit to 1 tsp/5 mL.)

HEALTH TIP

Beans and rice are commonly served for breakfast throughout Latin America. This recipe has the spicy flavors of onion and garlic, to give you a spirited start to your day. The recipe can be made ahead and reheated. Serve with a scrambled egg cooked in a greased nonstick pan, with salsa and cucumbers.

Food Choices	Large Meal	Small Meal
Carbohydrate	2	1½
Protein	2	1
Fat	1	1

Your Breakfast Menu	Large Meal (370 calories)	Total Carbs	Net Carbs	Small Meal (250 calories)	Total Carbs	Net Carbs
Mexican Rice & Beans	¾ cup (175 mL)	33	28	½ cup (125 mL)	22	19
Scrambled egg	2 large	0	0	1 large	0	0
Salsa	2 tbsp (30 mL)	2	1	2 tbsp (30 mL)	2	1
Sliced cucumbers	6 slices	1	1	6 slices	1	1
Café Almondo	1 cup (250 mL)	2	1	1 cup (250 mL)	2	1
		38 g	**31 g**		**27 g**	**22 g**

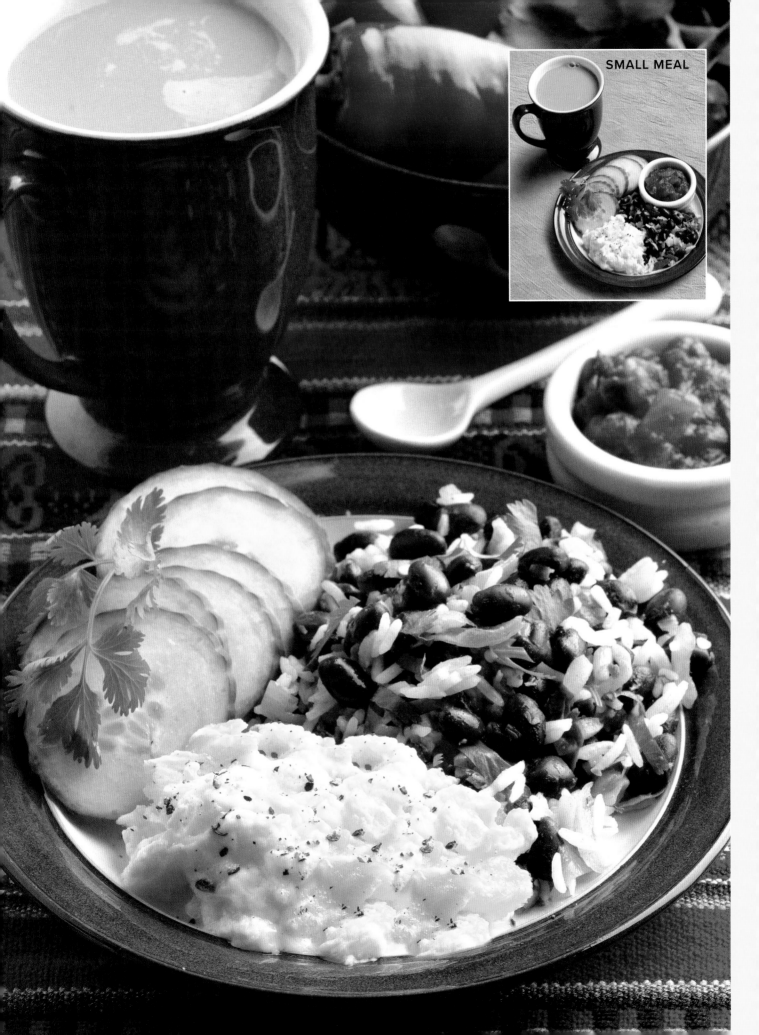

SMALL MEAL

Fast-Food Breakfast

If you are tempted to eat breakfast at a fast-food restaurant or coffee shop, then carefully choose your meal. Portion sizes are often large or extra large. Meal items are layered with ingredients, which means more fat, sugar, salt and calories. Ask for their nutrient guides, or visit their websites. Then you can check which items would fit into your large-meal breakfast of 370 calories or your small-meal breakfast of 250 calories.

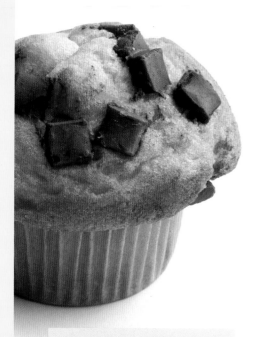

FOOD CHARTS

See page 296: Bagel Breakfast.

How calories add up

Muffins and donuts: Muffins have become so large that they are exploding with calories. Typically, a donut has 200 to 400 calories, while a fast-food muffin has 300 to 500 calories! Your lowest-calorie choice may be the old-fashioned cake donut, at about 200 calories, rather than a muffin.

Bagels: One large bagel is equal to four slices of regular bread, or 300 calories. A large buttered bagel has 400 to 500 calories, and if you add cream cheese it goes up to 500 to 650 calories.

Tea biscuits: A tea biscuit can have 150 to 300 calories, depending on its size. With a tablespoon of butter spread on, you add 135 more calories.

Croissant: A standard-size croissant has 200 to 300 calories, but if you eat a double-croissant sandwich with sausage, egg and cheese, expect 500 calories.

Burritos: A plain breakfast burrito has about 400 calories; a supersize breakfast burrito has 600 to 800 calories.

Beverages: Large-size specialty cappuccinos have 500 calories or more. Juices come in large containers, so are high in calories from sugar ("natural" sugar and, in some cases, extra added sugar).

Food Choices	Large Meal	Small Meal
Carbohydrate	3½	2
Protein	1	1
Fat	1	0

Your Breakfast Menu	Large Meal (370 calories)	Total Carbs	Net Carbs	Small Meal (250 calories)	Total Carbs	Net Carbs
Entrée	1-egg English muffin with cheese and bacon (or fast food cheeseburger)	27	25	1-egg English muffin with cheese, no butter (or fast-food hamburger / no cheese, or chicken fajita)	28	26
Apple juice	¾ cup (175 mL)	21	21	–	–	–
Coffee or tea with single milk, low-calorie sweetener	1 cup (250 mL)	1	1	1 cup (250 mL)	1	1
		49 g	**47 g**		**29 g**	**27 g**

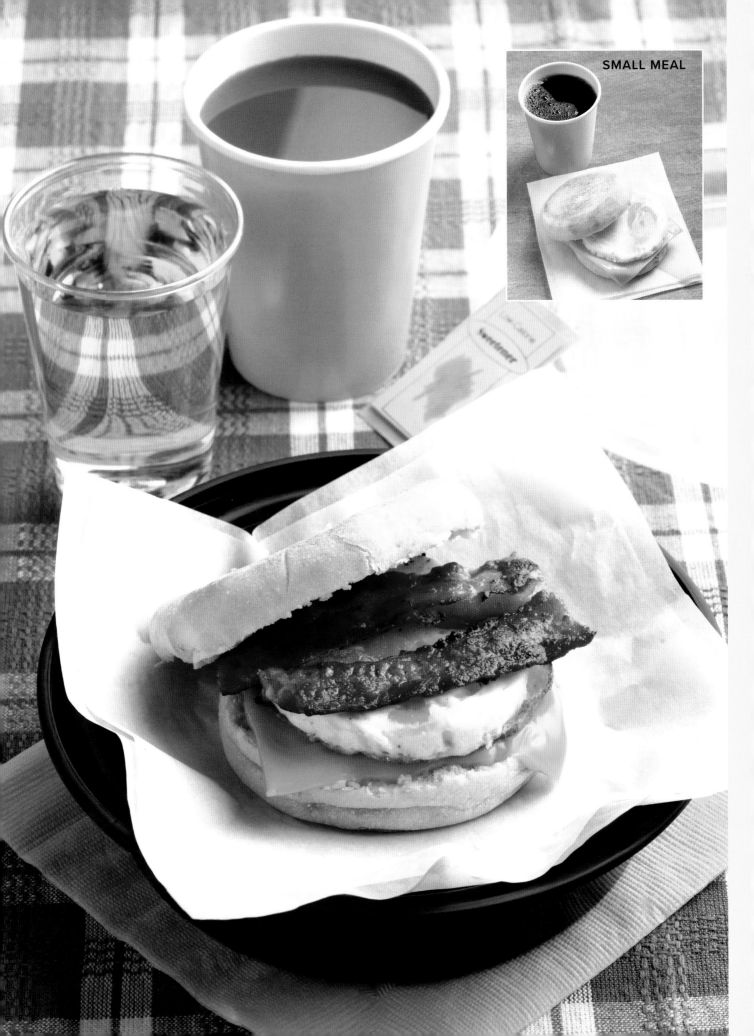

SMALL MEAL

Granola Combo

This combo of fruit, yogurt and protein-rich granola can be enjoyed at home or carried with you to work.

OPTIONS

This homemade granola has protein and healthy fats from sunflower seeds and nuts. If you want to substitute a store-bought granola or cereal, measure a portion equal to 150 calories for the large meal or 110 calories for the small meal.

FOOD CHARTS

See page 292: Cold Cereal.

Crunchy Nut Granola

Makes 10 cups (2.5 L)

½ cup (125 mL) shelled sunflower seeds

¾ cup (175 mL) sweetened flaked coconut

¼ cup (60 mL) wheat germ

¼ cup (60 mL) ground flax seeds (flaxseed meal)

1 cup (250 mL) chopped or sliced almonds, walnuts or pecans

4 cups (1 L) large-flake old-fashioned rolled oats

½ cup (125 mL) corn syrup

3 tbsp (45 mL) olive oil or vegetable oil

1 tsp (5 mL) vanilla

1 tsp (5 mL) almond extract or coconut extract

2 cups (500 mL) crisp rice or round oat cereal

½ cup (125 mL) raisins or other dried fruit, chopped

PER ½ CUP (125 ML)	
Calories	221
Carbohydrate	29 g
Fiber	4 g
Net carbs	25 g
Protein	6 g
Fat, total	10 g
Fat, saturated	2 g
Cholesterol	0 mg
Sodium	52 mg

1. In a large bowl, mix sunflower seeds, coconut, wheat germ, ground flax seeds, nuts and oats.
2. In a small bowl, combine corn syrup, oil, vanilla and almond or coconut extract.
3. Add syrup mixture to dry ingredients. Make sure any wet lumps are well blended in.
4. Place granola in a large casserole dish and bake on middle rack at 350°F (180°C) for 30 to 35 minutes, or until slightly toasted. During baking, remove the pan from the oven *every 10 minutes* and stir, so that the granola cooks evenly.
5. Once toasted, remove from the oven. Immediately transfer to a metal bowl or pot; otherwise, the granola may stick to the bottom of the hot pan as it sits to cool. Stir once or twice as it's cooling. Once cooled, add cereal and raisins. Store in an airtight container.

Food Choices	Large Meal	Small Meal
Carbohydrate	3½	2½
Fat	2	1

Your Breakfast Menu	Large Meal (370 calories)	Total Carbs	Net Carbs	Small Meal (250 calories)	Total Carbs	Net Carbs
Berries and chopped fruit (fresh or frozen)	1½ cups (375 mL)	20	15	1 cup (250 mL)	13	10
Greek yogurt (0 to 2%), flavored, less sugar	¾ cup (175 mL)	9	8	¾ cup (175 mL)	9	8
Crunchy Nut Granola	½ cup (125 mL)	29	25	¼ cup (60 mL)	15	13
Tea or coffee	1 cup (250 mL)	1	1	1 cup (250 mL)	1	1
		59 g	**49 g**		**38 g**	**32 g**

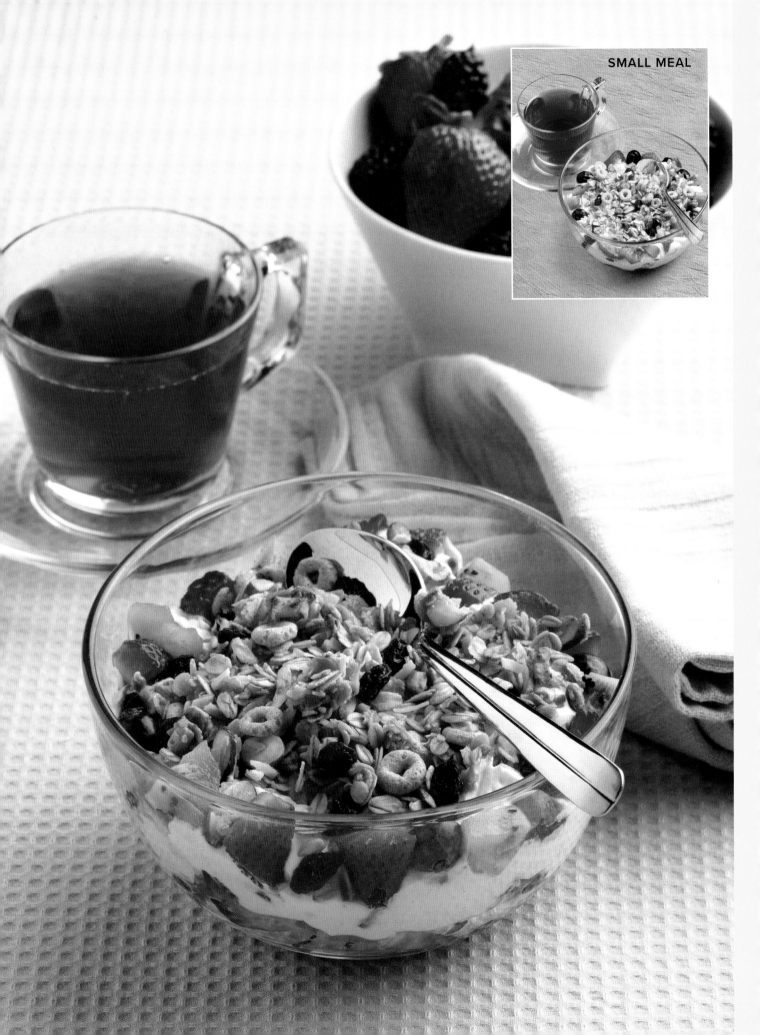

SMALL MEAL

Prairie Quiche

Prairie Quiche has a bread-crumb crust, which is much lower in calories, carbs and fat than a traditional pastry crust. This delicious quiche takes about 45 minutes to prepare and cook, so it's perfect when you have a carefree morning ahead.

OPTIONS

Four- or 5-blend shredded cheese

Where shredded cheese is an ingredient in recipes, you can use a 4- or 5-cheese blend, which may include Cheddar, mozzarella, Parmesan and specialty cheeses.

Prairie Quiche

Makes 2 large or 3 small servings

1 tsp (5 mL) margarine or butter, to generously grease the casserole

⅓ cup (75 mL) dry bread crumbs

2 eggs

2 slices raw bacon, fat partly trimmed off, chopped, or 2 slices turkey bacon

½ cup (125 mL) skim milk

Pinch of black pepper

¾ cup (175 mL) sweet red pepper or broccoli (or a combination), chopped into small pieces

½ cup (125 mL) shredded cheese

PER ½ QUICHE	
Calories	318
Carbohydrate	21 g
Fiber	2 g
Net carbs	20 g
Protein	20 g
Fat, total	17 g
Fat, saturated	7 g
Cholesterol	214 mg
Sodium	628 mg

1. Grease the sides and bottom of a 6-inch (15 cm) casserole dish with margarine or butter. Spread bread crumbs on the bottom of the casserole dish.
2. In a bowl, combine eggs, chopped bacon, milk, pepper and vegetables. Pour on top of bread crumbs. Top with shredded cheese.
3. Bake in oven on the middle rack at 400°F (200°C) for 25 minutes.
4. Once cooked, remove from the oven and let sit for 5 minutes. Gently remove slices with an egg turner.

A small glass of orange, apple, grapefruit or cranberry juice is served with the Prairie Quiche. Juice is an excellent source of vitamin C, but has little of the fiber found in fresh fruit. For an occasional breakfast choice, have a small glass of juice instead of fresh fruit. (See page 15.)

Food Choices	Large Meal	Small Meal
Carbohydrate	2	2
Protein	2	1
Fat	1	1

Your Breakfast Menu	Large Meal (370 calories)	Total Carbs	Net Carbs	Small Meal (250 calories)	Total Carbs	Net Carbs
Quiche	½ of the recipe	21	19	⅓ of the recipe	14	13
Orange juice, unsweetened	½ cup (125 mL)	13	13	½ cup (125 mL)	13	13
		34 g	**32 g**		**27 g**	**26 g**

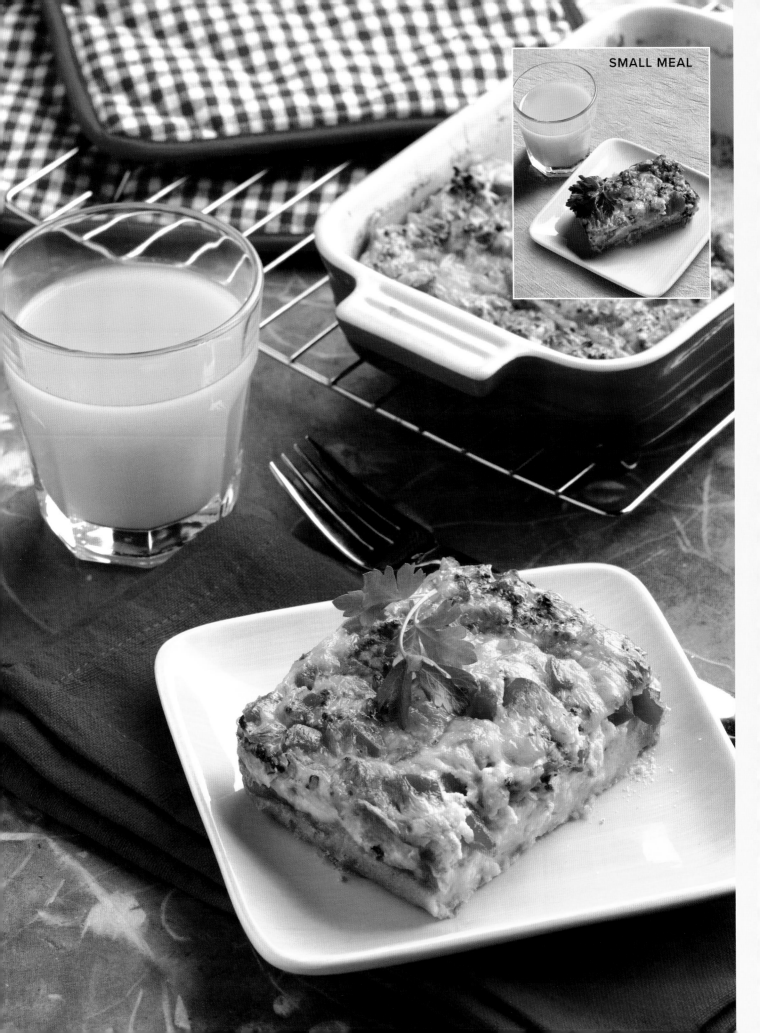

SMALL MEAL

Irish Currant Cake

FOOD FACT

This yummy cake is an adaptation of traditional Irish soda bread. The recipe uses currants, which are dried from a small seedless variety of grape. (You can replace the currants with raisins.)

HEALTH TIP

When you cook with a cast-iron pan or pot, your food becomes enriched with the iron.

OPTIONS

Papaya is a tropical fruit rich in potassium and vitamins A and C. An alternative would be a similar portion of cantaloupe.

Food Choices	Large Meal	Small Meal
Carbohydrate	3½	3
Protein	1	0
Fat	1	1

Irish Currant Cake
Makes 10 slices

2 cups (500 mL) flour
½ tsp (2 mL) salt
1½ tsp (7 mL) baking powder
½ tsp (2 mL) baking soda
⅓ cup (75 mL) sugar
¾ cup (175 mL) dried currants
1 egg
1 cup (250 mL) buttermilk (if you don't have buttermilk, start with 2 tbsp/25 mL vinegar and add skim or 1% milk to make up 1 cup/250 mL)
¼ cup (60 mL) butter, melted

PER SLICE	
Calories	206
Carbohydrate	35 g
Fiber	2 g
Net carbs	33 g
Protein	5 g
Fat, total	4 g
Fat, saturated	3 g
Cholesterol	32 mg
Sodium	260 mg

1. In a bowl, mix together flour, salt, baking powder, baking soda and sugar. Sift out any lumps.
2. Add currants to the dry ingredients and toss until they are well coated in flour.
3. In a small bowl, beat egg with a fork. Add the buttermilk and the melted butter to egg and stir with fork.
4. Add this milk mixture to the dry ingredients and blend until all the flour is mixed in.
5. Turn batter into a greased 10-inch (25 cm) cast-iron pan, a 9- by 5-inch (2 L) loaf pan or a 7½-inch (18 cm) square baking pan. Or drop as 12 biscuits onto a greased cookie sheet.
6. Bake at 350°F (180°C) for 30 to 40 minutes, until golden brown. Cool slightly. If baked in a pan, turn pan upside down onto a plate and the cake will fall out. Let it sit for a few minutes, then turn it over again and slice it, serving it still warm.

Your Breakfast Menu	Large Meal (370 calories)	Total Carbs	Net Carbs	Small Meal (250 calories)	Total Carbs	Net Carbs
Irish Currant Cake	1 slice	35	33	1 slice	35	33
Piece of cheese	1 oz (30 g)	0	0	–	0	0
Jam or marmalade	2 tsp (10 mL) regular	9	9	1 tsp (5 mL) regular or 2 tsp (10 mL) light	5	0
Papaya with lime juice	½ small	7	6	½ small	7	6
Tea or coffee	1 cup (250 mL)	1	1	1 cup (250 mL)	1	1
		52 g	**49 g**		**48 g**	**40 g**

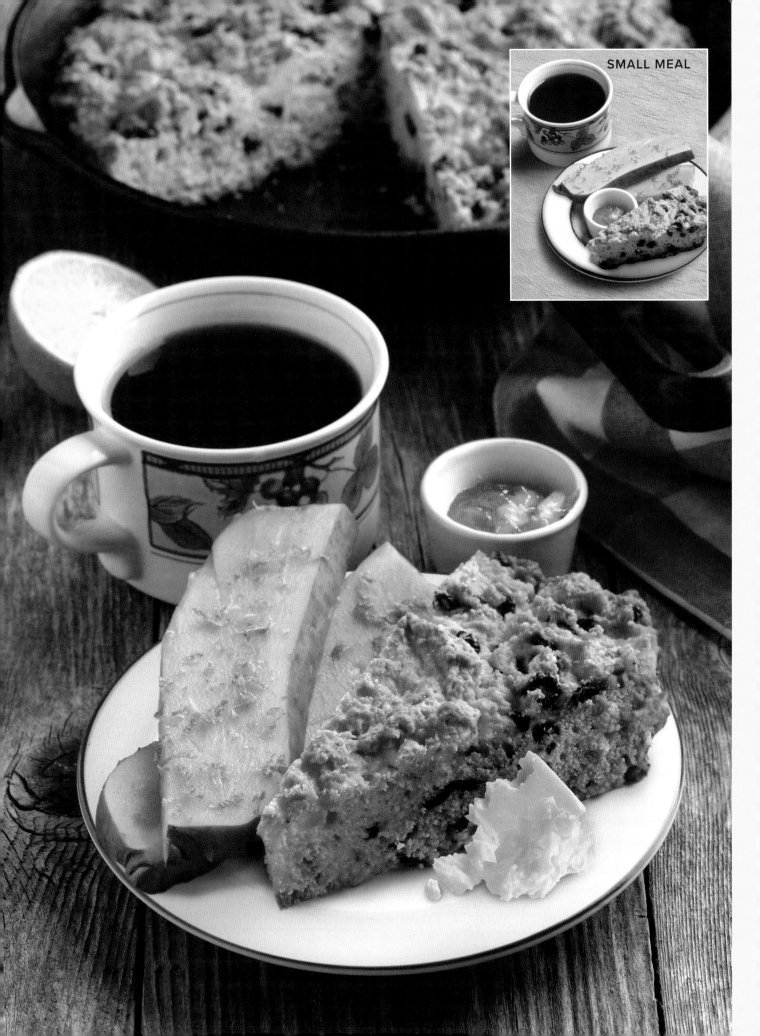

SMALL MEAL

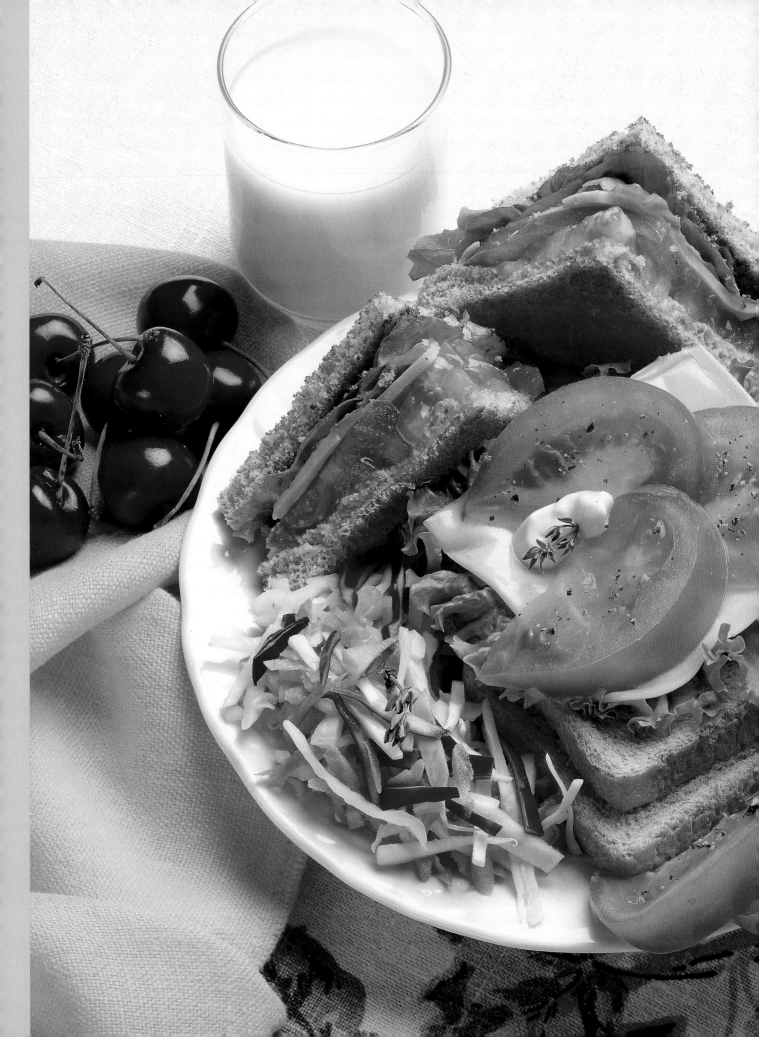

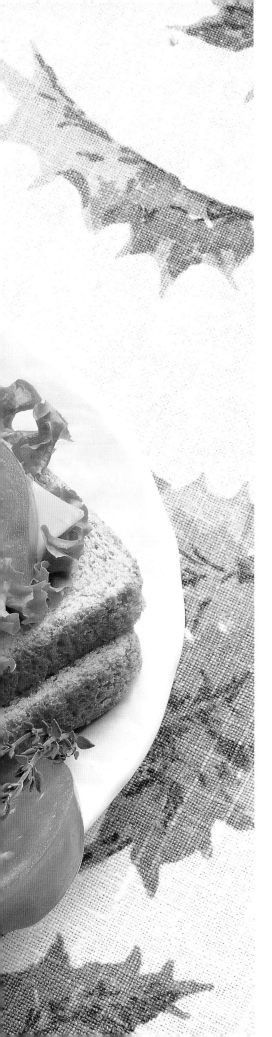

Lunch Meals

- Each large lunch has **520 calories**
  Total carbs: 90 g or less | Net carbs: 80 g or less

- Each small lunch has **400 calories**
  Total carbs: 70 g or less | Net carbs: 60 g or less

LUNCH 1

Sandwich with Milk

There are many fillings for sandwiches, for example, roast beef (as shown in the photograph) or other lean meat, chicken or turkey breast, cheese, egg or fish. For a lower-salt option, choose home-cooked meat instead of deli meats. Tuna, salmon or sardine sandwiches are also great choices; see Lunch 11.

Include some kind of vegetable on the side, such as radishes, celery, slices of tomato or sweet pepper.

Cantaloupe or any other type of fruit serving is good with this meal.

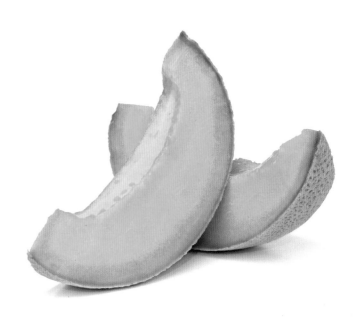

OPTIONS

Instead of light mayonnaise:
- 1 tsp (5 mL) of relish or mustard, or
- 1 tbsp (15 mL) of salsa

Instead of 1 cup (250 mL) of milk:
- 1 cup (250 mL) buttermilk
- ¾ cup (175 mL) of low-fat yogurt
- a slice of cheese
- 1 cup (250 mL) of fortified unsweetened soy beverage
- 1 cup (250 mL) of fortified unsweetened almond beverage (lower in protein and calories)

Food Choices	Large Meal	Small Meal
Carbohydrate	5	4
Protein	2	1
Fat	1	1

Your Lunch Menu	Large Meal (520 calories)	Total Carbs	Net Carbs	Small Meal (400 calories)	Total Carbs	Net Carbs
Meat sandwich	1½ sandwiches	43	38	1 sandwich	29	26
• bread, light rye	3 slices	0	0	2 slices	0	0
• roast beef	2 oz (60 g)	1	1	1 oz (30 g)	1	1
• light mayonnaise	1 tbsp (15 mL)	0	0	1 tbsp (15 mL)	0	0
• lettuce	2 large leaves	0	0	2 large leaves	0	0
Radishes	3	0	0	3	0	0
Cantaloupe	½ small (1½ cups/375 mL diced)	18	16	½ small (1½ cups/375 mL diced)	18	16
Skim or 1% milk	1 cup (250 mL)	12	12	1 cup (250 mL)	12	12
		74 g	**67 g**		**60 g**	**55 g**

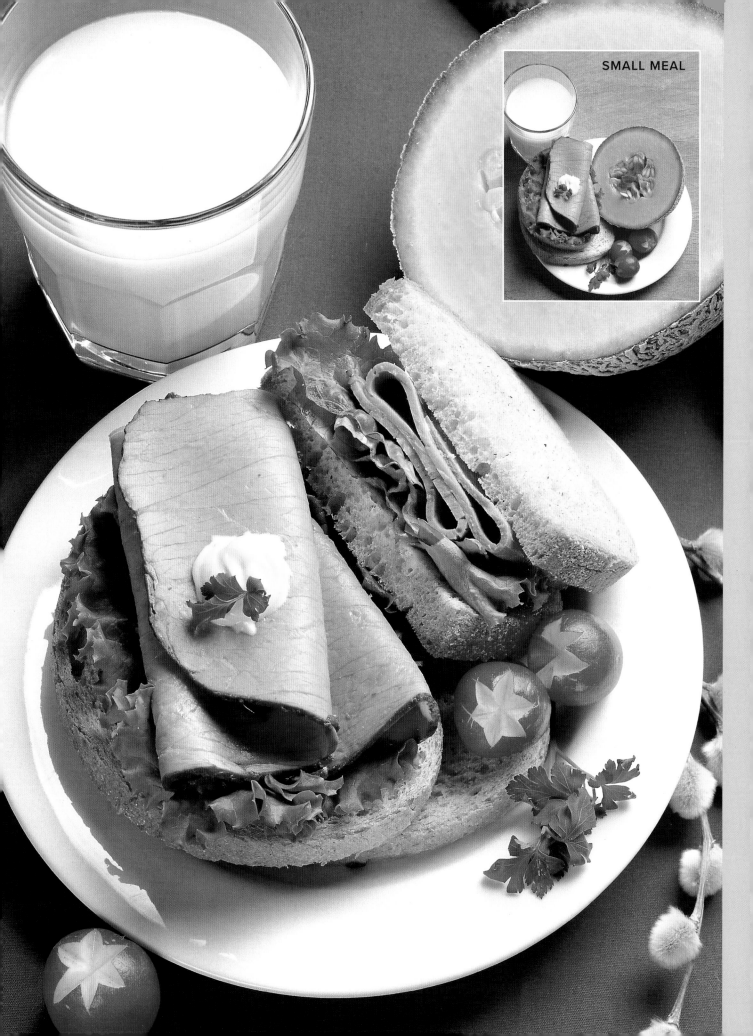

SMALL MEAL

Beans & Toast

Open a can of brown beans, warm them up and serve a portion of them, as shown, with toast and raw vegetables.

OPTIONS

If you don't have any celery, choose a sliced tomato or 1/2 cup (125 mL) of tomato or vegetable juice.

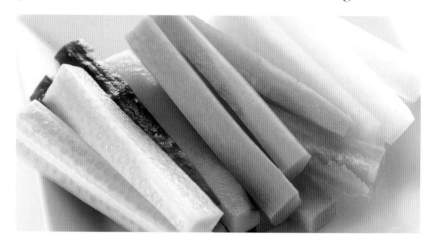

OPTIONS

Instead of a Frozen Yogurt Bar

Check the labels of small ice cream bars. Choose the ones that have 100 calories or less and are about 2 fl oz (60 mL).

Frozen Yogurt Bars are a light and easy-to-make dessert.

Frozen Yogurt Bars

Makes 8 bars

2 cups (500 mL) plain
   skim milk yogurt
1/2 tsp (5 mL) diet (sugar-free)
   fruit-flavored drink crystals

1. Mix the crystals with the yogurt.
2. Pour into containers and freeze. The bars will be ready to eat in 2 to 3 hours.

PER BAR	
Calories	32
Carbohydrate	5 g
Fiber	0 g
Net carbs	5 g
Protein	3 g
Fat, total	0 g
Fat, saturated	0 g
Cholesterol	1 mg
Sodium	46 mg

Food Choices	Large Meal	Small Meal
Carbohydrate	4	3
Protein	2	1
Fat	2	2

Your Lunch Menu	Large Meal (520 calories)	Total Carbs	Net Carbs	Small Meal (400 calories)	Total Carbs	Net Carbs
Canned baked beans	1 cup (250 mL)	54	44	1/2 cup (125 mL)	27	22
Toast	1 1/2 slices	24	21	1 1/2 slices	24	21
Margarine	2 tsp (10 mL)	0	0	2 tsp (10 mL)	0	0
Celery sticks	2 stalks	3	2	2 stalks	3	2
Frozen Yogurt Bar	1	5	5	1	5	5
		86 g	**72 g**		**59 g**	**50 g**

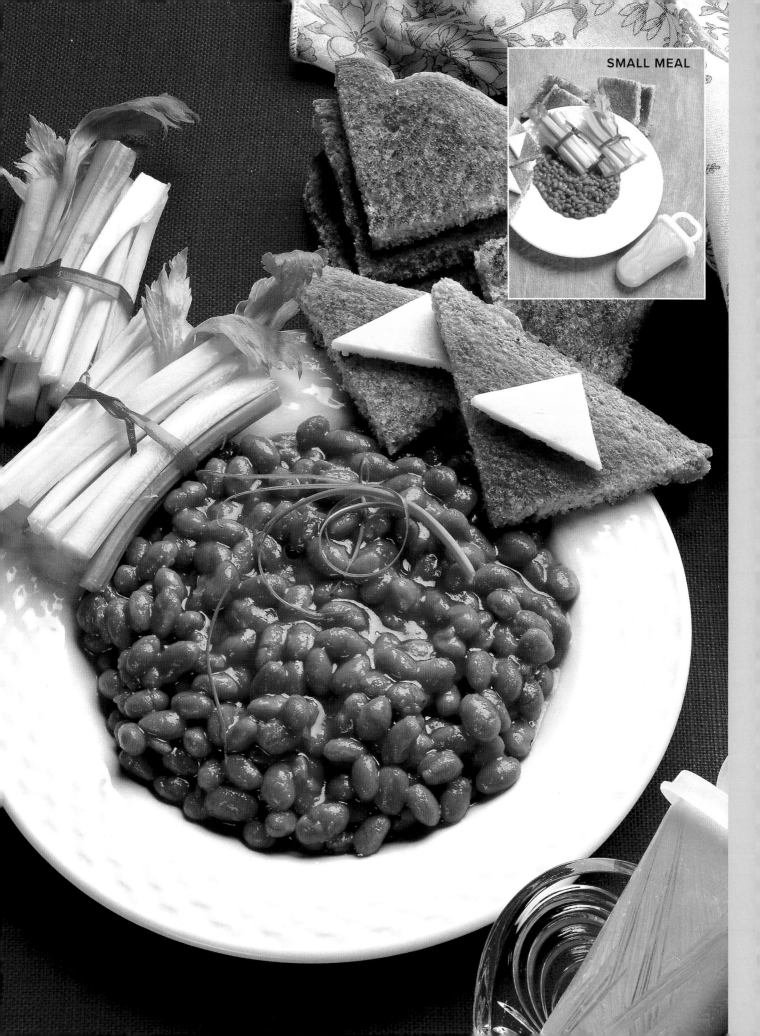

SMALL MEAL

Chicken Soup & Bagel

OPTIONS

Instead of both salmon and cream cheese, top your bagel with any of these:

- 1 oz (30 g) or one thin slice of cheese or meat such as ham or turkey. Limit high-fat meats like bologna and salami.
- ¼ cup (60 mL) canned fish
- 2 tbsp (30 mL) peanut butter

Chicken Rice Soup

Makes 7½ cups (1.9 L)

2 medium carrots, chopped
1 medium onion, chopped
2 stalks celery, chopped
¼ cup (60 mL) rice (uncooked)
1 package (2 oz/60 g) of dried chicken noodle soup mix
½ tsp (2 mL) of dried dill
6 cups (1.5 L) of water

1. Chop carrots, onion and celery.
2. Put all ingredients in a medium pot.
3. Cover and gently boil for about 20 minutes, until carrots are cooked. Stir occasionally.

It is important to note that the bagel in this meal is a 3-inch (7.5 cm) bagel weighing 2 oz (60 g), and it equals two slices of bread. Larger bagels can equal four or more slices of bread.

The bagel is served with light cream cheese, and salmon, tomato and onion. For a change, try smoked salmon (lox).

PER 1 CUP (250 ML)	
Calories	67
Carbohydrate	13 g
Fiber	1 g
Net carbs	12 g
Protein	2 g
Fat, total	1 g
Fat, saturated	0 g
Cholesterol	6 mg
Sodium	316 mg

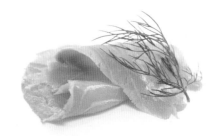

Food Choices	Large Meal	Small Meal
Carbohydrate	4½	3
Protein	1	1
Fat	1	½

Your Lunch Menu	Large Meal (520 calories)	Total Carbs	Net Carbs	Small Meal (400 calories)	Total Carbs	Net Carbs
Chicken Rice Soup	1½ cups (375 mL)	20	18	1½ cups (375 mL)	20	18
Soda crackers	2	4	4	2	4	4
Bagel	1 (or 2 slices bread)	31	30	½ (or 1 slice bread)	15	14
Light cream cheese (20%)	2 tbsp (30 mL)	1	1	1 tbsp (15 mL)	1	1
Canned pink or red salmon	¼ cup (60 mL)	0	0	¼ cup (60 mL)	0	0
Tomato	½ medium	2	1	½ medium	2	1
Sliced onion	2 slices	2	0	2 slices	2	0
Orange	1 medium	15	13	1 medium	15	13
		75 g	67 g		59 g	51 g

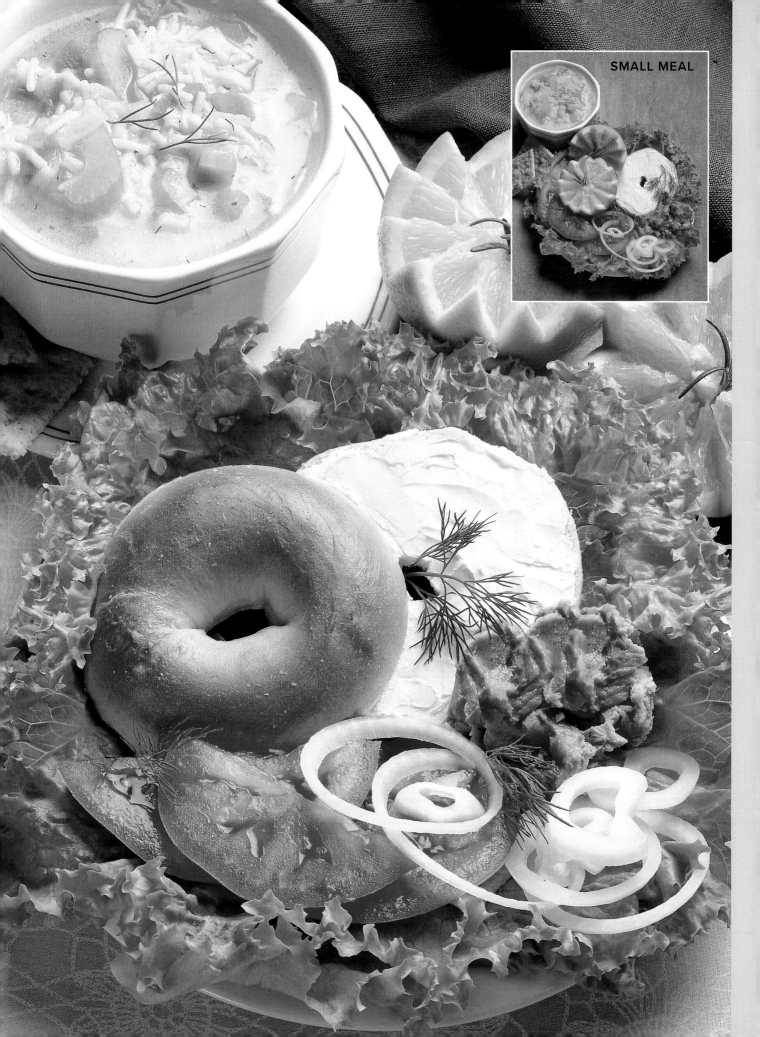

SMALL MEAL

4

Toasted Cheese & Tomato Sandwich

Restaurant or store-bought coleslaw usually has a lot of fat and sugar in the dressing. Try this healthy recipe.

OPTIONS

Mayonnaise has about the same calories as margarine or butter. Light mayonnaise or calorie-reduced margarine has one-third the calories or less. These light brands have fewer than 45 calories in 1 tbsp (15 mL).

Coleslaw

Makes 6½ cups (1.6 L)

4 cups (1 L) shredded cabbage

4 medium carrots, grated

4 stalks celery, finely chopped

1 small onion, finely chopped,
    or 2 green onions, chopped

3 tbsp (45 mL) light mayonnaise

1 tbsp (15 mL) sugar

¼ cup (60 mL) vinegar

¼ tsp (1 mL) garlic powder

Salt and pepper, to taste

PER ½ CUP (125 ML)	
Calories	33
Carbohydrate	5 g
Fiber	1 g
Net carbs	4 g
Protein	1 g
Fat, total	1 g
Fat, saturated	0 g
Cholesterol	1 mg
Sodium	47 mg

1. Chop cabbage in fine strips, grate carrots, and finely chop celery and onion. Mix these together in a large bowl.
2. In a small bowl, mix mayonnaise, sugar, vinegar, garlic powder, salt and pepper. Add to cabbage. Mix well.
3. Cover and put in the fridge. This will keep well for one week.

Food Choices	Large Meal	Small Meal
Carbohydrate	4½	3½
Protein	1	½
Fat	½	½

Your Lunch Menu	Large Meal (520 calories)	Total Carbs	Net Carbs	Small Meal (400 calories)	Total Carbs	Net Carbs
Toasted cheese & tomato sandwich	1½ sandwiches			1 sandwich		
• bread (whole wheat)	3 slices	49	42	2 slices	32	27
• cheese	1½ slices	2	2	1 slice	2	2
• tomato	1 large	7	5	1 medium	7	5
• lettuce	1 to 2 leaves	0	0	1 to 2 leaves	0	0
• light mayonnaise	2 tsp (10 mL)	1	1	2 tsp (10 mL)	1	1
Coleslaw (or raw veggies)	½ cup (125 mL)	5	4	½ cup (125 mL)	5	4
Cherries	½ cup (125 mL)	8	7	½ cup (125 mL)	8	7
Skim or 1% milk	½ cup (125 mL)	6	6	½ cup (125 mL)	6	6
		78 g	67 g		61 g	52 g

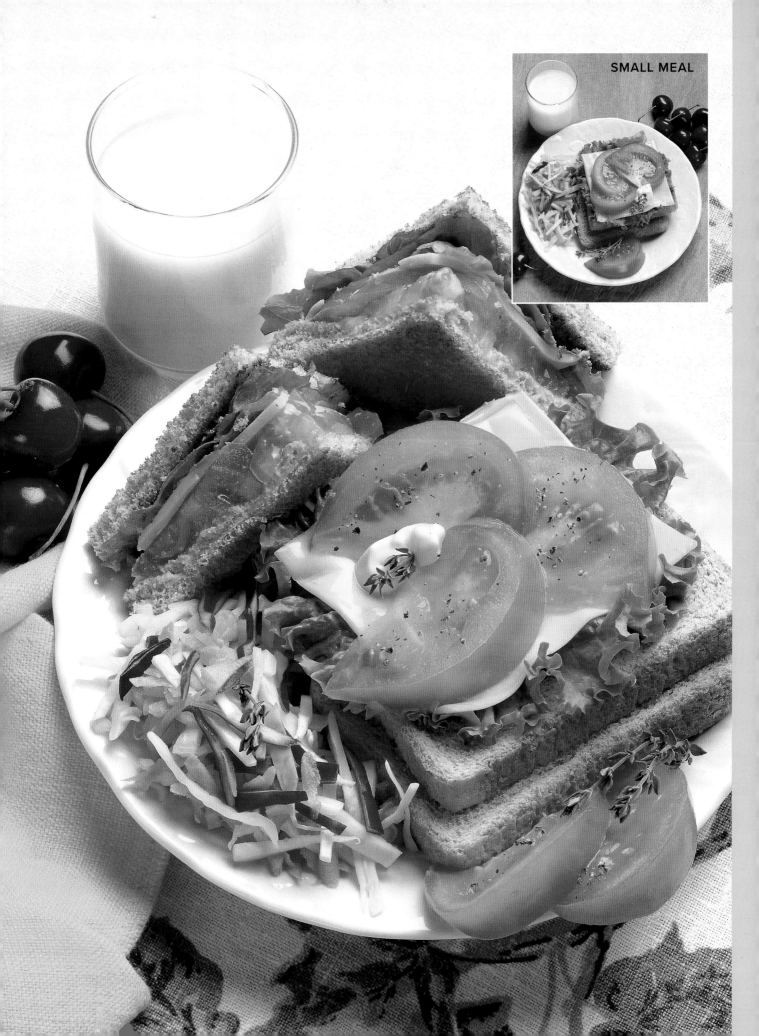

SMALL MEAL

LUNCH 5

Cold Plate with Soup

"Instant" Cup-of-Soups are fast and easy and may be a favorite for you but they are ridiculously high in salt. We recommend you remove half of the salty spice mix before putting it in your mug. See recipe below.

Reduced-Salt Instant Cup-of-Soup

Makes 1 cup (250 mL)

1 package of instant vegetable soup mix (this recipe based on a 1.9 oz/54 g box of four)

1 cup (250 mL) boiling water

PER CUP (250 ML)	
Calories	36 g
Carbohydrate	6 g
Fiber	0 g
Net Carbs	6 g
Protein	2 g
Fat, total	1 g
Fat, saturated	0 g
Cholesterol	4 mg
Sodium	240 mg

1. Place a small sifter over a bowl. Open up your package of soup and pour the soup into the sifter. Sift out ¾ tbsp (3 mL) of the spice mix (this is half of the spice mix).
2. Add the soup spice mix and dehydrated vegetables remaining in your sifter into your mug.
3. Add the boiling water; stir. Let stand for 1 minute to allow the noodles and vegetables to soften.

A standard Cup-of-Soup will have about 650 mg of sodium, and this Reduced Salt version has 240 mg. Make your own homemade soup with no-salt-added broth with lots of your favorite vegetables, herbs and spices, and dried noodles added.

OPTIONS

Instead of the small bun shown, you could have a slice of bread, half an English muffin, one small bran muffin, four melba toasts or seven soda crackers.

If you don't usually eat cottage cheese, have a slice of cheese instead.

For a less salty choice than dill pickle, choose sliced cucumber in vinegar.

Food Choices	Large Meal	Small Meal
Carbohydrate	3½	3½
Protein	4	2

Your Lunch Menu	Large Meal (520 calories)	Total Carbs	Net Carbs	Small Meal (400 calories)	Total Carbs	Net Carbs
Reduced-Salt Instant Cup-of-Soup	1 cup (250 mL)	6	6	1 cup (250 mL)	6	6
Cold plate						
• 1% or 2% cottage cheese	1 cup (250 mL)	6	6	½ cup (125 mL)	3	3
• peaches, canned or fresh	2 halves	17	15	2 halves	17	15
• dill pickle	1 medium	3	2	1 medium	3	2
• lettuce	5 large leaves	1	1	5 large leaves	1	1
• tomato	1 medium	6	5	1 medium	6	5
• green onions	4	4	2	4	4	2
• whole wheat bun (small)	1	16	14	1	16	14
• margarine or butter	1 tsp (5 mL)	0	0	—	—	—
• arrowroot biscuits	3	12	12	3	12	12
		71 g	63 g		68 g	60 g

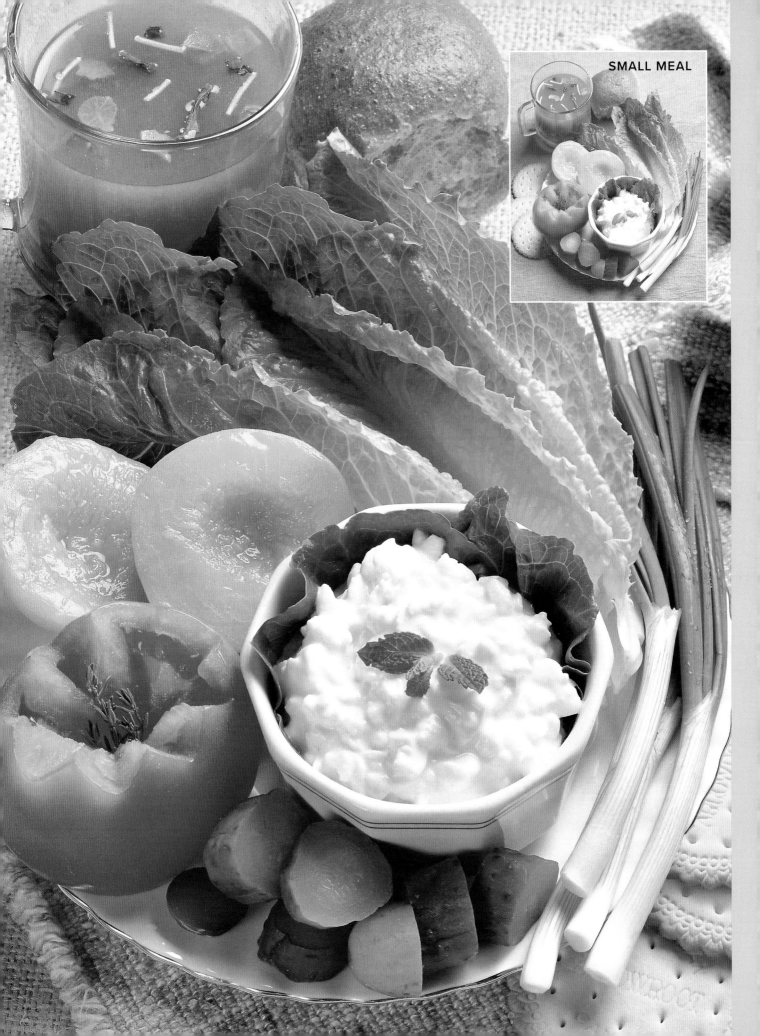

SMALL MEAL

Peanut Butter & Banana Sandwich

OPTIONS

Karen's dad's favorite Sunday lunch was a peanut butter and onion sandwich. If you like onions, use as many as you like on your peanut butter sandwich. Then have your fruit on the side.

The classic peanut butter and banana sandwich is made on white bread, but you may want to make yours on whole grain or your own favorite bread choice.

We just had to include the classic peanut butter and banana sandwich — fast, easy and delicious.

Peanut butter also goes well with jam or honey. Limit the jam or honey to 1 tsp (5 mL), or 2 tsp (10 mL) of diet jam. Still have $\frac{1}{2}$ banana or any other fruit choice on the side.

Choose vegetable juice and carrot sticks as shown, or other fresh vegetables.

You may have either $\frac{3}{4}$ cup (175 mL) of light yogurt or 1 cup (250 mL) of low-fat milk.

HEALTH TIPS

Yogurt ideas

- Did you know? Regular fruit-flavored yogurt may have 3 or more teaspoons (12 g) of sugar added in $\frac{1}{2}$ cup (125 mL). A yogurt made with a low-calorie sweetener (such as sucralose, acesulfame potassium or aspartame) will cut out this extra sugar.

- Greek yogurt is a healthy choice with higher protein and lower carbs, but you should still buy low-fat (0%, 1% or 2% at the most).

- Mix one container of plain skim milk yogurt with one container of regular fruit yogurt. It will then have $1\frac{1}{2}$ tsp (6 g) of sugar in $\frac{1}{2}$ cup (125 mL).

- Make up your own fruit yogurt simply by adding fruit to a low-fat plain yogurt.

Food Choices	Large Meal	Small Meal
Carbohydrate	$4\frac{1}{2}$	$3\frac{1}{2}$
Protein	1	$\frac{1}{2}$

Your Lunch Menu	Large Meal (520 calories)	Total Carbs	Net Carbs	Small Meal (400 calories)	Total Carbs	Net Carbs
Peanut Butter & Banana Sandwich	$1\frac{1}{2}$ sandwiches			1 sandwich		
• white bread	3 slices	46	44	2 slices	30	29
• peanut butter	$1\frac{1}{2}$ tbsp (22 mL)	5	3	1 tbsp (15 mL)	3	2
• small banana	$\frac{1}{2}$	12	11	$\frac{1}{2}$	12	11
Carrot sticks	1 medium carrot	5	4	1 medium carrot	5	4
Tomato or vegetable juice	$\frac{1}{2}$ cup (125 mL)	5	4	$\frac{1}{2}$ cup (125 mL)	5	4
Greek yogurt (0 to 2%), flavored, less sugar	$\frac{1}{2}$ cup (125 mL)	6	5	$\frac{1}{2}$ cup (125 mL)	6	5
		79 g	71 g		61 g	55 g

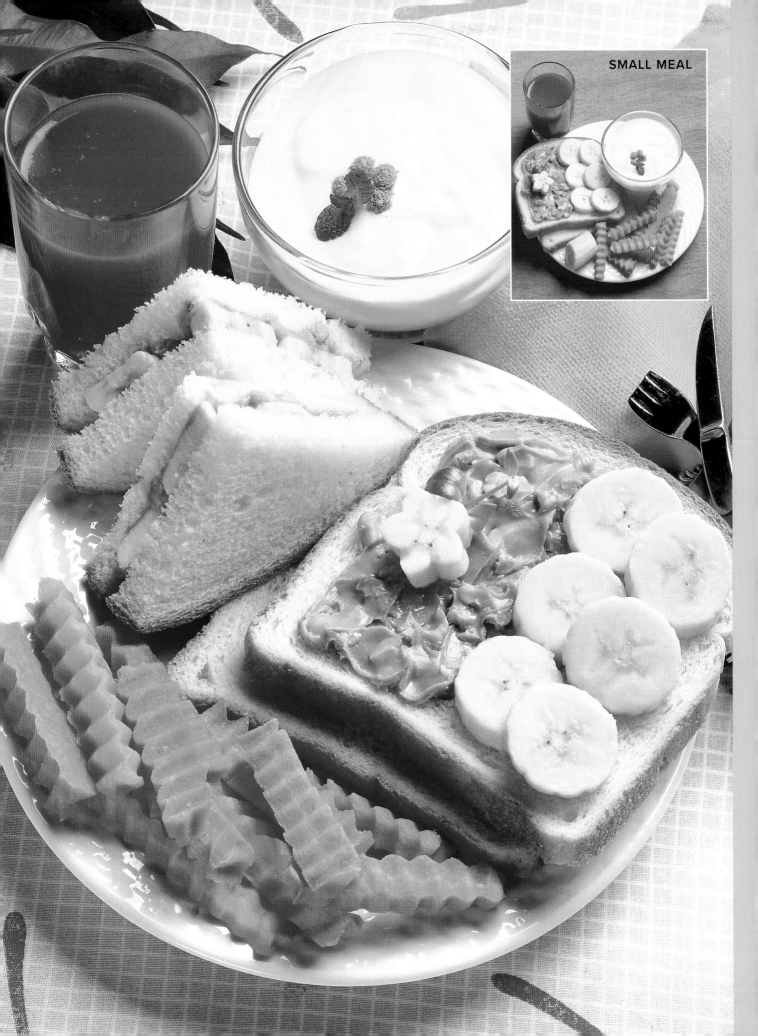

SMALL MEAL

LUNCH 7

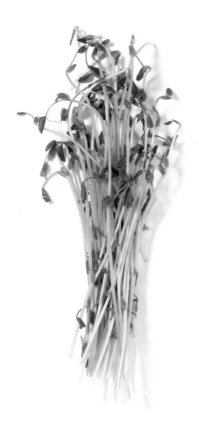

Pita Sandwich

Fill your pita with lots of vegetables!

Try these vegetables in your pita:

- lettuce and tomatoes
- bean sprouts and alfalfa sprouts
- grated carrots
- chopped green pepper
- spinach, arugula or other greens

Try one of these in your pita instead of the cheese and ham:

- ½ cup (125 mL) water-packed tuna or salmon
- ½ cup (125 mL) 1% cottage cheese
- 3 oz (85 g) firm tofu, chopped
- 2 tbsp (30 mL) peanut butter
- ½ small avocado, sliced
- ⅓ cup (75 mL) hummus

(Portions are for the large meal.)

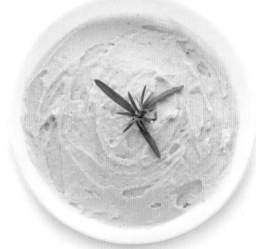

Food Choices	Large Meal	Small Meal
Carbohydrate	4	3
Protein	2	1½

Your Lunch Menu	Large Meal (520 calories)	Total Carbs	Net Carbs	Small Meal (400 calories)	Total Carbs	Net Carbs
Pita	1 (6-inch/15 cm)	33	32	1 (6-inch/15 cm)	33	32
• lettuce	¼ cup (60 mL) chopped	0	0	¼ cup (60 mL) chopped	0	0
• tomato	½ medium	2	1	½ medium	2	1
• bean sprouts	¼ cup (60 mL)	2	2	¼ cup (60 mL)	2	2
• carrots	½ small	3	2	½ small	3	2
• green pepper	2 tbsp (30 mL) chopped	1	1	2 tbsp (30 mL) chopped	1	1
• ham, lean	1 oz (30 g)	0	0	1 oz (30 g)	0	0
• Cheddar cheese, shredded	¼ cup (60 mL)	0	0	2 tbsp (30 mL)	0	0
Plums	2 medium	15	13	1 medium	8	7
Skim or 1% milk	½ cup (125 mL)	6	6	½ cup (125 mL)	6	6
Gingersnap cookies	2	11	11	–	–	–
		73 g	**68 g**		**55 g**	**51 g**

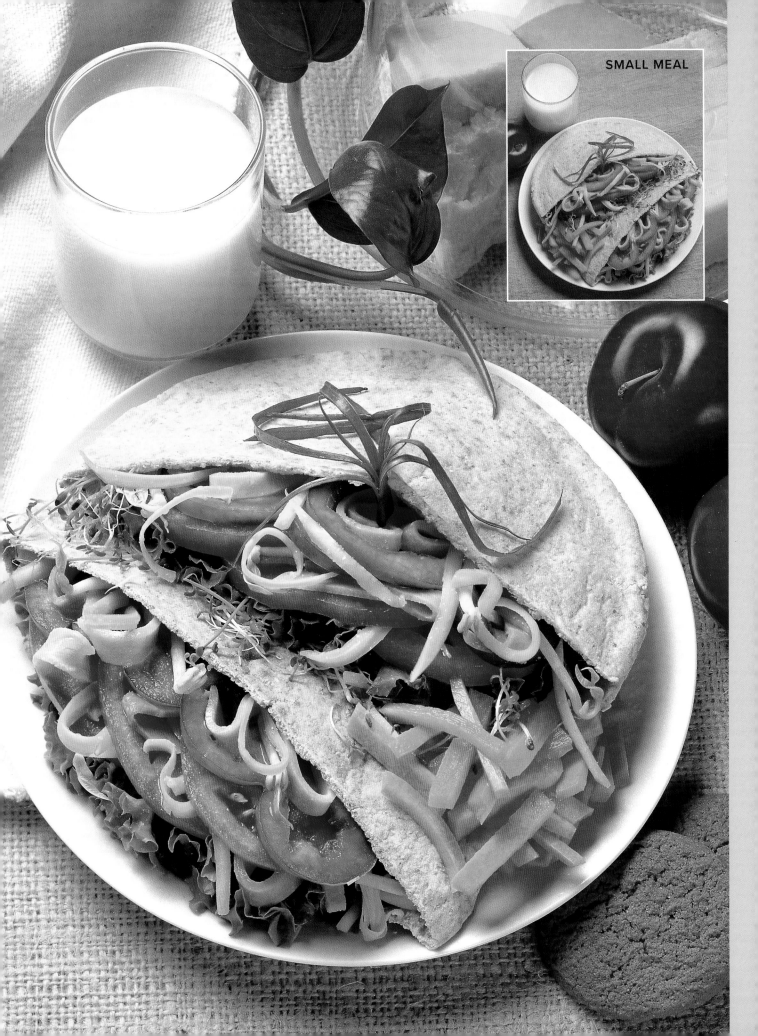

SMALL MEAL

Chef's Salad, Bun & Soup

HEALTH TIPS

When you order a salad in a restaurant, ask for low-fat salad dressing on the side. If you don't, your salad will come soaked in fat and may be just as greasy as your neighbor's order of fries.

In restaurants, salads often are served with high-fat garlic toast. You might want to consider asking for a plain bun or crackers or bread sticks instead.

Whether you're at home or in a restaurant, you may want to have a salad with a bun and soup for your lunch.

Chef's Salad

Makes 2 servings

2 cups (500 mL) chopped lettuce

2 medium tomatoes, sliced

Other vegetables, such as onions, green peppers, celery, radishes or carrots

1 apple, sliced

2 slices (2 oz/60 g) sliced chicken, meat or cheese, or fish

2 eggs, hard boiled and sliced

2 tbsp (30 mL) low-fat croutons

1. Toss vegetables and apple. Place the meat or cheese and egg on top. Add croutons.

PER SERVING	
Calories	243
Carbohydrate	21 g
Fiber	4 g
Net carbs	17 g
Protein	13 g
Fat, total	13 g
Fat, saturated	6 g
Cholesterol	208 mg
Sodium	229 mg

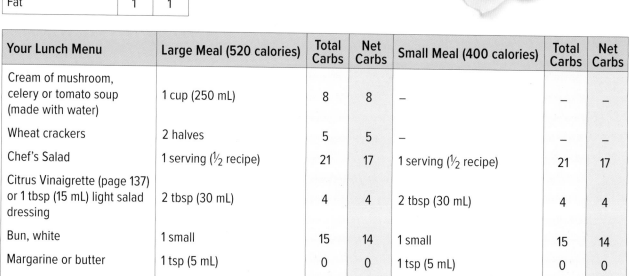

Food Choices	Large Meal	Small Meal
Carbohydrate	3	2
Protein	2	2
Fat	1	1

Your Lunch Menu	Large Meal (520 calories)	Total Carbs	Net Carbs	Small Meal (400 calories)	Total Carbs	Net Carbs
Cream of mushroom, celery or tomato soup (made with water)	1 cup (250 mL)	8	8	–	–	–
Wheat crackers	2 halves	5	5	–	–	–
Chef's Salad	1 serving (½ recipe)	21	17	1 serving (½ recipe)	21	17
Citrus Vinaigrette (page 137) or 1 tbsp (15 mL) light salad dressing	2 tbsp (30 mL)	4	4	2 tbsp (30 mL)	4	4
Bun, white	1 small	15	14	1 small	15	14
Margarine or butter	1 tsp (5 mL)	0	0	1 tsp (5 mL)	0	0
		53 g	**48 g**		**40 g**	**35 g**

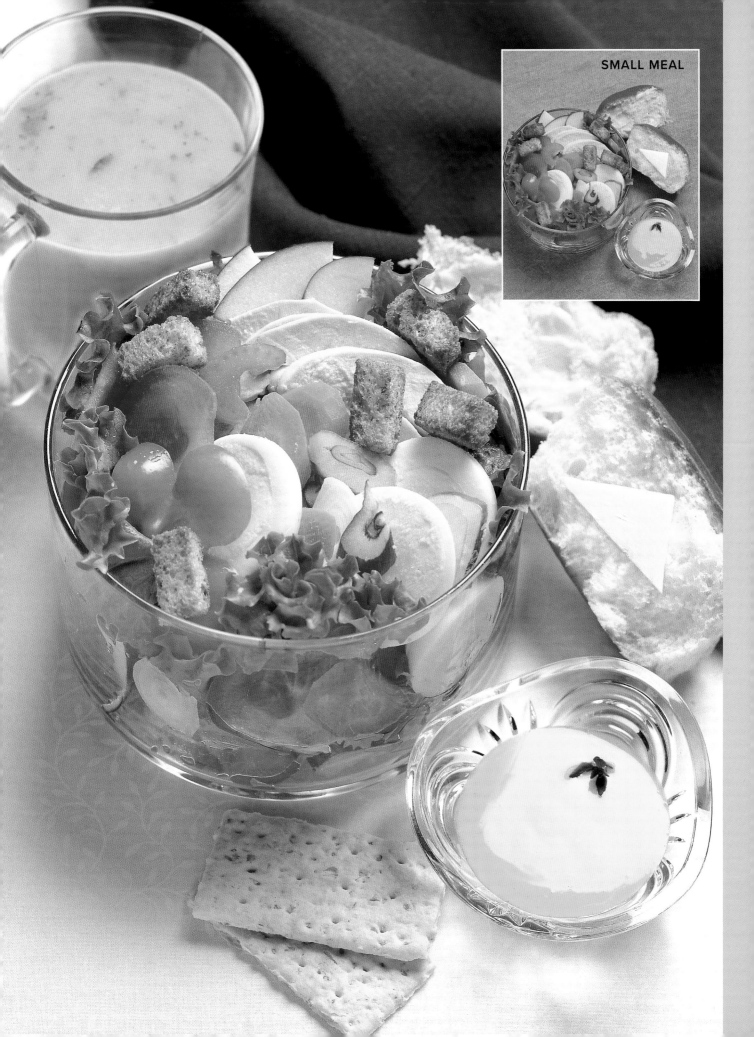

SMALL MEAL

French Onion Soup

French onion soup is easy to make at home with this recipe.

Other hearty soups are canned split pea or bean soup, or homemade hamburger soup (see recipe on page 132).

French Onion Soup

Makes 4 servings

3 packets (each 0.2 oz/4.5 g)
    reduced-salt beef bouillon mix

4 cups (1 L) water

2 medium onions, thinly sliced

4 slices white bread, toasted

4 oz (125 g) Swiss or mozzarella cheese
    (this is equal to 4 slices of cheese,
    each 4 inches/10 cm square)

PER SERVING	
Calories	218
Carbohydrate	23 g
Fiber	2 g
Net carbs	21 g
Protein	11 g
Fat, total	9 g
Fat, saturated	5 g
Cholesterol	27 mg
Sodium	621 mg

1. In a pot, add bouillon mix, water and sliced onions. Bring to a boil. Turn down heat and simmer for 15 minutes, until onions are soft.
2. Pour soup into four ovenproof bowls.
3. Cut dry toast into cubes. Put 1 full slice of cubed toast onto each bowl of soup. Place a slice of Swiss cheese on top of the bread.
4. Broil in the oven until the cheese bubbles.

Serve soup with a tossed salad with light salad dressing and a pear and, for the large meal, a slice of rye bread.

RECIPE TIP

Another way to make this soup is to use one package of dried onion soup mix. This package of soup would replace the bouillon and the onions.

For a low-salt diet

Use 3 cups (750 mL) of no-salt-added beef broth to replace the beef bouillon and water.

Food Choices	Large Meal	Small Meal
Carbohydrate	3	2
Protein	1	1
Fat	1	–

Your Lunch Menu	Large Meal (520 calories)	Total Carbs	Net Carbs	Small Meal (400 calories)	Total Carbs	Net Carbs
French Onion Soup	1 serving	23	21	1 serving	23	21
Tossed salad	Large	7	6	Large	7	6
Citrus Vinaigrette (page 137) or 1 tbsp (15 mL) light salad dressing	2 tbsp (30 mL)	4	4	2 tbsp (30 mL)	4	4
Rye bread	1 slice	15	13	–	–	–
Margarine	1 tsp (5 mL)	0	0	–	–	–
Pear	1 medium	26	21	1 medium	26	21
		75 g	**65 g**		**60 g**	**52 g**

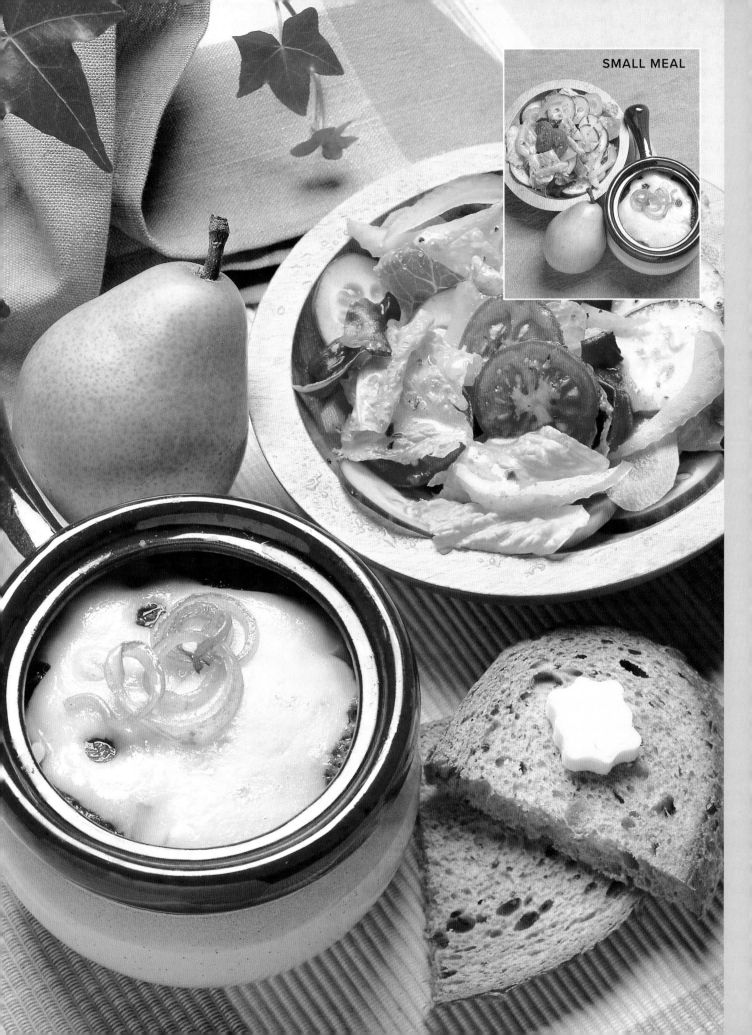

SMALL MEAL

Quesadilla

A quesadilla is a flour tortilla folded in half and lightly fried, with a combination of food in the middle. Be creative with every one you make — the combinations are endless. Include sliced avocado or some kind of protein, such as cooked meat, chicken, bacon, canned tuna, canned salmon or beans, along with cheese and salsa.

FOOD FACTS

How big is 1 ounce (30 g) of cheese or meat?

- cut from a 3½-inch (8.5 cm) block of cheese, it's a ½-inch (1 cm) thick piece
- 1¼-inch (3 cm) cube of cheese or meat
- One slice from a 4- by 4-inch (10 by 10 cm) package of sliced meat or cheese
- ⅓ small (5½ oz/156 g) can of minced chicken or ham

Quesadilla

Each quesadilla:

1 8-inch (20 cm) flour tortilla

1 oz (30 g) cooked chicken or meat, sliced or cut into small pieces

2 tbsp (30 mL) shredded cheese

1 tbsp (15 mL) salsa (or several slices of fresh tomato)

½ tsp (2 mL) margarine, olive oil or other vegetable oil

1 tbsp (15 mL) light sour cream or Greek yogurt

PER QUESADILLA	
Calories	300
Carbohydrate	32 g
Fiber	2 g
Net carbs	30 g
Protein	16 g
Fat, total	11 g
Fat, saturated	4 g
Cholesterol	40 mg
Sodium	508 mg

1. Fold tortilla in half, then open it up and cover half of the tortilla with meat, cheese and salsa. Close by folding the top half over.
2. Lightly coat your tortilla with margarine or oil (using a pastry brush, if you have one).
3. In a frying pan, cook over medium heat until lightly browned on both sides.
4. Remove from pan and cut in half or into quarters. Serve with sour cream or Greek yogurt on the side.

Low-calorie add-ins for your quesadilla

- a few olives
- sliced onions
- pickled hot peppers or banana peppers
- chopped fresh parsley or cilantro
- shredded lettuce or greens (add after the quesadilla is cooked)

Food Choices	Large Meal	Small Meal
Carbohydrate	4	3
Protein	2	1½

Your Lunch Menu	Large Meal (520 calories)	Total Carbs	Net Carbs	Small Meal (400 calories)	Total Carbs	Net Carbs
Quesadilla	1½	48	45	1	32	30
Sweet pepper or raw veggies	1 cup (250 mL)	6	4	1 cup (250 mL)	6	4
Chocolate pudding, no sugar added	3¾-oz (106 g) container	13	13	3¾-oz (106 g) container	13	13
		67 g	**62 g**		**51 g**	**47 g**

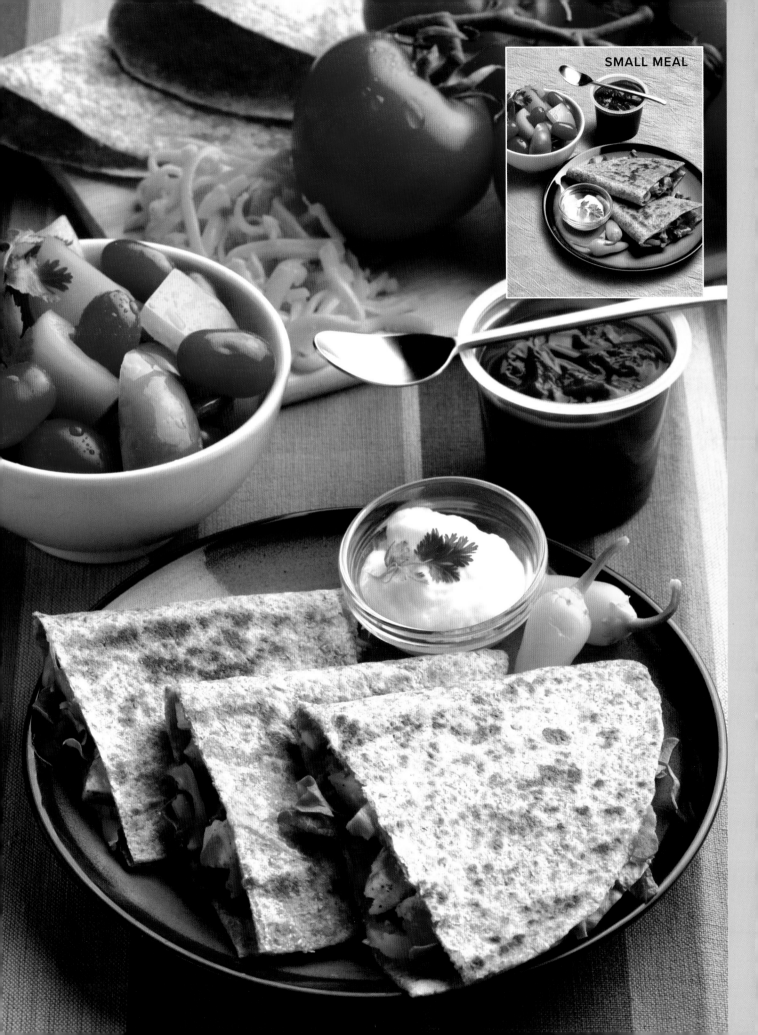

SMALL MEAL

LUNCH 11

Tuna Sandwich

Fish has two great benefits: it is the best source of the most important omega-3 fat, called DHA and EPA, and it is an excellent dietary source of vitamin D. See page 18 for other sources of omega-3 fats.

OPTIONS

Flavored tunas

For those of you who are not so fond of fish, you may like the flavored single-serving cans of tuna. One small tin (3 oz/85 g) is equal to half a can of regular tuna. If the tuna is canned in oil, you don't need to add any mayonnaise.

A tuna sandwich is a smart and easy way to eat one serving of fish. Choose canned fish or leftover mashed fish for your sandwiches. Salmon and sardines are also excellent choices, and their soft fish bones give you calcium. Pickled herring is a favorite Scandinavian fish option for a sandwich.

Fish and seafood are very nutritious, so try to eat two servings a week. In this book, you'll find six fish or seafood dinners, two lunch meals with fish and several snack ideas to bring fish into your weekly diet.

If you love avocado, then mash some up with the fish instead of mayonnaise.

Possible additions to your fish sandwich
- chopped celery
- chopped or thinly sliced dill pickles
- sliced onion
- alfalfa sprouts
- sliced olives or hot pepper pickles
- green pickle relish
- mustard or horseradish

Serve your sandwich with a glass of milk and a small fruit of your choice.

Food Choices	Large Meal	Small Meal
Carbohydrate	5	4
Protein	2	1½
Fat	1	½

Your Lunch Menu	Large Meal (520 calories)	Total Carbs	Net Carbs	Small Meal (400 calories)	Total Carbs	Net Carbs
Tuna sandwich	1½ sandwiches			1 sandwich		
• bread, whole wheat or whole grain	3 slices	47	40	2 slices	31	26
• tuna, canned in water, drained	⅔ of a 6-oz (170 g) can	0	0	½ of a 6-oz (170 g) can	0	0
• light mayonnaise	1 tbsp (15 mL)	1	1	2 tsp (10 mL)	1	1
• chopped celery and alfalfa sprouts	As desired	1	1	As desired	1	1
Skim or 1% milk	1 cup (250 mL)	12	12	1 cup (250 mL)	12	12
Apple	1 small	15	13	1 small	15	13
		76 g	**67 g**		**60 g**	**53 g**

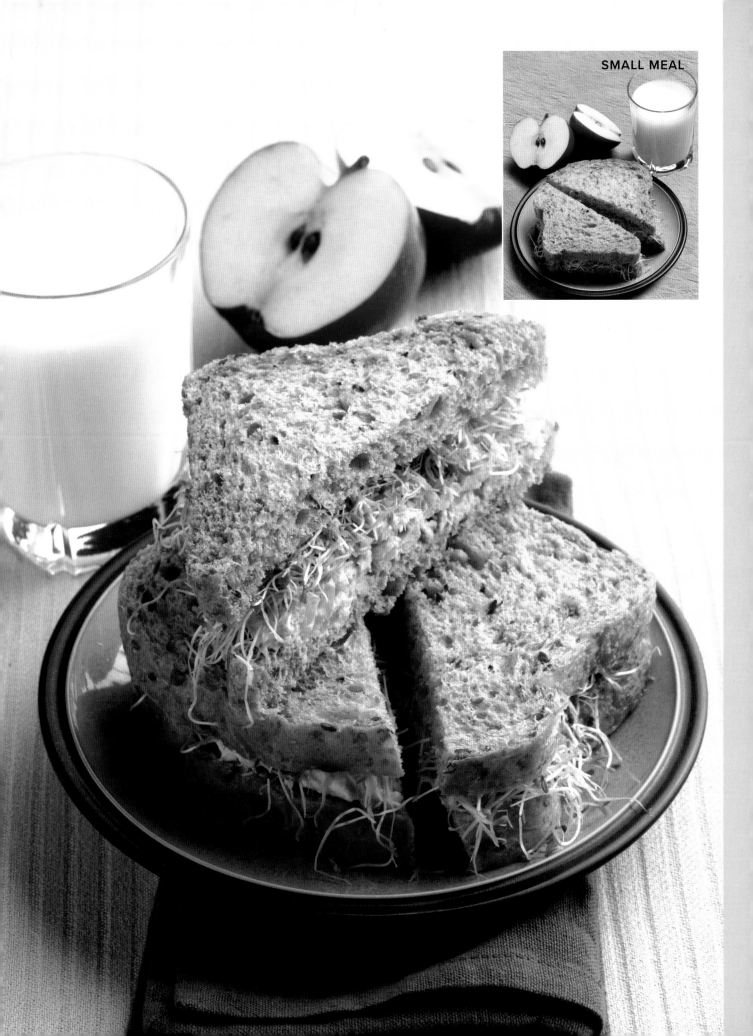

SMALL MEAL

LUNCH 12

Cheese & Crackers

A quick and easy lunch at home or work is cheese and crackers, an apple and a few pecans or almonds. Voilà — a variety of food groups!

Nuts provide protein and have heart-healthy fats. Because of their calories, just a few nuts are included in this lunch.

If you have a bit more time, you can chop your choice of fruit into bite-size pieces, toss them in a bowl with a sprinkle of grated lemon or lime rind and top with a spoonful of yogurt.

This lunch is complemented with a cup of hot iced tea (sugar-free iced tea mix blended with boiling water).

Portions of cheese, crackers and nuts

When choosing your crackers and cheese varieties, keep in mind that manufacturers vary their products and portion sizes, which can change the calories. There are also variations between brand-name and no-name food products. It's a good idea to read the "Nutrition Facts" on the label.

Then select the right portion. For example, for the large meal cracker portion, 120 calories would be about 12 soda crackers, or 5 Breton-type wheat crackers, or 3 flavored rice cakes, or a combination of these 3 types.

HEALTH TIP

Food groups

To get a healthy balance of nutrients, choose foods from three or more food groups at every meal. For information about the food groups, and photographs, see pages 13–19.

FOOD CHARTS

See page 313: Cheese and Crackers.

Food Choices	Large Meal	Small Meal
Carbohydrate	3½	2½
Protein	1½	1
Fat	1½	1

Your Lunch Menu	Large Meal (520 calories)	Total Carbs	Net Carbs	Small Meal (400 calories)	Total Carbs	Net Carbs
Cheese	180-calorie portion	1	1	120-calorie portion	0	0
Crackers, whole wheat or whole grain	160-calorie portion	29	24	110-calorie portion	21	17
Fruit	1½ cups (375 mL)	30	24	1½ cups (375 mL)	30	24
Nuts	75-calorie portion	2	1	50-calorie portion	1	1
Sugar-free iced tea	1 cup (250 mL)	1	1	1 cup (250 mL)	1	1
		63 g	51 g		53 g	43 g

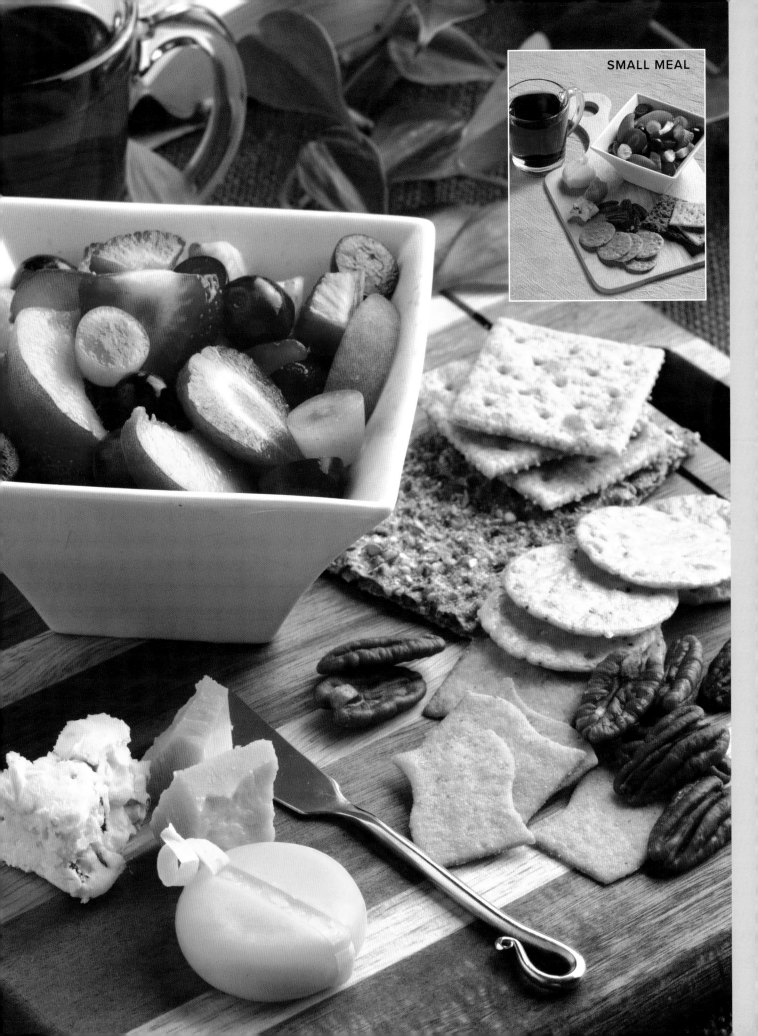

SMALL MEAL

Frozen Entrée or Leftovers

FOOD TIP

Dinner Leftovers = An Environmental Choice

On pages 104 and 105 are some dinner meals from this book that can be easily downsized to make a lunch entrée for the next day. Buy reusable microwavable bowls and plates with lids, and use last night's dinner leftovers to make lunch meals that can be frozen and reheated as you need them. These lunch meals will have less salt and additives than store-bought frozen entrées. Store-bought frozen entrées also have throwaway packaging. Help make a difference to the environment by using your own bowls and plates most often.

Store-Bought Frozen Entrées

An occasional choice

To complete your frozen entrée or leftover meal and to boost your vitamins, have some raw vegetables on the side and a fruit.

For the large meal:
Select a frozen entrée with less than 420 calories

You will be able to choose from a wide variety of the regular meals. Select ones that are lower in fat, sugar and salt. Some of the chicken or beef pot pies are less than 420 calories but have more fat and salt. If you choose a light TV dinner under 300 calories, add either a slice of bread or a small bun, pudding or a glass of milk, in addition to your vegetables and fruit.

For the small meal:
Select a frozen entrée with less than 300 calories

You will need to choose from the light selection of frozen entrées. One pizza pop, pizza pocket or mini pizza will generally fit into this calorie range. Remember to include vegetables and a fruit of your choice.

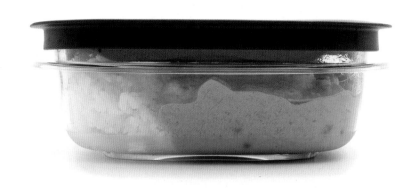

Food Choices	Large Meal	Small Meal
Carbohydrate	4½	3½
Protein	2	1
Fat	1	1

Your Lunch Menu	Large Meal (520 calories)	Total Carbs	Net Carbs	Small Meal (400 calories)	Total Carbs	Net Carbs
Frozen entrée or leftovers: • store-bought or • leftovers from dinner	up to 420 calories or portions as shown in chart	53	50	up to 300 calories or portions as shown in chart	36	34
Carrots	10 baby carrots or 1 medium	6	5	10 baby carrots or 1 medium	6	5
Banana	1 small (4-inch/10 cm) piece	16	15	1 small (4-inch/10 cm) piece	16	15
		75 g	**70 g**		**58 g**	**54 g**

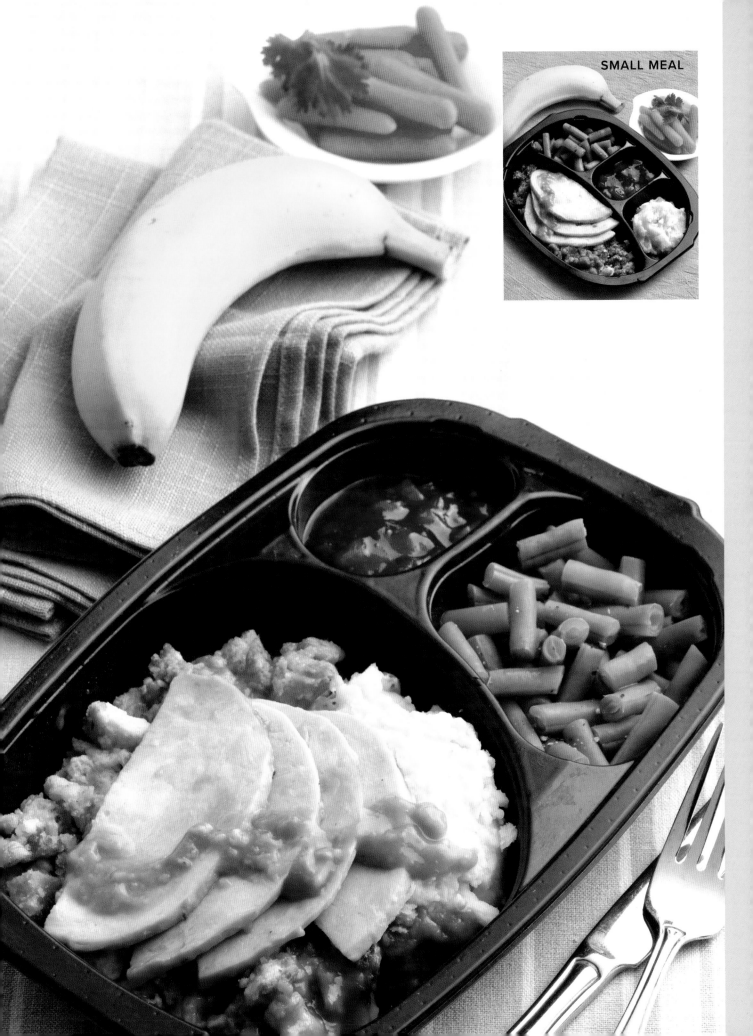

SMALL MEAL

Turn Dinner Leftovers into an Easy Lunch

➤ Add a green salad or raw vegetables to your lunch.

		Large Lunch Serving of Dinner Leftovers (about 420 calories)	Total Carbs	Net Carbs	Small Lunch Serving of Dinner Leftovers (about 300 calories)	Total Carbs	Net Carbs
Dinner 1:	Baked chicken Potato Mixed vegetables	3 oz (90 g) 1 medium ½ cup (125 mL)	47	41	2 oz (60 g) ½ medium ½ cup (125 mL)	30	25
Dinner 2:	Cooked spaghetti Spaghetti Meat Sauce	1½ cups (375 mL) ¾ cup (175 mL)	72	65	1 cup (250 mL) ½ cup (125 mL)	48	43
Dinner 4:	Roast beef Horseradish Roasted potatoes Low-Salt Gravy Beets	3 oz (90 g) 2 tsp (10 mL) 1 large 2 tbsp (30 mL) ½ cup (125 mL)	58	50	2 oz (60 g) 2 tsp (10 mL) 1 medium 2 tbsp (30 mL) ½ cup (125 mL)	45	39
Dinner 6:	Hamburger Soup	2¾ cups (675 mL)	50	44	2 cups (500 mL)	36	32
Dinner 7:	Beans & Wieners Tossed salad Citrus Vinaigrette	1 cup (250 mL) Large 1 tbsp (15 mL)	62	50	¾ cup (175 mL) Large 1 tbsp (15 mL)	49	40
Dinner 10:	Baked ham Sweet potato	4 oz (125 g) 1 large	47	44	3 oz (90 g) 1 medium	37	32
Dinner 11:	Beef Stew Boiled potatoes	2 cups (500 mL) ½ medium	56	48	1⅓ cups (325 mL) ½ medium	47	41
Dinner 13:	Sausages Cornbread	4 links 1½ pieces	33	31	3 links 1 piece	22	21
Dinner 14:	Chili Con Carne Rice	1 cup (250 mL) ⅔ cup (150 mL)	58	50	¾ cup (175 mL) ⅓ cup (75 mL)	37	31
Dinner 15:	Perogies Garlic sausage	5 + 1 tsp (5 mL) margarine 1½ oz (45 g)	60	55	4 1 oz (30 g)	41	37
Dinner 17:	Turkey, white Turkey, dark meat Low-Fat Mashed Potatoes Low-Fat Gravy Peas and carrots	2 oz (60 g) 2 oz (60 g) 1 cup (250 mL) ¼ cup (60 mL) ½ cup (125 mL)	50	45	3 oz (90 g) — ½ cup (125 mL) ¼ cup (60 mL) ½ cup (125 mL)	31	28
Dinner 18:	Baked Macaroni & Cheese	1¾ cups (425 mL)	54	52	1¼ cups (300 mL)	39	37
Dinner 19:	Pork chop Applesauce Boiled potatoes	3 oz (90 g) ¼ cup (60 mL) 6 small	45	41	3 oz (90 g) 2 tbsp (30 mL) 3 small	23	21

	Large Lunch Serving of Dinner Leftovers (about 420 calories)	Total Carbs	Net Carbs	Small Lunch Serving of Dinner Leftovers (about 300 calories)	Total Carbs	Net Carbs
Dinner 20: Bean and Meat Filling Cheese, shredded Brown rice	1 cup (250 mL) 2 tbsp (30 mL) ⅓ cup (75 mL)	39	30	¾ cup (175 mL) 2 tbsp (30 mL) ⅓ cup (75 mL)	33	26
Dinner 21: Chicken Curry Stew Whole wheat bread	1¾ cups (300 mL) 1 slice	46	38	1½ cup (375 mL) —	26	21
Dinner 23: Sun Burgers Mixed vegetables	2 burgers 1 cup (250 mL)	55	41	1½ burgers ¾ cup (175 mL)	41	30
Dinner 25: Hamburger Noodle Dish	1½ cups (375 mL)	57	53	1 cup (250 mL)	38	35
Dinner 26: Pizza Skim milk	1 large slice 1 cup (250 mL)	53	50	1 medium slice 1 cup (250 mL)	43	40
Dinner 28: Stir-Fry Rice	2 cups (500 mL) 1 cup (250 mL)	69	63	1½ cups (375 mL) ⅔ cup (150 mL)	48	43
Dinner 30: Shish Kebab Rice	1 made with 4 meat cubes ⅔ cup (150 mL)	35	33	1 made with 3 meat cubes ⅓ cup (75 mL)	21	19
Dinner 31: Chicken leg Tandoori Sauce Rice, basmati	2 small ¼ cup (60 mL) ⅓ cup (75 mL)	20	19	1 small 2 tbsp (30 mL) ⅓ cup (75 mL)	20	19
Dinner 32: Swiss Steak and sauce Potatoes	4 oz (125 g) ½ medium	23	20	3 oz (90 g) ½ medium	21	19
Dinner 33: Thai Chicken Rice noodles or pasta	1 cup (250 mL) ⅔ cup (150 mL)	49	46	¾ cup (175 mL) ⅓ cup (75 mL)	30	28
Dinner 36: Beef Parmesan Pasta sauce Cheese, shredded, low-fat Low-Fat Mashed Potatoes	1 patty ¼ cup (60 mL) 2 tbsp (30 mL) ½ cup (125 mL)	30	27	1 patty ¼ cup (60 mL) 2 tbsp (30 mL) —	11	9
Dinner 38: Pork Chop Casserole with sauce Rice	1 chop 1 cup (250 mL)	51	49	1 chop ⅔ cup (150 mL)	36	35
Dinner 39: Shrimp Linguini Sauce Linguini	1 cup (250 mL) 1 cup (250 mL)	54	51	¾ cup (175 mL) ½ cup (125 mL)	30	28
Dinner 40: Chicken Cordon Bleu Mashed sweet potato	1 medium piece ½ cup (125 mL)	35	30	1 large piece ⅓ cup (75 mL)	23	20

LUNCH 14

Avocado Salad & Bruschetta

Avocado Salad

Makes 2 servings

2 cups (500 mL) lettuce pieces or greens
1 medium tomato, cut into wedges
1 apple, thinly sliced
1 avocado, sliced
¼ cup (60 mL) shredded cheese
Grated lime rind and a drizzle of lime juice

PER ½ RECIPE	
Calories	268
Carbohydrate	23 g
Fiber	8 g
Net carbs	15 g
Protein	7 g
Fat, total	19 g
Fat, saturated	5 g
Cholesterol	10 mg
Sodium	140 mg

1. Toss all ingredients.
2. Top with your favorite low-fat salad dressing.

This is a low-fat version of a traditional Italian bruschetta.

Bruschetta

For each slice:

½-inch (1 cm) slice of French baguette
   (or ½ slice of regular bread)
1 tsp (5 mL) salsa or low-fat pasta sauce
1 to 2 tsp (5 to 10 mL) of toppings such as:
  • sliced olives or capers
  • pickled or fresh garlic cloves,
    chopped or whole
  • chopped fresh or dried herbs,
    such as cilantro, basil or chives
2 tsp (10 mL) thinly sliced, crumbled or shredded cheese

PER SLICE	
Calories	40
Carbohydrate	5 g
Fiber	0 g
Net carbs	5 g
Protein	2 g
Fat, total	2 g
Fat, saturated	1 g
Cholesterol	2 mg
Sodium	123 mg

1. Place bread pieces on a cookie sheet. Under the grill, toast the top side of the bread slices.
2. Remove cookie sheet from the oven. To each slice of bread add the salsa, toppings and cheese. Put the bread slices back in the oven to grill the cheese.

HEALTH TIP

Avocados are nutrient-rich

Avocados have a mild flavor and a smooth texture, and are low in carbohydrates. They have healthy monounsaturated fat — the kind that helps lower the bad LDL cholesterol in your blood. They are also rich in vitamin E, an important antioxidant, and folic acid, a B vitamin.

Food Choices	Large Meal	Small Meal
Carbohydrate	2	1½
Protein	½	½
Fat	4	3½

Your Lunch Menu	Large Meal (520 calories)	Total Carbs	Net Carbs	Small Meal (400 calories)	Total Carbs	Net Carbs
Avocado Salad	1 serving	23	15	1 serving	23	15
Light salad dressing	2 tbsp (30 mL)	5	5	1 tbsp (15 mL)	3	3
Bruschetta	5 baguette slices	24	22	3 baguette slices	14	13
		52 g	**42 g**		**40 g**	**31 g**

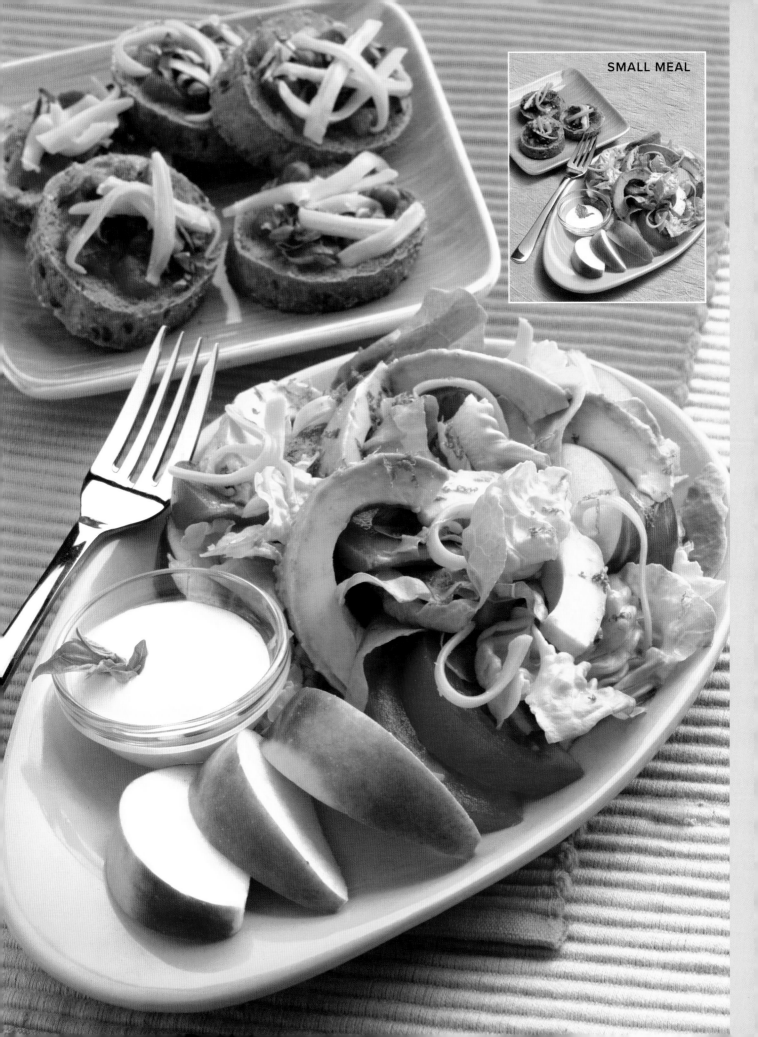

SMALL MEAL

LUNCH 15

Crab Cakes

Baltimore Maryland, Dr. Shomali's hometown, is famous for crab cakes. Here's a recipe we've adapted from his friend Sally.

Maryland Crab Cakes

Makes 6 crab cakes
(½ cup/125 mL raw mixture per crab cake)

1 egg
¼ cup (60 g) mayonnaise
1 tbsp (15 mL) fresh parsley, chopped
    (or 2 tsp/10 mL dried)
2 tsp (10 mL) prepared or Dijon or
    prepared mustard
2 tsp (10 mL) Worcestershire sauce
1 tsp (5 mL) Old Bay seasoning
1 tsp (5 mL) lemon juice, fresh
1 lb (500 g) fresh chunky crab meat
⅔ cup (150 mL) soda cracker crumbs (14 crackers)
2 tbsp (30 mL) butter, melted, to grease the baking sheet
    and remainder to brush on patty before baking
Lemon wedge, on the side

PER CRAB CAKE	
Calories	180
Carbohydrate	6 g
Fiber	0 g
Net Carbs	6 g
Protein	13 g
Fat, total	8 g
Fat, saturated	1 g
Cholesterol	63 mg
Sodium	582 mg

1. In a large bowl, whisk together egg, mayonnaise, parsley, mustard, Worcestershire sauce, Old Bay, lemon juice and salt. Place crab meat on top, followed by cracker crumbs. With a rubber spatula or large spoon, very gently fold together.
2. Cover tightly and refrigerate for at least 30 minutes or up to 1 day, to chill the mixture so it can be shaped.
3. Preheat oven and generously grease a rimmed baking sheet with the some of the butter.
4. Using a ½ cup (125 mL) measuring cup, portion the crab cake mixture into six mounds and gently form into cakes on the baking sheet. Brush each lightly with melted butter.
5. Bake at 450°F (232°C) for 12 to 14 minutes or until lightly browned around the edges and on top. Drizzle each with fresh lemon juice and serve warm.

Salmon cakes

If you don't have fresh or frozen crab available, you can make salmon cakes instead. These are also delicious! A calorie replacement for the 1 lb (500 g) of fresh crab meat would be one can of canned sockeye salmon (7.5 oz/213 g). This will make six salmon cakes.

Grilled vegetables

One cup (250 mL) of your favorite vegetables plus a medium cob of corn (large meal) or ½ cob of corn (small meal). Toss with 1 tbsp (15 mL) oil or butter for the large serving, or 2 tsp (10 mL) oil for small serving. Sprinkle with dried oregano and no-added salt herb spice blend. Grill in the oven with the crab cakes, on their own baking sheet, until tender.

Food Choices	Large Meal	Small Meal
Carbohydrate	3	2
Protein	2	2
Fat	3	2

Your Lunch Menu	Large Meal (520 calories)	Total Carbs	Net Carbs	Small Meal (400 calories)	Total Carbs	Net Carbs
Maryland Crab Cake	1 crab cake	6	5	1 crab cake	6	5
Cocktail Sauce	2 tbsp (30 mL)	10	9	2 tbsp (30 mL)	10	9
Grilled corn	1 medium cob	38	34	½ medium cob	19	17
Grilled vegetables	1 cup (250 mL)	5	4	1 cup (250 mL)	5	4
		59 g	**52 g**		**40 g**	**35 g**

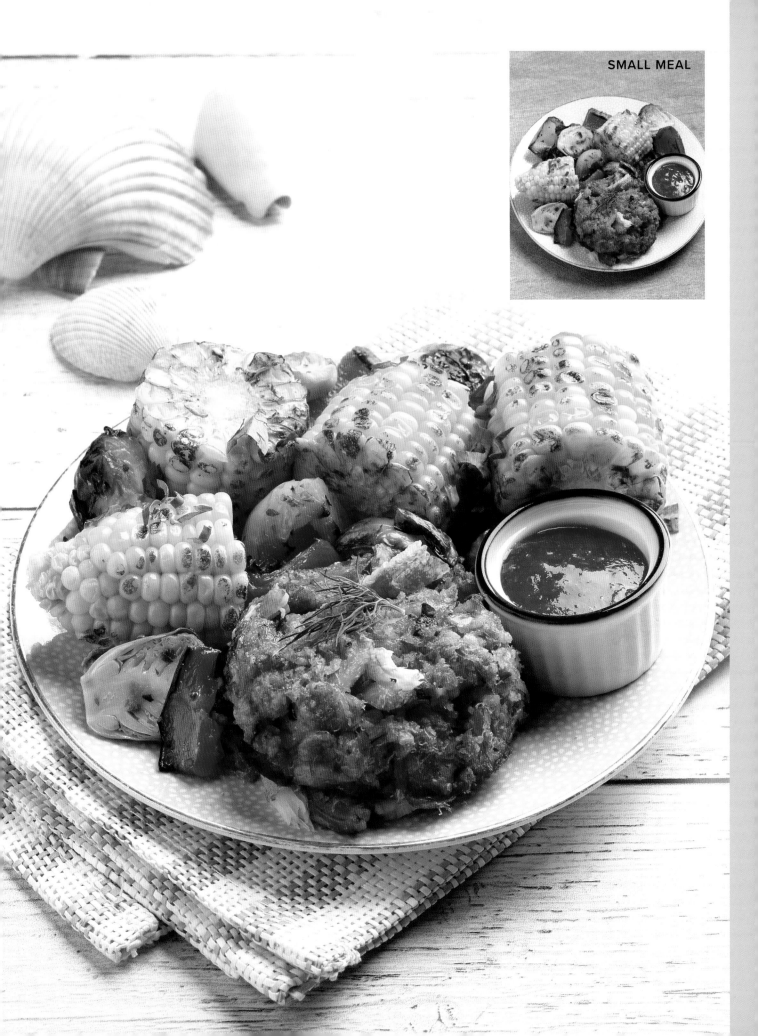

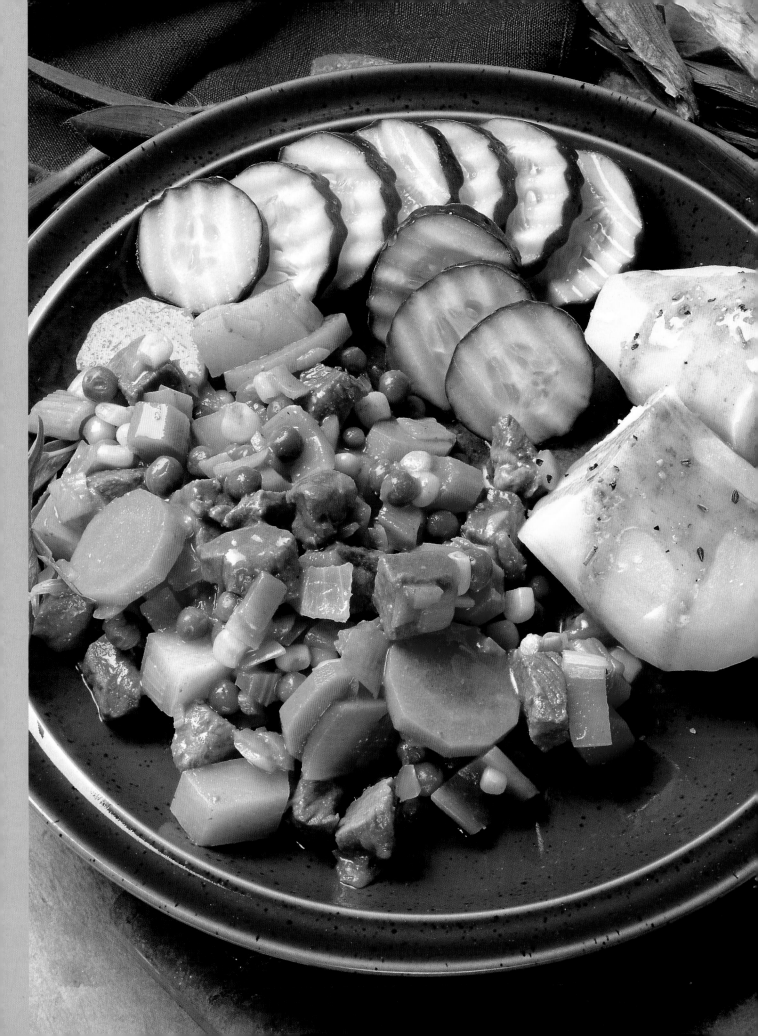

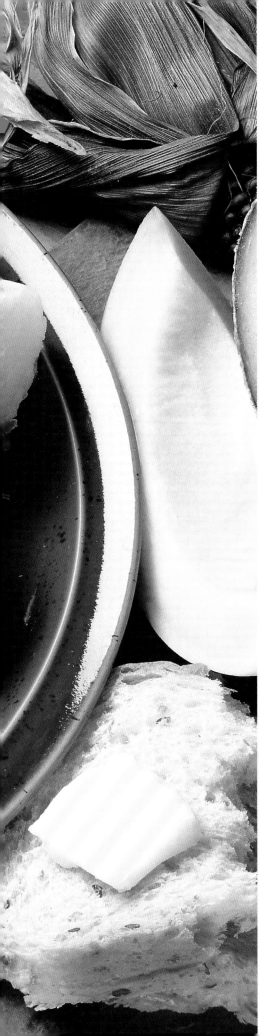

Dinner Meals

- Each large dinner has **730 calories**
  total carbs: 110 g or less | net carbs: 100 g or less
- Each small dinner has **550 calories**
  total carbs: 90 g or less | net carbs: 80 g or less

DINNER 1

Baked Chicken & Potato

RECIPE TIP

Chicken Spice Mix

Makes enough for many meals. Put 2 tsp (10 mL) oregano and 1 tsp (5 mL) each thyme, paprika, pepper and chili powder in a jar with a tight lid. Mix well. Sprinkle the mixture on the skinless chicken.

It is important to remove the fatty chicken skin. Sprinkle on this salt-free and sugar-free Chicken Spice Mix — see Recipe Tip, left.

In a pan, bake the chicken pieces in a 350°F (180°C) oven for about an hour. Or grill on the barbecue. Chicken is cooked when the meat moves easily when pierced with a fork, and the juices have no trace of pink. Or cook to 170°F (75°C) measured with an instant-read thermometer.

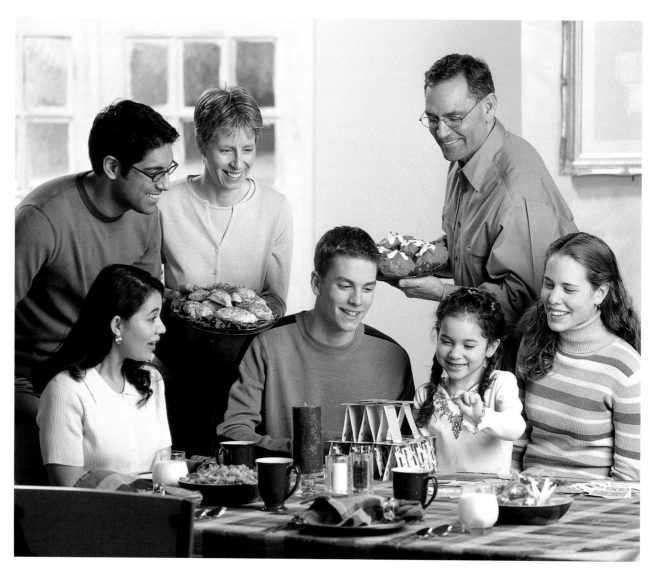

Compare the fat and carbohydrate content of fast-food chicken with this home-baked chicken, which has the skin and fat removed.

The breast of baked chicken shown in the **small** meal photograph has:
- 1 tsp (5 mL) of fat
- no sugar
- no carbs

The same piece of chicken, if battered and deep-fried at a fast-food restaurant, would have:
- 4 tsp (20 mL) of fat
- 3 tsp (15 mL) of sugar or starch equals 12 g of carbs

Have your potato plain, with 1 tsp (5 mL) of butter or margarine, or with 1 tbsp (15 mL) of low-fat sour cream or plain Greek yogurt.

The vegetables that go with this meal are celery, radishes and frozen mixed vegetables.

Easy-to-make pudding from a box

Light puddings sweetened with a low-calorie sweetener are often marked as "fat-free." You can tell they are diet mixes because they are a lot lighter in weight than the regular. The same is true for diet gelatin. Make your puddings with skim milk. The puddings are a good source of calcium and have fewer calories than regular puddings. Butterscotch pudding has been chosen for this meal, but you can choose your own favorite flavor.

FOOD CHARTS

See page 299 for information on choosing chicken.

OPTIONS

Instead of frozen mixed vegetables, you could choose one of these vegetables with similar carbs:
- peas
- carrots
- parsnips
- beets
- turnips
- winter squash (orange-colored)

Instead of pudding, you could choose 1 cup (250 mL) low-fat milk.

Food Choices	Large Meal	Small Meal
Carbohydrate	4	3
Protein	5	3½

Your Dinner Menu	Large Meal (730 calories)	Total Carbs	Net Carbs	Small Meal (550 calories)	Total Carbs	Net Carbs
Baked chicken	1½ breasts (5 oz/150 g, cooked)	0	0	1 breast (3½ oz/100 g, cooked)	0	0
Baked potato, with skin	1 large or 1½ medium	55	50	1 medium	35	32
Light sour cream	1½ tbsp (22 mL)	3	3	1 tbsp (15 mL)	2	2
Mixed vegetables	¾ cup (175 mL)	18	14	¾ cup (175 mL)	18	14
Radishes	4	1	1	4	1	1
Celery	1 stalk	1	0	1 stalk	1	0
Light butterscotch pudding	½ cup (125 mL)	12	12	½ cup (125 mL)	12	12
		90 g	**80 g**		**69 g**	**61 g**

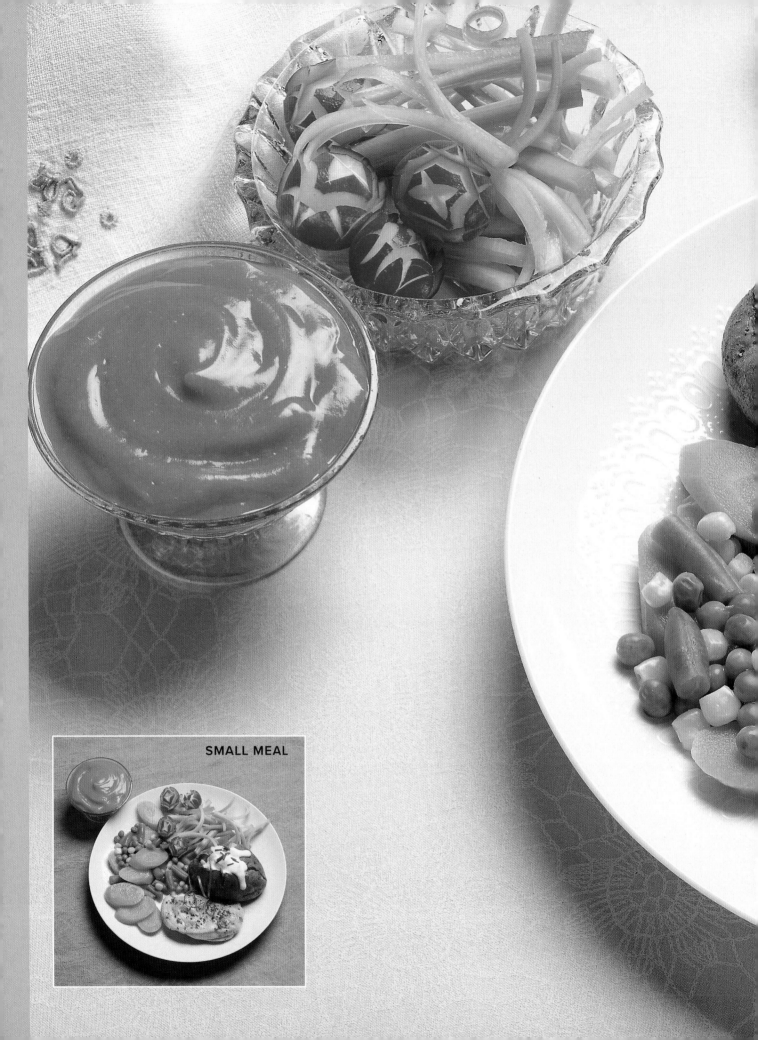

SMALL MEAL

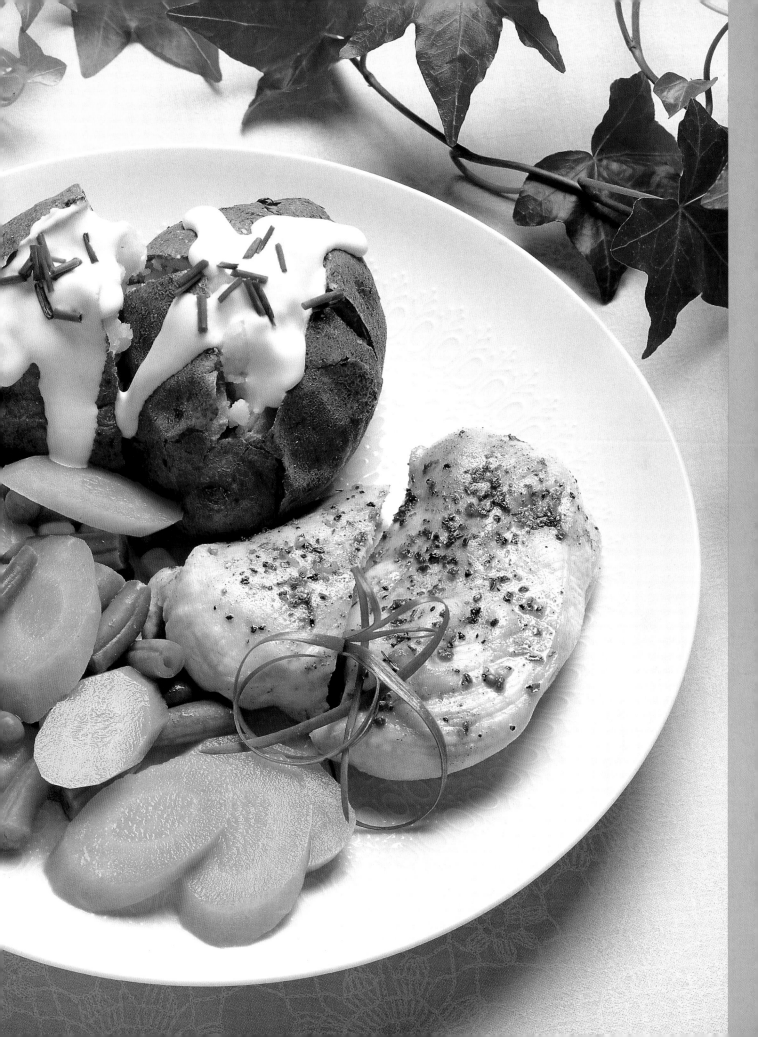

DINNER 2

Spaghetti & Meat Sauce

Spaghetti and meat sauce is an easy-to-make favorite. You can double this recipe and freeze the extra. When you have no dinner planned, it's great to have a container of spaghetti sauce in the freezer.

Spaghetti Meat Sauce

Makes 6 cups (1.5 L) of sauce

1 lb (500 g) lean ground beef
1 medium onion, chopped
28 oz (796 mL) can tomatoes
1 cup (250 mL) water
1 small tin (5½ oz/156 mL) tomato paste
½ tsp (2 mL) garlic powder or
    2 cloves garlic, chopped
2 bay leaves (remove before serving)
½ tsp (2 mL) chili powder
1 tsp (5 mL) dried oregano
1 tsp (5 mL) dried basil
¼ tsp (1 mL) paprika
⅛ tsp (0.5 mL) ground cinnamon
⅛ tsp (0.5 mL) ground cloves
1 cup (250 mL) chopped vegetables, such as
    green pepper, celery or mushrooms

PER 1 CUP (250 ML)	
Calories	200
Carbohydrate	17 g
Fiber	4 g
Net carbs	13 g
Protein	17 g
Fat, total	8 g
Fat, saturated	3 g
Cholesterol	40 mg
Sodium	296 mg

1. Brown the ground beef. Drain off as much fat as you can.
2. Add the rest of the ingredients.
3. Bring to a boil, then turn down heat. Cover and simmer for about 1 hour. Stir every now and then so the sauce doesn't stick. Add extra water if it gets too thick.
4. Serve over hot spaghetti, with grated Parmesan cheese.

Use regular or whole wheat spaghetti. Add dry spaghetti to a pot of boiling water, stir and cook for about 10 minutes. Drain off water.

Whole wheat or whole grain pasta

While not as traditional in Italian cuisine, you might want to try a pasta with more fiber. Per cup (250 mL) of cooked pasta it has an extra 2 grams of fiber, which reduces the net carbs and can feel more filling for the same amount.

RECIPE TIP

For a meatless spaghetti sauce, make this recipe according to the directions but do not add the ground beef (omit step 1). For protein for the large meal, sprinkle 5 tbsp (75 mL) of shredded cheese or 3 tbsp (45 mL) of sunflower seeds or chopped nuts on top of your cooked spaghetti and sauce. Use a little less for the small meal.

FOOD FACT

Store-bought spaghetti sauces (in jars or cans) can have a lot of added fat, sugar, salt or starch. For example, 1 cup (250 mL) of some meatless spaghetti sauces have 2 tsp (10 mL) of added fat and 4 tsp (16 g) of added sugar or starch. If you do buy spaghetti sauce, look for one labeled as "light."

For your beverage, would you like a glass of red or white wine with your pasta? A 5-oz (140 mL) glass of red table wine has 125 calories, 4 carbs and 4 net carbs (no fiber), no protein or fat, and 12% alcohol.

Light gelatin has few calories and is a good dessert choice after a big meal. It takes only a few minutes to make, but must be left in the fridge for about 2 hours to set. If you find the boxed diet gelatins are costly, try this easy-to-make recipe.

Light Gelatin

Makes 2 cups (500 mL)

1 envelope (¼ oz/7 g)
    unflavored gelatin

½ package regular drink mix
    (such as Kool-Aid)

1 cup (250 mL) cold water

1 cup (250 mL) boiling water

Low-calorie sweetener equal to
    ¼ cup (60 mL) sugar (use a bit less
    or more, to suit your taste)

PER ½ CUP (125 ML)	
Calories	13
Carbohydrate	2 g
Fiber	0 g
Net carbs	2 g
Protein	2 g
Fat, total	0 g
Fat, saturated	0 g
Cholesterol	0 mg
Sodium	19 mg

1. Soften the unflavored gelatin in ½ cup (125 mL) cold water.
2. Add the drink mix and 1 cup (250 mL) boiling water. Stir until gelatin is all mixed in.
3. Add ½ cup (125 mL) cold water and low-calorie sweetener.
4. Chill until firm (about 2 hours).

OPTIONS

Another low-calorie dessert is store-bought "no sugar added" popsicles.

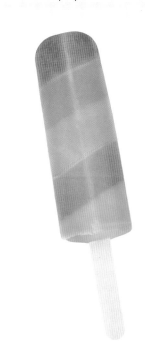

Food Choices	Large Meal	Small Meal
Carbohydrate	4	3
Protein	2½	1½

Your Dinner Menu	Large Meal (730 calories)	Total Carbs	Net Carbs	Small Meal (550 calories)	Total Carbs	Net Carbs
Spaghetti, cooked	1½ cups (375 mL)	59	55	1½ cups (375 mL)	59	55
Meat sauce	1¼ cups (300 mL)	22	17	¾ cup (175 mL)	13	10
Parmesan cheese	1 tbsp (15 mL)	0	0	1 tbsp (15 mL)	0	0
Cooked carrots	½ cup (125 mL)	8	6	½ cup (125 mL)	8	6
Salad	Medium	5	4	Medium	5	4
Oil and vinegar dressing (2 parts oil, 1 part vinegar)	1 tbsp (15 mL)	0	0	½ tbsp (7 mL)	0	0
Almond beverage	1 cup (250 mL)	1	0	½ cup (125 mL)	1	0
Light gelatin	½ cup (125 mL)	2	2	½ cup (125 mL)	2	2
		97 g	84 g		88 g	77 g

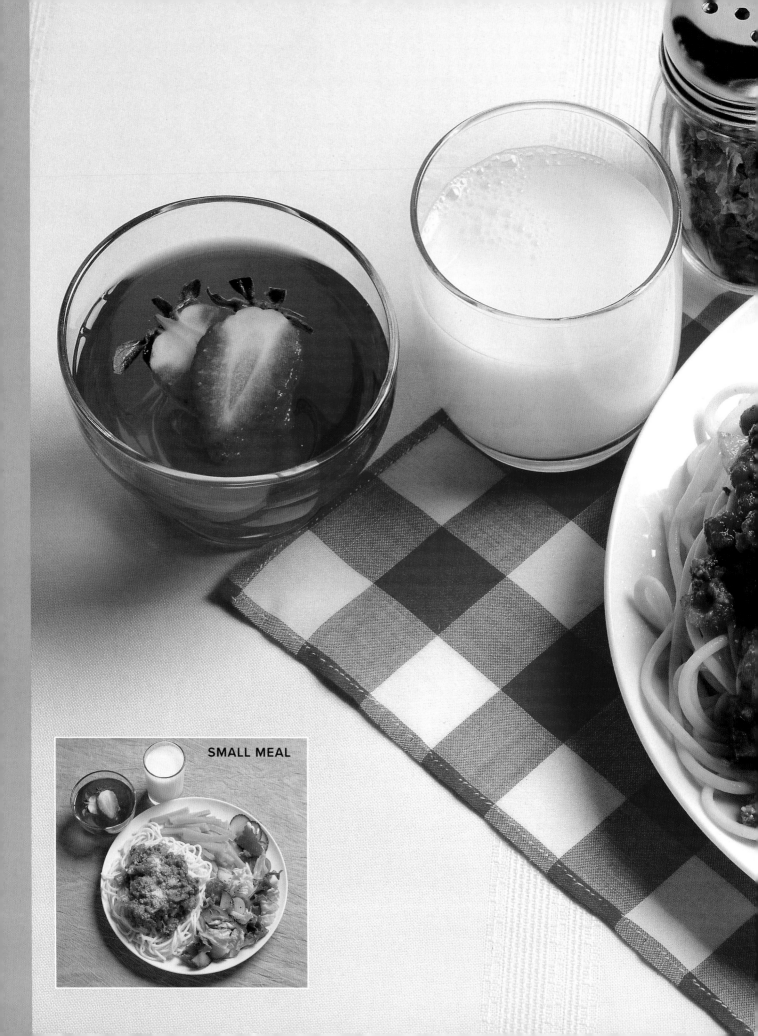

SMALL MEAL

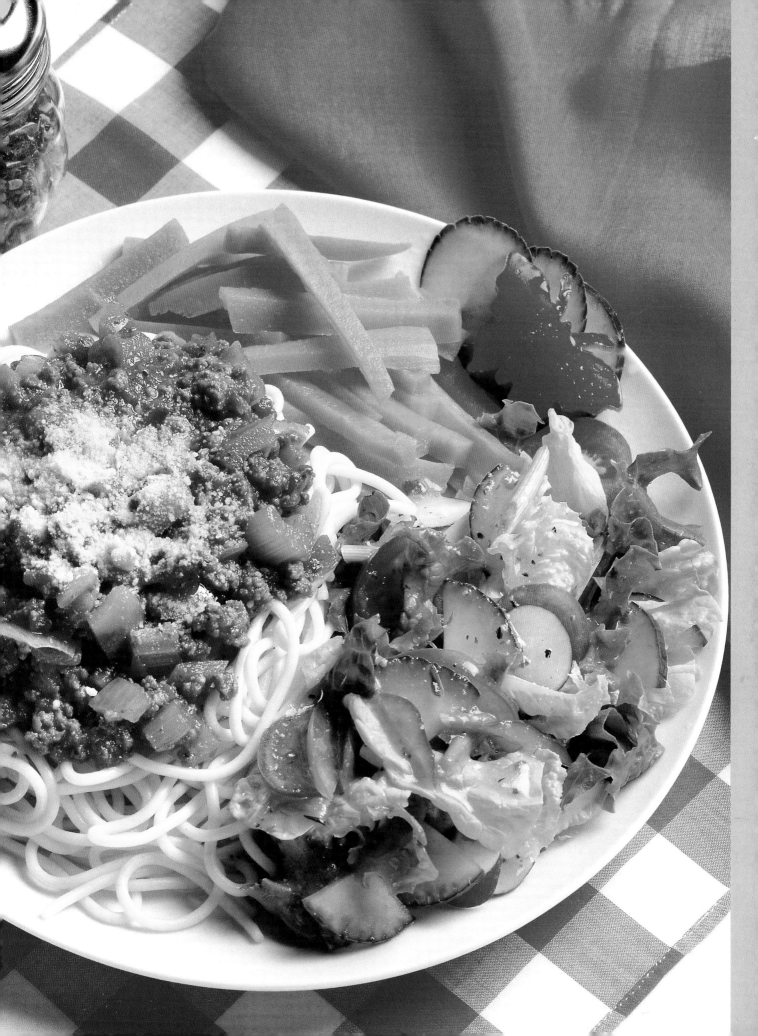

DINNER 3

FOOD FACTS
Low-fat fish:
- bluefish
- catfish
- cod
- haddock
- perch
- pickerel
- red snapper
- sole
- tilapia

High-fat fish (good sources of healthy omega-3 fats):
- mackerel
- salmon
- sardines
- trout
- tuna
- herring

Eat a bit less of the high-fat fish.

These spices go well with fish:
- allspice
- basil
- Cajun spice
- curry
- dill
- mustard
- oregano
- parsley
- thyme
- Old Bay seasoning

Fish with Rice

The fish may be broiled or baked in an oven at 350°F to 400°F (180°C to 200°C). The fish shown in the photograph is red snapper, and it was baked and lightly brushed with margarine. Fish can also be microwaved, steamed, grilled on the barbecue, or fried in a nonstick pan (with just a little fat). If you are cooking fish in your oven or on your barbecue, you can wrap it in foil. Fish is good with spices, onions and vegetables wrapped up in the foil too.

Before cooking fish

Poke it with a fork and sprinkle with lemon juice or dry wine, and your favorite spices.

The secret to great-tasting fish is to not overcook it. Fish is cooked when it flakes easily.

Rice

For this meal, cook brown rice along with a handful of wild rice. Cook according to directions on the brown rice package, omitting any salt.

Cooked white and brown rice both have about 210 calories per cup (250 mL). Brown rice is a good choice, as it has almost 3 grams of fiber per cup, while white rice has just over half a gram. Converted rice (also called parboiled) such as Uncle Ben's Original Converted Rice, long-grain (brown or white) and basmati rice have a lower glycemic index. This means they raise blood sugar slower than short-grain white rice.

Vegetables

This meal is served with peas, a sweet vegetable, and with yellow or green beans, which are less sweet. See page 149 for a list of low-calorie vegetables.

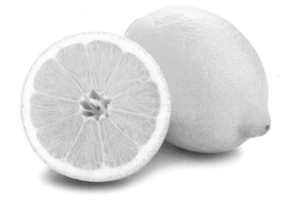

Fruit Milkshake

Makes 2 cups (500 mL)

1 cup (250 mL) skim milk

½ cup (125 mL) frozen or fresh fruit
of your choice

1 tbsp (15 mL) sugar or equal amount
of low-calorie sweetener

PER 1 CUP (250 ML)	
Calories	79
Carbohydrate	16 g
Fiber	1 g
Net carbs	15 g
Protein	4 g
Fat, total	0 g
Fat, saturated	0 g
Cholesterol	2 mg
Sodium	52 mg

1. Pour milk in a mixing bowl or a blender. Place mixing bowl or blender in your freezer for 30 minutes.

2. Take bowl or blender out of the freezer. Add fruit and sugar (or low-calorie sweetener) to the milk. Mix in blender for about 30 seconds. If you don't have a blender, mix in bowl with beaters until thick and frothy. Serve right away.

RECIPE TIPS

If you increase the size of the recipe, you will need to freeze the milk for longer.

This milkshake is easy to make. It is so thick and good, you won't believe it's made with skim milk!

Food Choices	Large Meal	Small Meal
Carbohydrate	4½	3½
Protein	6	4
Fat	1	1

Your Dinner Menu	Large Meal (730 calories)	Total Carbs	Net Carbs	Small Meal (550 calories)	Total Carbs	Net Carbs
Fish with lemon slice	6 oz (175 g), cooked	0	0	4 oz (125 g), cooked	0	0
Margarine (to cook fish)	1 tsp (5 mL)	0	0	1 tsp (5 mL)	0	0
Brown rice, cooked	1 cup (250 mL)	45	42	⅔ cup (150 mL)	30	28
Green peas	½ cup (2 mL)	11	7	½ cup (2 mL)	11	7
Yellow beans	1 cup (250 mL)	10	7	1 cup (250 mL)	10	7
Fruit Milkshake	1 cup (250 mL)	16	15	1 cup (250 mL)	16	15
Kiwi	1 medium	11	8	1 medium	11	8
		93 g	**79 g**		**78 g**	**65 g**

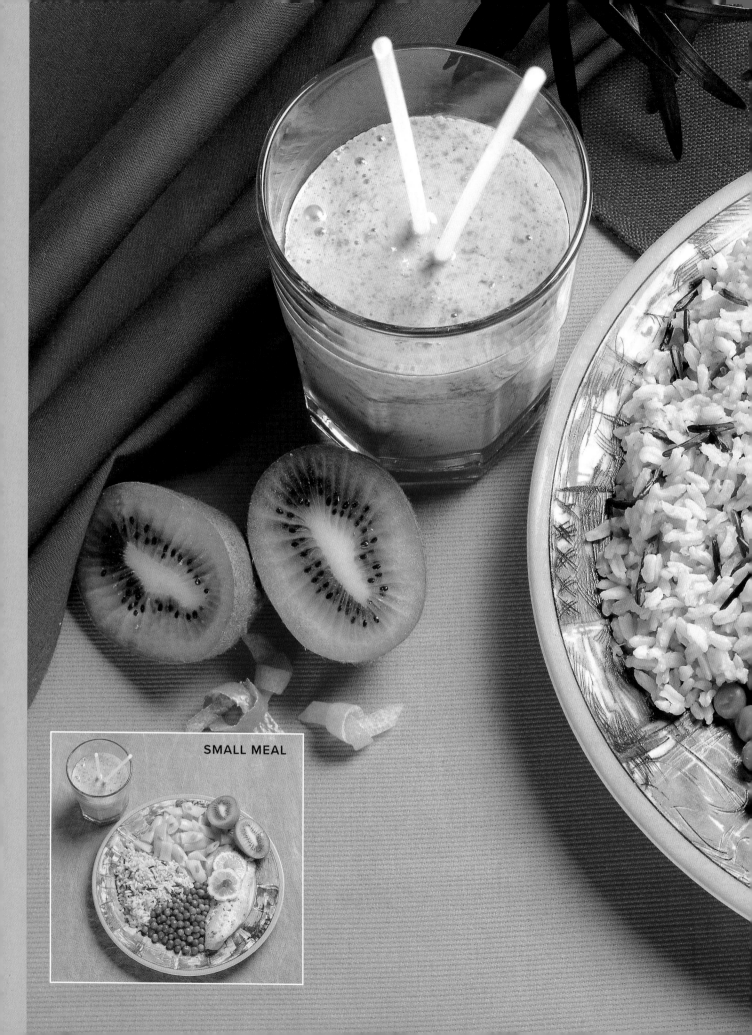

SMALL MEAL

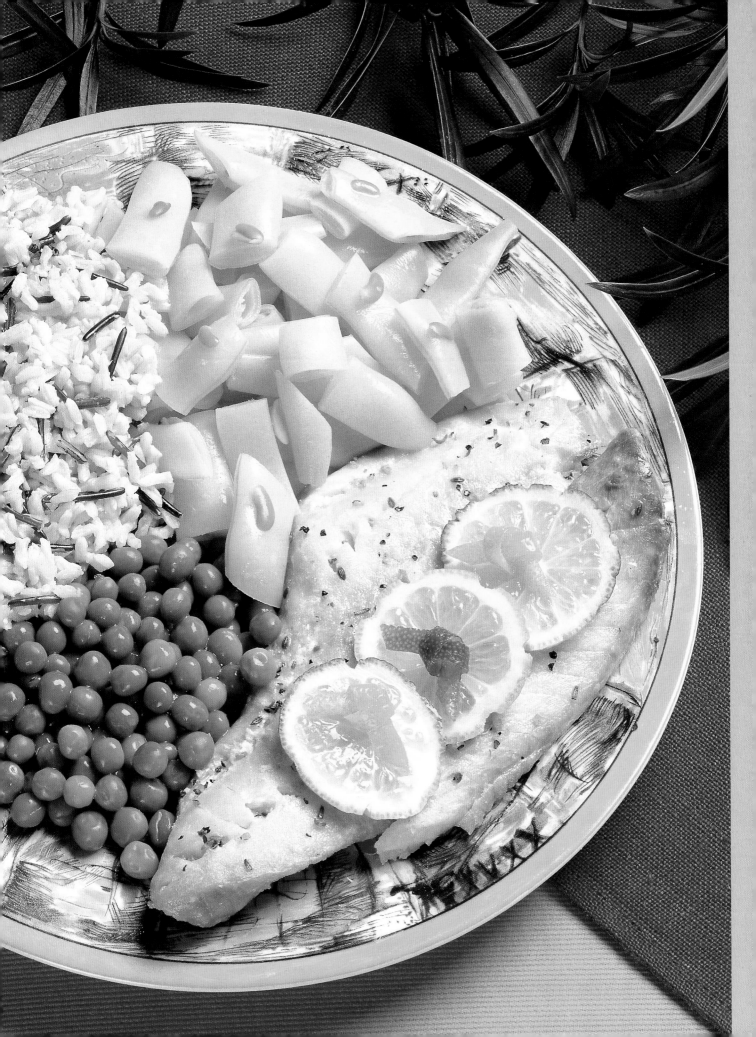

Roast Beef

Here's a great way to cook a tender cut of roast:

- Place your roast on a rack in a roasting pan, with no lid. Add 1 cup (250 mL) of water to the pan. Sprinkle with pepper but not salt (salt tends to dry out the roast).
- Roast in a hot 500°F (260°C) oven for 30 minutes.
- Reduce heat to 275°F (140°C). Leave roast uncovered and cook for another 1½ hours for a 5-pound (2.4 kg) roast.

For medium done, cook to 145°F (62°C) measured with an instant-read thermometer placed into the thickest part of the roast.

> If cooking a less expensive, tougher cut of meat, you will need to use a moist cooking method to make the meat tender. See sidebar for cooking tips.

Once your roast is cooked, remove it from your pan, cover and put to the side. Add 1 cup (250 mL) of water to the pan and scrape the meat bits off the bottom of the pan. Use this to make the gravy below.

Low-Salt Gravy

Makes 2⅓ cups (575 mL)

Beef bits in roasting pan (see above)

1 to 2 packets (4.5 g each) reduced-salt beef bouillon mix (use chicken bouillon if making gravy for poultry) or 1 tsp (5 mL) onion soup mix

1 tbsp (15 mL) finely chopped onion

2 cups (500 mL) liquid made from either fat-free meat juice, potato water or other vegetable water

¼ cup (60 mL) flour, cornstarch or instant blending flour

½ cup (125 mL) cold water

1. Add beef bouillon, onion and liquid to your pan with the beef bits. Bring to a boil.
2. In a jar, mix flour or cornstarch with the cold water. Tighten the lid and shake well. Add this mixture slowly to the hot juice and cook at medium heat. Stir often with a whisk until thick and smooth, about 5 minutes.

PER ¼ CUP (60 ML)	
Calories	81
Carbohydrate	4 g
Fiber	0 g
Net carbs	4 g
Protein	3 g
Fat, total	5 g
Fat, saturated	4 g
Cholesterol	0 mg
Sodium	93 mg

RECIPE TIPS

Tender cuts of roast

The roast you choose will likely depend on your budget.

- Ribeye roast is an excellent roast for special occasions; it is more marbled with fat.
- A top lean cut is tenderloin roast.
- Other lean cuts are sirloin tip, top round and top sirloin.

Less tender cuts of roast

Less expensive inside round and outside round roasts are tougher, so need slow, extended cooking. Roast with lid on and several cups of water added to the pan, or cook in a slow cooker according to slow cooker directions.

OPTIONS

You can also buy low-fat gravy mix packages, to which you add only water. These should have fewer than 10 calories in a serving. Look for one that says it is low in calories; it may be called "au jus" (with juice). The sodium content will be about 600 mg per ¼ cup (60 mL).

The oven-roasted potatoes are peeled and cooked for an hour on a nonstick or greased pan. Coat your potatoes with an oil-free Italian dressing or sprinkle with spices.

Have beets as shown, or carrots, turnips, corn, peas, or any other vegetable.

For dessert have the rhubarb with either ice cream, sherbet, frozen yogurt or ice milk.

Stewed Rhubarb
Makes 1³⁄₄ cups (425 mL)

4 cups (1 L) rhubarb (fresh or frozen), cut into 1-inch (2.5 cm) pieces
2 tbsp (30 mL) water
½ tsp (2 mL) sugar-free drink mix (either strawberry or raspberry)
Dash of cinnamon

PER 1 CUP (250 ML)	
Calories	64
Carbohydrate	15 g
Fiber	5 g
Net carbs	10 g
Protein	3 g
Fat, total	1 g
Fat, saturated	0 g
Cholesterol	0 mg
Sodium	21 mg

1. Put the rhubarb and water in a heavy pot and cook at low temperature on the stove. Add water as needed. Cook for about 15 minutes, or until soft.
2. Take off the stove and, while still warm, add sugar-free drink mix and cinnamon.
3. Have it warm or cool. Keep in the fridge.

RECIPE TIPS
Vegetables such as beets or carrots are also good when lightly oiled and baked on a pan in the oven.

OPTIONS
This rhubarb is also nice as a dessert or a snack served warm on a piece of toast.

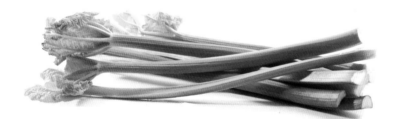

Food Choices	Large Meal	Small Meal
Carbohydrate	4	3
Protein	5	3

Your Dinner Menu	Large Meal (730 calories)	Total Carbs	Net Carbs	Small Meal (550 calories)	Total Carbs	Net Carbs
Roast Beef	5 oz (150 g), cooked	0	0	3 oz (90 g), cooked	0	0
Horseradish	1 tbsp (15 mL)	2	1	1 tbsp (15 mL)	2	1
Baked onions	3 small or 1 medium	3	3	3 small or 1 medium	3	3
Roasted potatoes	1 large	47	42	1 medium	34	31
Low-Salt Gravy	¼ cup (60 mL)	4	4	2 tbsp (30 mL)	2	2
Beets	½ cup (125 mL)	8	6	½ cup (125 mL)	8	6
Salad	Small	3	3	Small	3	3
Oil-free Italian salad dressing	1 tbsp (15 mL)	2	2	1 tbsp (15 mL)	2	2
Stewed Rhubarb	1 cup (250 mL)	15	10	1 cup (250 mL)	15	10
Ice cream	¼ cup (60 mL)	9	9	¼ cup (60 mL)	9	9
		93 g	80 g		78 g	67 g

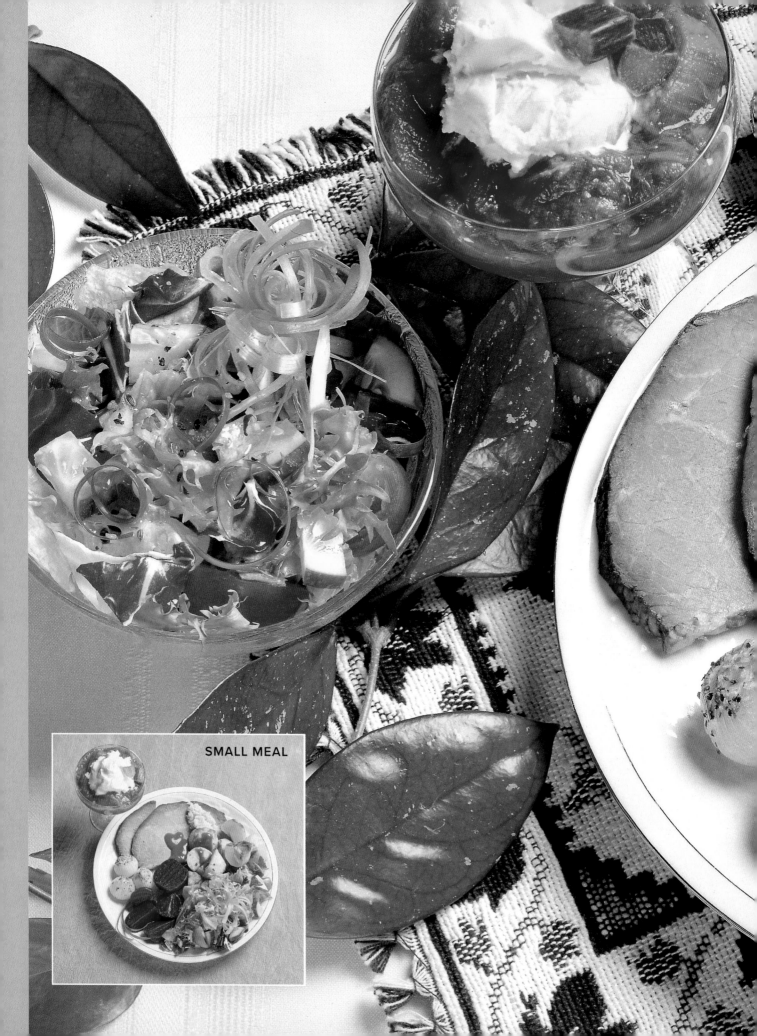

SMALL MEAL

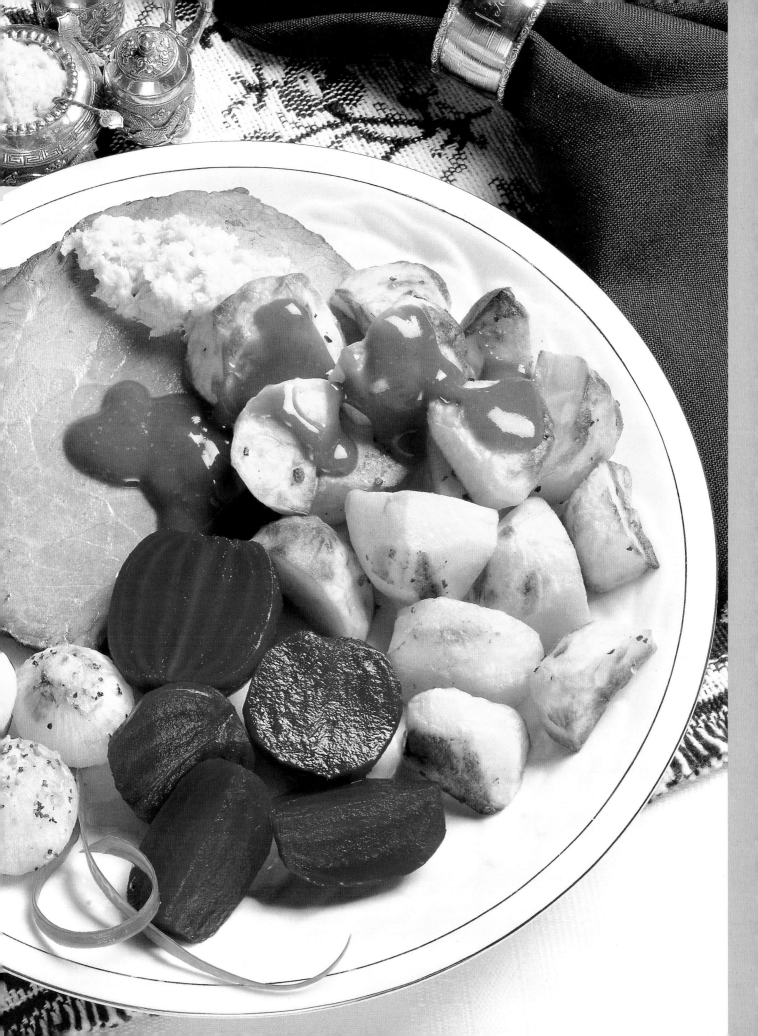

DINNER 5

Cold Plate Dinner

This is one of Karen's mom's favorite light and easy meals. It includes fresh vegetables, fish and cheese, plus rice pudding for dessert.

Fish choices include canned (or leftover cooked and chilled) salmon, tuna, sardines, shrimp, crab or lobster. Red (sockeye) salmon, rich in healthy omega-3 fat, is included with this meal. If you don't like fish, replace it with two eggs or 2 oz (60 g) roasted chicken.

Your starch may be a whole wheat bun, two slices of whole-grain bread, or eight melba toasts. Add any number and variety of fresh vegetables.

OPTIONS

You can replace 2 oz (60 g) of regular-fat cheese (32% fat) with:

- ½ cup (125 mL) of 1% or 2% cottage cheese

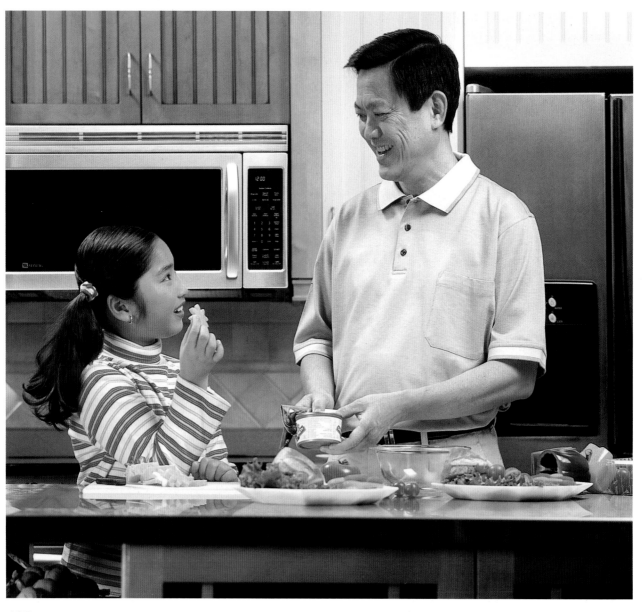

This rice pudding for dessert is good warm or cold.

Rice Pudding

Makes four 1-cup (250 mL) servings

1 egg

1½ cups (375 mL) skim milk

2 tbsp (30 mL) sugar (or low-calorie
 sweetener, if desired)

½ tsp (2 mL) ground cinnamon

½ tsp (2 mL) vanilla

2 cups (500 mL) cooked rice
 (brown or white)

¼ cup (60 mL) raisins

1. In a large bowl, beat the egg, milk, sugar or sweetener,
   cinnamon and vanilla. Use a spoon or whisk.
2. Stir in rice and raisins.
3. Pour into lightly greased baking dish.
4. Bake at 350°F (180°C) for 45 minutes, or until the center
   is set.

PER 1 CUP (250 ML)	
Calories	216
Carbohydrate	42 g
Fiber	2 g
Net carbs	40 g
Protein	8 g
Fat, total	2 g
Fat, saturated	1 g
Cholesterol	48 mg
Sodium	69 mg

OPTIONS

Instead of the rice pudding you could have a slice of banana bread, light pudding, a small dish of sherbet or frozen yogurt, or a serving of fresh fruit.

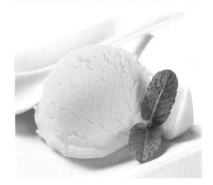

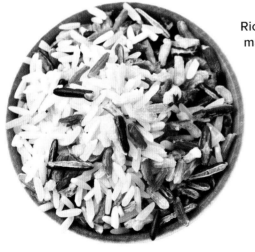

Rice pudding can be made with different types of rice.

Food Choices	Large Meal	Small Meal
Carbohydrate	4	3½
Protein	4	3
Fat	½	–

Your Dinner Menu	Large Meal (730 calories)	Total Carbs	Net Carbs	Small Meal (550 calories)	Total Carbs	Net Carbs
Cold Plate Dinner						
• lettuce or spinach	A plateful	1	1	A plateful	1	1
• tomato	½ medium	3	2	½ medium	3	2
• green & red pepper	5 rings	2	1	5 rings	2	1
• cucumber	4 thick slices	1	1	4 thick slices	1	1
• radishes	2 large	1	1	2 large	1	1
• salmon	½ cup (125 mL)	0	0	½ cup (125 mL)	0	0
• regular Cheddar cheese	2 oz (60 g)	1	1	1 oz (30 g)	0	0
• bun, whole wheat	1	23	20	1	23	20
• margarine	½ tsp (2 mL)	0	0	–	–	–
Rice Pudding	1 cup (250 mL)	42	40	¾ cup (175 mL)	31	30
		74 g	**67 g**		**62 g**	**56 g**

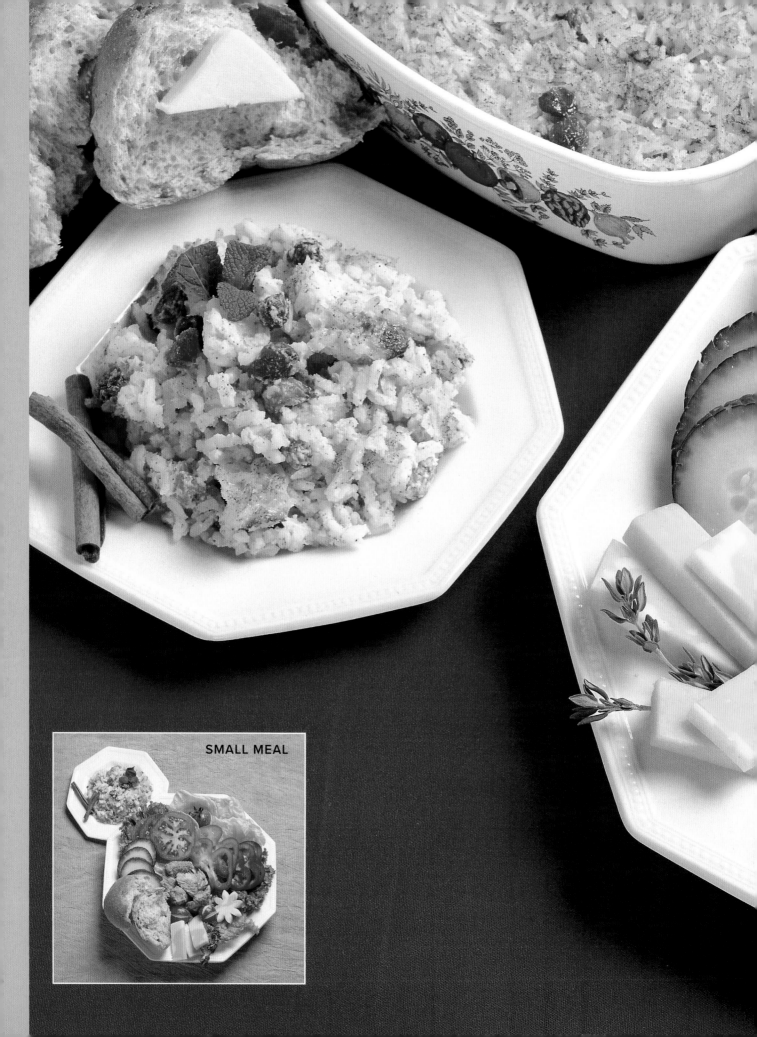

SMALL MEAL

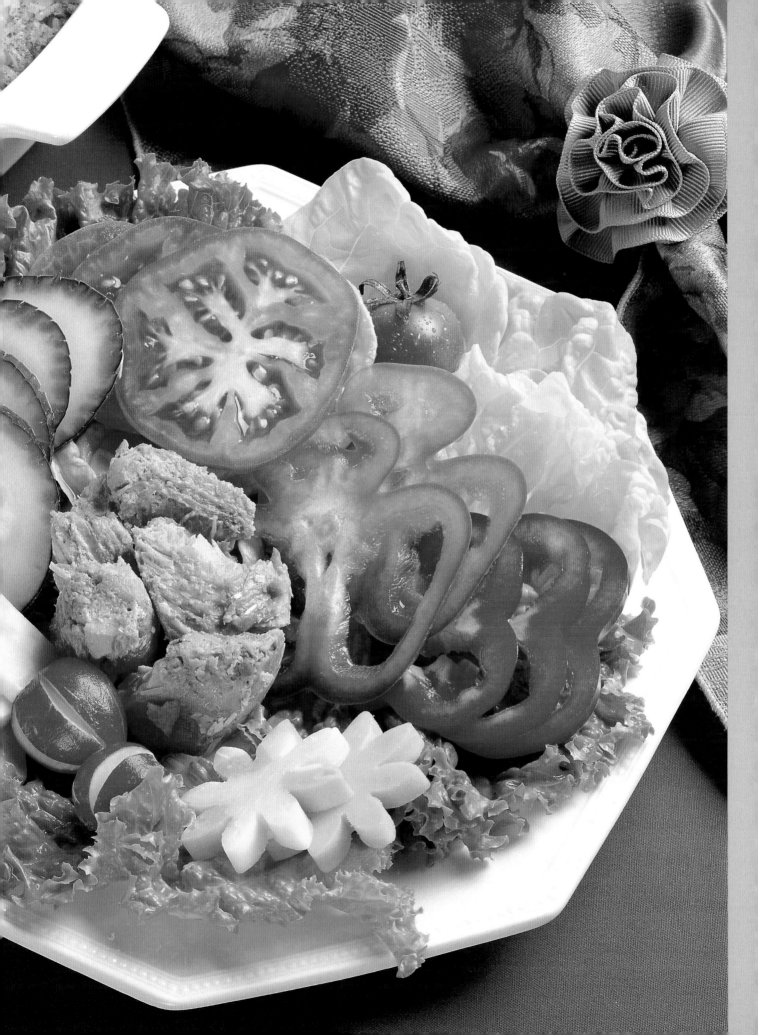

DINNER 6

Hamburger Soup & Bannock

This delicious meal is a favorite among North American Indigenous people. The great thing about this soup is that it is a meal all in one. Freeze any leftovers.

Hamburger Soup

Makes 10 cups (2.5 L)

1 lb (500 g) lean ground beef
  (or chopped or ground wild meat)
1 medium onion, chopped
4 cloves garlic, finely chopped,
  or 1 tsp (5 mL) garlic powder
19 oz (540 mL) can tomatoes
10 oz (284 mL) can tomato soup
1 tsp (5 mL) Worcestershire sauce
¼ tsp (1 mL) black pepper
4 cups (1 L) water
½ to 1 packet (2.25 to 4.5 g) reduced-salt beef bouillon mix
3 medium carrots, peeled and sliced
1 cup (250 mL) chopped cabbage
1½ cups (375 mL) frozen corn or 12 oz (341 mL) can
  corn kernels
¼ cup (60 mL) dry macaroni

PER 1½ CUPS (375 ML)	
Calories	229
Carbohydrate	27 g
Fiber	3 g
Net carbs	24 g
Protein	16 g
Fat, total	7 g
Fat, saturated	3 g
Cholesterol	36 mg
Sodium	456 mg

1. In a large heavy pot on the stove, brown ground beef. Drain off fat.
2. Add onions and garlic, and cook at low heat until onions are soft.
3. Add tomatoes, tomato soup, Worcestershire sauce, pepper, water and bouillon mix.
4. Bring to a boil, cover and simmer for 30 minutes.
5. Add vegetables and macaroni. Cover and simmer for another 30 minutes.

FOOD FACT

Canned vegetables and soup contain a lot of sodium, so you do not need to add salt to recipes that use them. If you are able to buy reduced-salt or low-sodium versions, such as tomato soup with 25% less salt or low-sodium canned tomatoes, they are good choices. In addition, plain frozen vegetables, such as frozen corn, have much less sodium than canned.

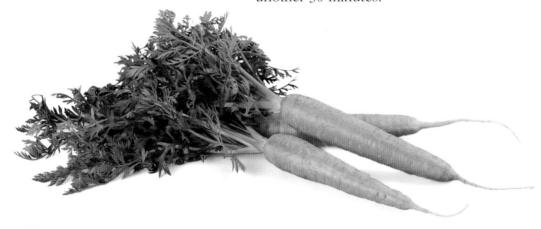

This bread is made without yeast and is easy to make. It is cooked in the oven or in a cast-iron frying pan.

Bannock

Makes one 9-inch (23 cm) bannock (or 10 pieces)

3 cups (750 mL) flour

1½ tsp (7 mL) baking powder

½ tsp (2 mL) salt

1 tbsp (15 mL) sugar

¼ cup (60 mL) vegetable oil, or other fat, melted

1¼ cups (300 mL) skim milk

PER 1 PIECE	
Calories	201
Carbohydrate	31 g
Fiber	1 g
Net carbs	30 g
Protein	5 g
Fat, total	6 g
Fat, saturated	0 g
Cholesterol	0 mg
Sodium	172 mg

1. In a large bowl, mix together flour, baking powder, salt and sugar.
2. Mix vegetable oil with the milk. Add this mixture to the flour. Mix with a spoon to make a soft dough.
3. Put this on a floured board or table. With your hands, flatten and shape it until it is one 9-inch (23 cm) piece.
4. Put on a nonstick or lightly greased cookie sheet. Bake in the oven at 375°F (190°C) for 20 minutes, or until lightly browned.
5. Cut into 10 pieces.

To cook bannock on your stove or campfire:

Make the bannock batter with only 2 tbsp (30 mL) of oil or other fat. Add an extra tbsp (15 mL) of milk to keep the batter soft. In the cast-iron pan, add 2 tbsp (30 mL) fat and fry the bannock for 10 minutes on each side at low heat. This fried bannock has the same amount of fat as it does when baked.

OPTIONS

Instead of the piece of bannock shown here, you may choose two slices of bread or one bun.

RECIPE TIP

I use milk instead of water in the bannock because the milk helps in the rising, adding flavor and good nutrition too.

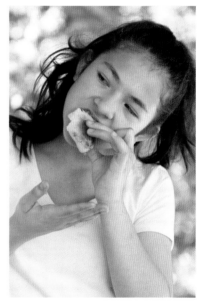

Food Choices	Large Meal	Small Meal
Carbohydrate	6	4½
Protein	1½	1½
Fat	3	2

Your Dinner Menu	Large Meal (730 calories)	Total Carbs	Net Carbs	Small Meal (550 calories)	Total Carbs	Net Carbs
Hamburger Soup	1½ cups (375 mL)	27	24	1½ cups (375 mL)	27	24
Bannock	2 pieces	63	61	1 piece	32	31
Margarine	1 tsp (5 mL)	0	0	1 tsp (5 mL)	0	0
Orange	1 medium	15	13	1 medium	15	13
		105 g	**98 g**		**74 g**	**68 g**

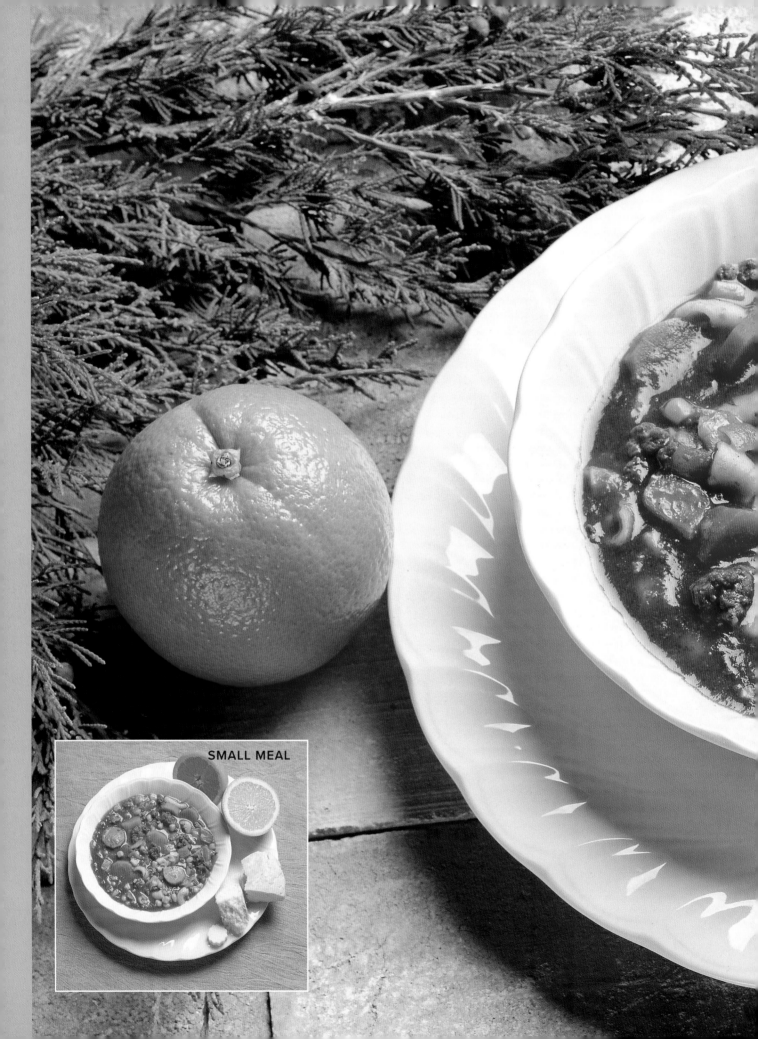

SMALL MEAL

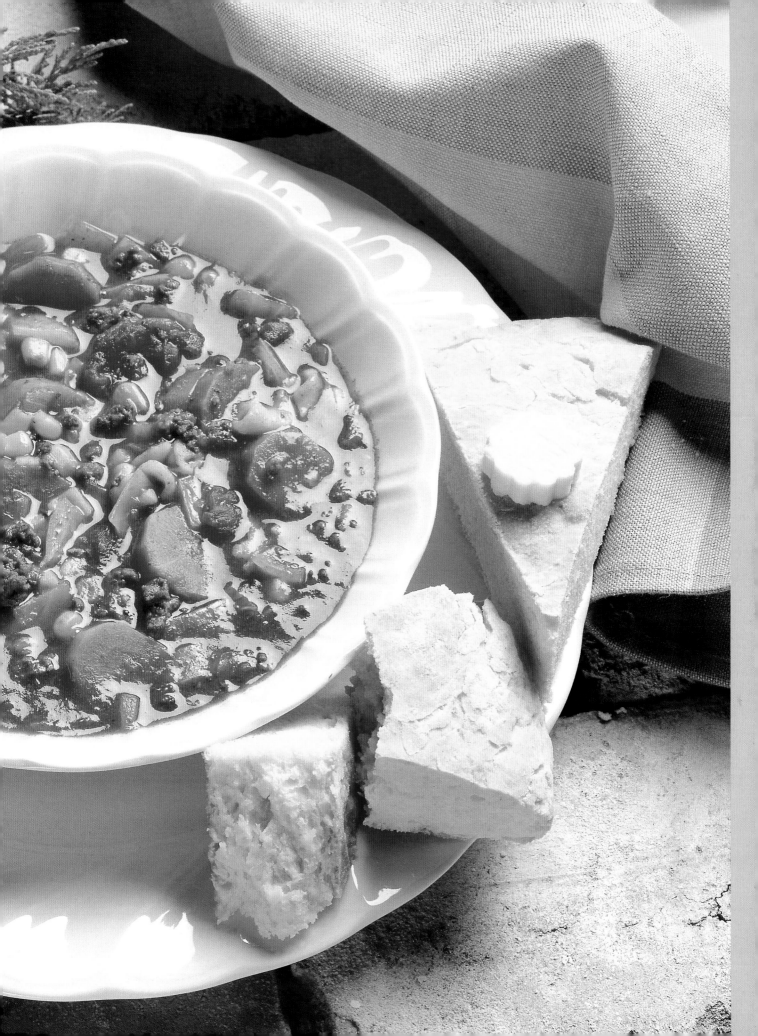

DINNER 7

Beans & Wieners

Beef or pork wieners are a favorite for many, but are high in fat and salt. This meal makes a few wieners go a long way. The beans are low-fat and give you protein and fiber.

OPTIONS

Turkey wieners are lower in fat than regular.

Tofu wieners are a vegetarian choice and are also lower in fat.

RECIPE TIPS

You can make Beans & Wieners with either the Home-Baked Beans or a can of brown beans.

Don't forget that canned beans contain a lot of sodium — about 850 mg per cup (250 mL). Home-Baked Beans are a healthier choice, at just 157 mg per cup.

Beans & Wieners

Makes 4 cups (1 L)

3 cups (750 mL) Home-Baked Beans or a 14-oz (398 mL) can of brown beans

3 regular wieners (each wiener weighs 1½ oz/45 g or less)

1. Place the beans in a pot or cooking dish.
2. Cut the wieners in slices and add to the beans.
3. Heat on the stove or in a microwave oven.

PER 1 CUP (250 ML)	
Calories	352
Carbohydrate	53 g
Fiber	11 g
Net carbs	42 g
Protein	19 g
Fat, total	8 g
Fat, saturated	3 g
Cholesterol	17 mg
Sodium	379 mg

Home-Baked Beans

Makes 4½ cups (1.125 L)

2 cups (500 mL) dry white beans (navy, small white or Great Northern)

1 medium onion, chopped

2 cloves garlic, finely chopped

1 tbsp (15 mL) dry mustard

¼ tsp (1 mL) black pepper

2 cups (500 mL) water

3 tbsp (45 mL) ketchup

2 tbsp (30 mL) molasses

Dash of hot pepper sauce (optional)

PER 1 CUP (250 ML)	
Calories	364
Carbohydrate	69 g
Fiber	15 g
Net carbs	54 g
Protein	20 g
Fat, total	2 g
Fat, saturated	0 g
Cholesterol	0 mg
Sodium	157 mg

1. Rinse the beans in cold water, removing any shriveled or discolored beans. Place in a pot with enough cold water to cover the beans.
2. Cover and bring to a boil over high heat; boil for 5 minutes. Remove from heat and let stand, covered, for 1 hour.
3. Drain the water from the beans and transfer beans to a casserole dish or bean pot. Mix in the remaining ingredients.
4. Cover and bake at 275°F (140°C) for 6 to 8 hours, or until beans are tender. Stir periodically and add extra water if the beans are drying out.

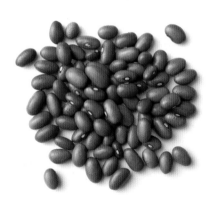

Serve Beans & Wieners with toast, and a tossed salad with Citrus Vinaigrette. If you use a store-bought salad dressing, make sure it's a light one. Look for the words "fat-free," "oil-free" or "calorie-reduced" on the label. It's a good choice if it has fewer than 30 calories per tbsp (15 mL). Some regular salad dressings have more than 100 calories per tablespoon.

Citrus Vinaigrette is an easy low-calorie, low-salt alternative to store-bought, and contains only 25 mg of sodium per tablespoon (15 mL), compared with over 200 mg in a typical fat-free dressing.

Citrus Vinaigrette

In a large jar (at least 16 oz/500 mL), combine ½ cup (125 mL) orange juice, ¼ cup (60 mL) water, ¼ cup (60 mL) vinegar, 2 tbsp (30 mL) honey, 2 tbsp (30 mL) lemon juice, ¼ tsp (1 mL) garlic powder, ¼ tsp (1 mL) salt and a dash of hot pepper sauce (optional). Shake well and store in the refrigerator for up to 7 days. Makes 1½ cups (375 mL).

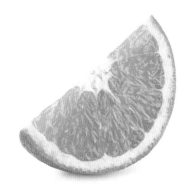

This dessert recipe is easy, thick and delicious.

Chocolate Mousse

Makes six ½-cup (125 mL) servings.

1½ cups (375 mL) skim milk
1 package (4-serving size) of light chocolate instant pudding mix
1 cup (250 mL) frozen light whipped topping, thawed until soft

1. In a medium bowl, pour the skim milk and then add pudding mix. Beat with a whisk or an electric mixer until thickened (about 2 minutes).
2. Fold in the thawed whipped topping until well blended (or if you want a marbled look, fold in the topping gently and don't fully mix). Pour into six dessert dishes, and serve.

PER ½ CUP (125 ML)	
Calories	79
Carbohydrate	11 g
Fiber	1 g
Net carbs	10 g
Protein	3 g
Fat, total	2 g
Fat, saturated	2 g
Cholesterol	1 mg
Sodium	253 mg

RECIPE TIP

You may want to make the chocolate mousse with regular pudding instead of light. By doing so, you will add an extra 2½ tsp (10 g) of sugar to each serving.

Food Choices	Large Meal	Small Meal
Carbohydrate	5	4
Protein	3	2
Fat	1	–

Your Dinner Menu	Large Meal (730 calories)	Total Carbs	Net Carbs	Small Meal (550 calories)	Total Carbs	Net Carbs
Beans & Wieners	1⅓ cups (325 mL)	71	56	1 cup (250 mL)	53	42
Toast	2 small or 1 regular slice	12	11	2 small or 1 regular slice	12	11
Margarine	1 tsp (5 mL)	0	0	–	–	–
Tossed salad	Large	6	4	Large	6	4
Citrus Vinaigrette	2 tbsp (30 mL)	4	4	2 tbsp (30 mL)	4	4
Chocolate Mousse	½ cup (125 mL)	11	10	½ cup (125 mL)	11	10
		104 g	85 g		86 g	71 g

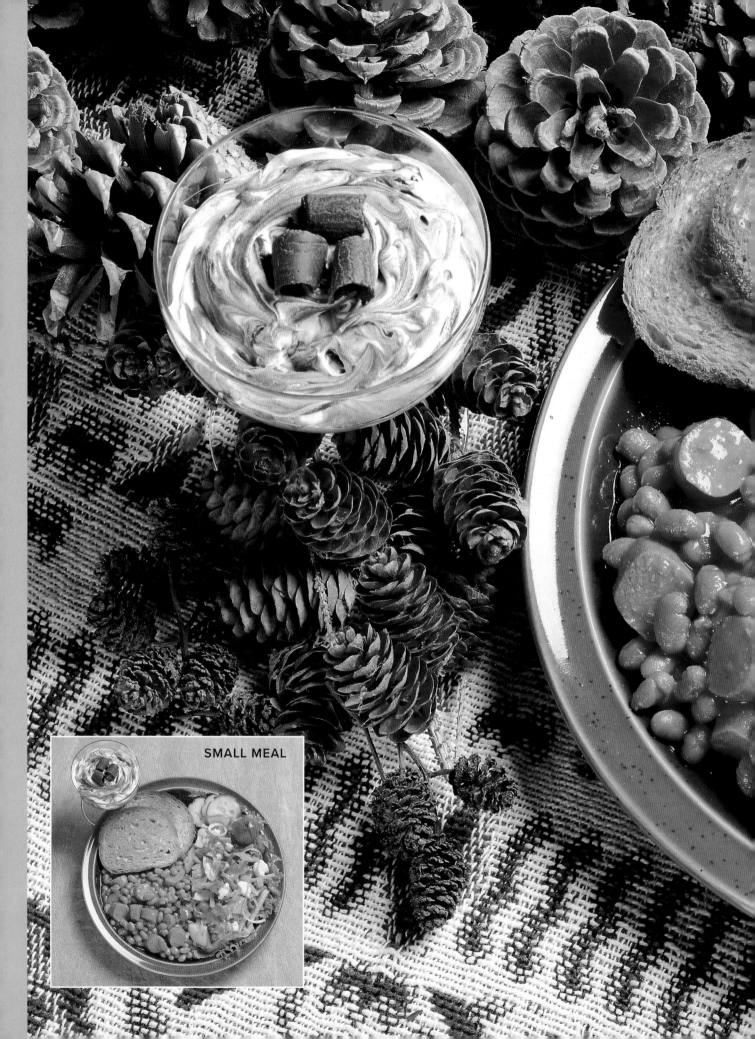

SMALL MEAL

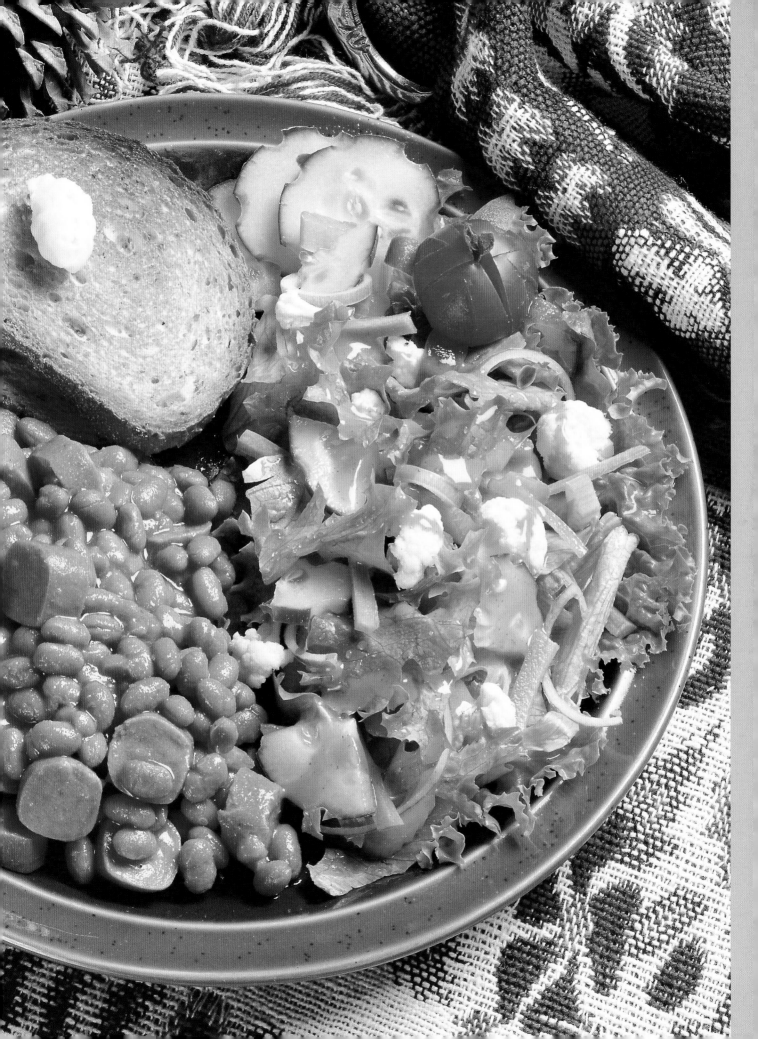

DINNER 8

Steak & Potato

The simplest way to cook a steak is to barbecue or broil it, or fry it in a very hot, heavy frying pan with a bit of water. If frying in a pan, cover with a lid to reduce fat spraying out. Cook for only about 4 minutes on each side.

RECIPE TIPS

Cuts of steak

As a general rule, the more expensive the steak, the more tender it will be to barbecue or cook on your stove.

Tender steaks may be sold as "grilling steaks." Examples are top sirloin, T-bone or rib eye.

Cheaper steaks will be tougher and will probably need pre-tenderizing and cooking in liquid. An example would be flank steak or "round" cuts.

If unsure of the cut, ask someone who works in the meat section of the grocery store.

Tips to make your steak more tasty and tender

- A tender cut of steak can be grilled as is and will be delicious. Try a sprinkle of Hy's Seasoning Salt (or your own favorite seasoning) applied before cooking and rubbed in. Or instead you can apply a barbecue sauce toward the end of grilling.
- For a low-salt alternative to commercial seasoning salt use the Spice Mix mixture below.
- Less tender steaks will need to be tenderized before cooking. It's helpful to pound with a tenderizing mallet or the edge of a plate. Then soak them overnight in the fridge in canned tomatoes with a small amount of added wine, wine vinegar, beer or soy sauce. The next day the steaks can be cooked slowly in the tenderizing liquid in a covered pan, or removed from the liquid and fried or barbecued.

Fresh mushrooms can be barbecued or broiled. Canned or fresh mushrooms can be cooked in a separate pan or added to the pan with the steak.

Spice Mix

Here is a spice mix you can make. Shake some on your meat, your potato or rice, and your vegetable.

2 tsp (10 mL) garlic powder
1 tsp (5 mL) dried basil
1 tsp (5 mL) dried oregano
1 tsp (5 mL) ground black pepper
1 tsp (5 mL) chili powder

PER ¼ TSP (1 ML)	
Calories	2
Carbohydrate	0 g
Fiber	0 g
Net carbs	0 g
Protein	0 g
Fat, total	0 g
Fat, saturated	0 g
Cholesterol	0 mg
Sodium	1 mg

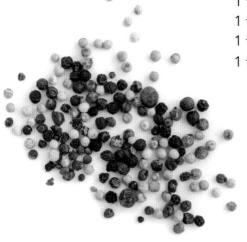

Serve the steak with Low-Fat Mashed Potatoes or with a boiled or baked potato.

Low-Fat Mashed Potatoes

Makes 2 cups (500 mL)

3 medium potatoes (about 1 lb/500 g)
⅓ cup (75 mL) skim or 1% milk

1. Wash and peel potatoes and cut into quarters.
2. Place potatoes in a large pot with enough water to cover. Bring to a boil, then reduce heat, cover and boil gently for about 20 minutes or until fork-tender.
3. Remove from heat, add milk and mash.

PER ½ CUP (125 ML)	
Calories	86
Carbohydrate	19 g
Fiber	1 g
Net carbs	18 g
Protein	2 g
Fat, total	0 g
Fat, saturated	0 g
Cholesterol	0 mg
Sodium	13 mg

RECIPE TIP

Make low-fat mashed potatoes by mashing the potatoes and adding only milk, and no butter or margarine. Add enough milk to make the potatoes creamy and smooth.

Brussels sprouts are healthy mini cabbages. If you don't have any, choose one of your own favorite vegetables.

Here's a little trick to help your smaller dessert portion seem like more: portion out your sherbet, ice cream or yogurt with a melon baller.

Cauliflower Mashed Potatoes

Use cauliflower instead of potatoes for a lower-carb alternative. Cook half a head of cauliflower until tender, place in a colander and drain off the hot water. Put the cauliflower back in your pot and add the ⅓ cup (75 mL) milk (you may need a little less) and mash. Salt and pepper to taste. Makes 2 cups (500 mL). Half a cup (125 mL) has 33 calories, 7 g of carbs (5 g of net carbs) and 3 g of protein.

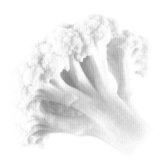

Food Choices	Large Meal	Small Meal
Carbohydrate	3½	2
Protein	5	3

Your Dinner Menu	Large Meal (730 calories)	Total Carbs	Net Carbs	Small Meal (550 calories)	Total Carbs	Net Carbs
Steak	5 oz (150 g), cooked	0	0	3 oz (90 g), cooked	0	0
Low-Fat Mashed Potatoes	1 cup (250 mL)	38	35	½ cup (125 mL)	19	18
Mushrooms	½ cup (125 mL)	4	2	½ cup (125 mL)	4	2
Brussels sprouts	¾ cup (175 mL)	8	4	¾ cup (175 mL)	8	4
Salad	Large	6	4	Large	6	4
Light salad dressing	1 tbsp (15 mL)	6	6	1 tbsp (15 mL)	6	6
Sherbet	½ cup (125 mL)	22	20	½ cup (125 mL)	22	20
		84 g	**71 g**		**65 g**	**54 g**

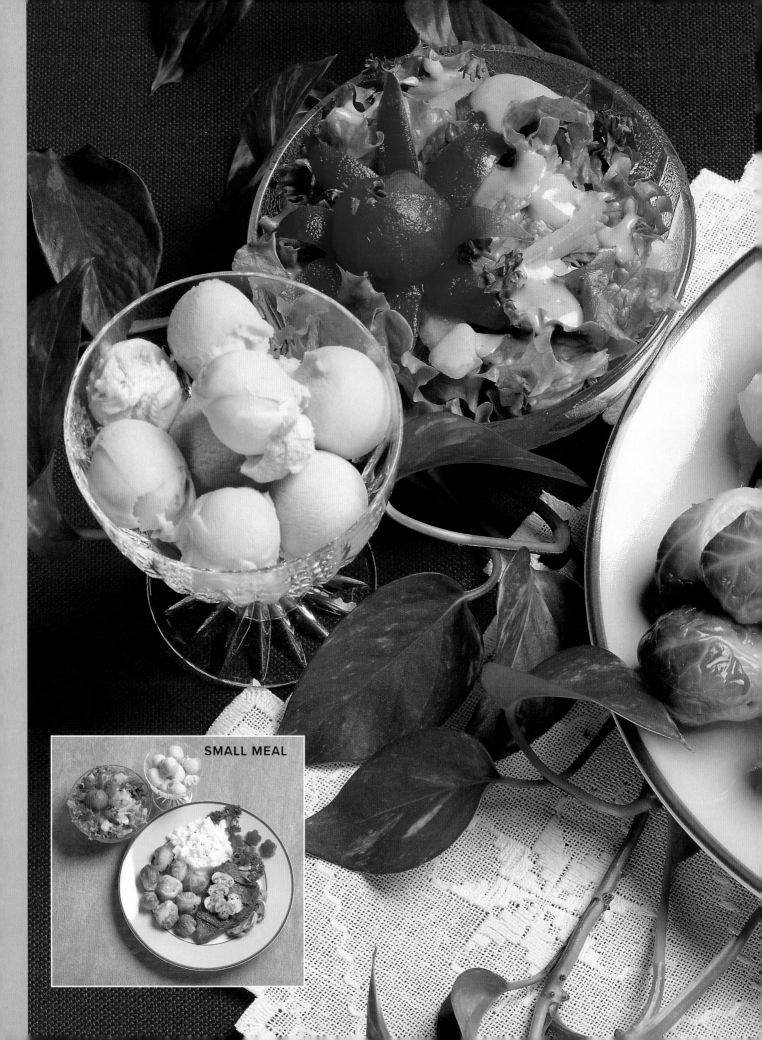

SMALL MEAL

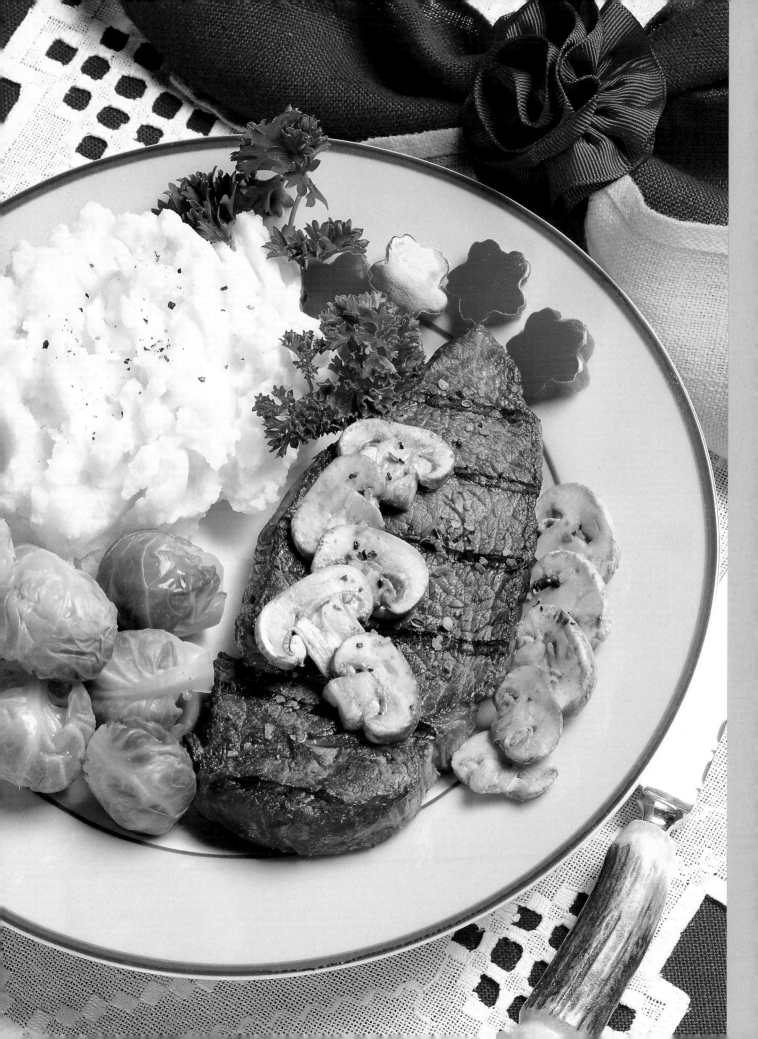

DINNER 9

Cheese Omelet

An omelet or scrambled eggs makes a great fast-and-easy nutritious dinner.

Cheese Omelet

2 eggs (large meal) or
  1 egg (small meal)
1 oz (30 g) (or 1 slice) cheese,
  cut into pieces or grated

1. In a small bowl, whisk the eggs. Pour into a nonstick pan.
2. Place the cheese on top.
3. Put a lid on and cook at low heat for about 5 minutes.
4. Fold in half.

The 1 tbsp (15 mL) of light cheese spread added to the broccoli has the same calories as 1 tsp (5 mL) of butter or margarine.

PER SMALL OMELET	
Calories	187
Carbohydrate	1 g
Fiber	0 g
Net carbs	1 g
Protein	13 g
Fat, total	14 g
Fat, saturated	8 g
Cholesterol	216 mg
Sodium	237 mg

RECIPE TIPS

Add this to your omelet:

- An extra egg white. The egg white has no cholesterol and only 20 calories. An egg yolk has 60 calories.

- Finely chopped onion, green onion or chives, celery and/or sweet pepper that you have precooked until soft in a bit of butter, margarine or oil.

- Fresh or dried herbs such as dill, parsley, basil or cilantro.

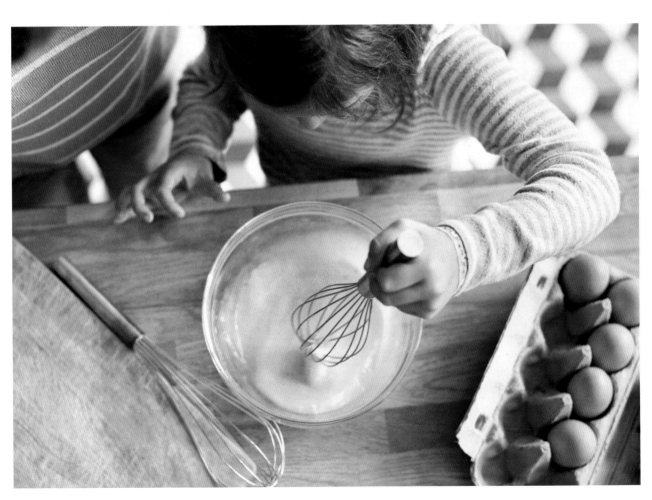

For dessert, enjoy one or two of these soft-textured oatmeal cookies. Or, in place of an oatmeal cookie, you could have a plain cookie such as a digestive or gingersnap.

Oatmeal Cookies

Makes 36 cookies

⅓ cup (75 mL) margarine
¾ cup (175 mL) packed brown sugar
1 egg
½ cup (125 mL) skim milk
1 tsp (5 mL) vanilla
1 cup (250 mL) flour
1 tsp (5 mL) baking powder
1 tsp (5 mL) baking soda
1 tsp (5 mL) ground cinnamon
1½ cups (375 mL) quick-cooking oats or large-flaked oats
1 cup (250 mL) raisins

PER COOKIE	
Calories	78
Carbohydrate	14 g
Fiber	1 g
Net carbs	13 g
Protein	1 g
Fat, total	2 g
Fat, saturated	0 g
Cholesterol	5 mg
Sodium	71 mg

1. In a large mixing bowl, mix together margarine, brown sugar and egg. Beat with a wooden spoon until smooth. Beat in the milk and vanilla.
2. In a medium bowl, mix together flour, baking powder, baking soda, cinnamon and rolled oats.
3. Add flour and oats to the large bowl. Stir well. Add raisins and stir again.
4. Drop small spoonfuls of batter onto a nonstick baking sheet or lightly greased regular cookie sheet. Batter will be sticky. Bake in a 375°F (190°C) oven for about 10 minutes, or until golden.

RECIPE TIP

To keep your nonstick pans and nonstick cookie sheets in good shape, use a plastic spatula or plastic spoon rather than a metal one. Store your nonstick pans so that other pots aren't scratching them; wrap in tea towels.

Food Choices	Large Meal	Small Meal
Carbohydrate	4	3
Protein	3	2
Fat	2½	1½

Your Dinner Menu	Large Meal (730 calories)	Total Carbs	Net Carbs	Small Meal (550 calories)	Total Carbs	Net Carbs
Cheese Omelet	1 large	1	0	1 small	1	0
Toast, whole wheat	2 slices	32	27	2 slices	32	27
Margarine	2 tsp (10 mL)	0	0	1 tsp (5 mL)	0	0
Broccoli	2 cups (500 mL) of pieces	10	7	2 cups (500 mL) of pieces	10	7
Light cheese spread	1 tbsp (15 mL)	1	1	1 tbsp (15 mL)	1	1
Oatmeal Cookies	2	27	26	1	14	13
		71 g	**61 g**		**58 g**	**48 g**

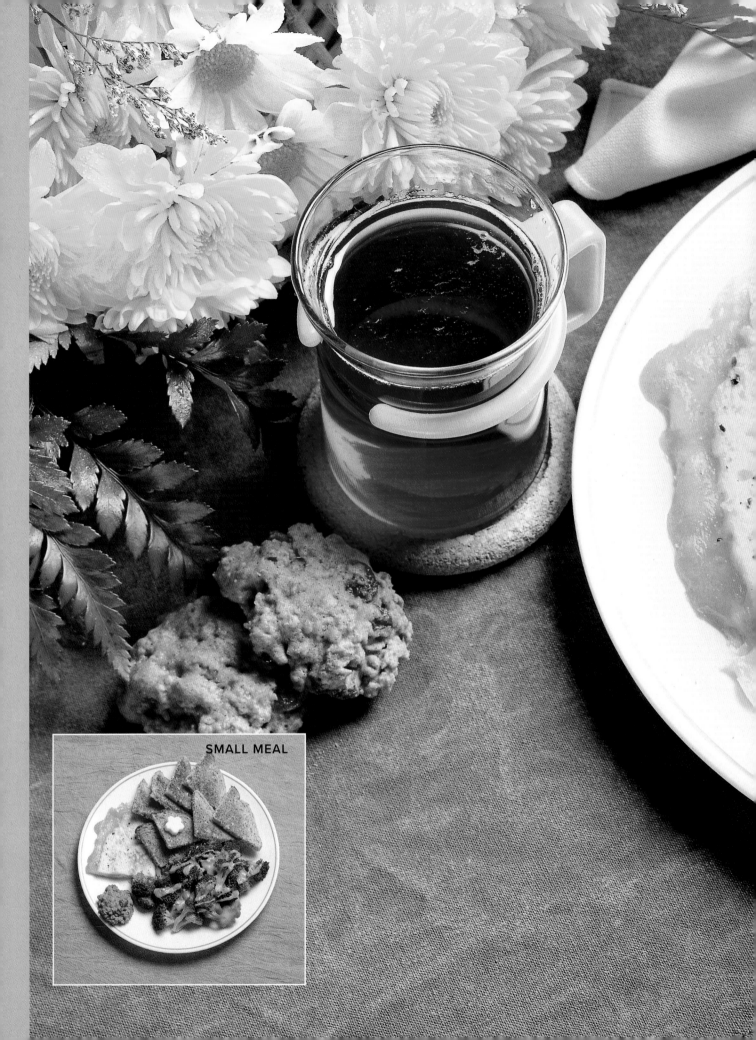

SMALL MEAL

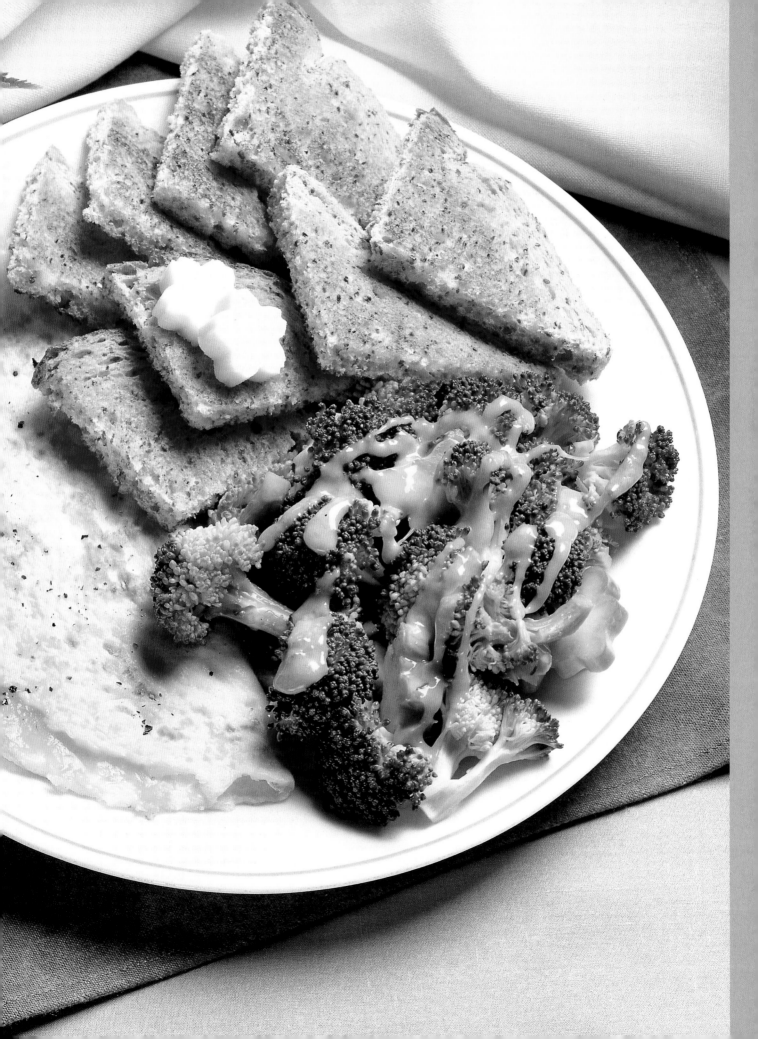

DINNER 10

Ham & Sweet Potato

For this meal, buy a cooking ham. Look for one that has the least amount of fat. Put the ham on a rack in a roasting pan. Bake your ham for about 25 minutes per pound (1½ hours per kg) at 325°F (160°C). If you are using a thermometer, cook to 160°F (71°C).

You can flavor and decorate the top of your ham by pushing about a dozen whole cloves into the outside of the ham. Add slices of pineapple on top of the ham for the last 30 minutes of the cooking.

A sweet potato has different vitamins and minerals than a regular potato, and it's nice for a change. Like orange squash and carrots, sweet potato is rich in vitamin A, which is important for healthy eyes. Since your oven is already on, cook it like a regular baked potato. Poke it with a fork and bake for 1 hour, or until tender.

Try these Seasoned Bread Crumbs sprinkled on your cauliflower. You can also sprinkle the Seasoned Bread Crumbs on other vegetables and on baked dishes.

Seasoned Bread Crumbs

Makes just over 1 cup (250 mL)

You can buy bread crumbs or make your own. To make your own, either crush the dry bread with a rolling pin or chop it in your blender.

1 cup (250 mL) dry bread crumbs
2 tbsp (30 mL) Parmesan cheese
1 tbsp (15 mL) dried parsley
1 tsp (5 mL) dried oregano
½ tsp (2 mL) garlic powder
⅛ tsp (0.5 mL) pepper

1. Mix ingredients together. Store Seasoned Bread Crumbs in the fridge or freezer.

PER 1 TSP (5 ML)	
Calories	10
Carbohydrate	2 g
Fiber	0 g
Net carbs	2 g
Protein	0 g
Fat, total	0 g
Fat, saturated	0 g
Cholesterol	0 mg
Sodium	24 mg

FOOD FACT

Hams have a small amount of either sugar or honey added. "Honey" ham does not have more sugar than regular ham, but all hams contain a lot of salt.

HEALTH TIP

Sweet potatoes are a powerhouse of vitamin A, which is important for good vision and healthy teeth, nails, hair, bones and glands. It also helps protect against infection and is an antioxidant (fighting cancer and heart disease). The deeper the orange color of the sweet potato, the richer the source of vitamin A. Sweet potatoes are also a good source of fiber, vitamin C and potassium.

RECIPE TIP

A sweet potato can also be cooked by:

- microwaving it on High for 10 minutes
- boiling it with the skin on (take off the skin, once it is cooked)

All vegetables are good choices but some, such as cauliflower and yellow beans, have a higher amount of fiber and water. This makes them especially low in carbs and calories.

Low-calorie vegetables

- asparagus
- green or yellow beans
- bean sprouts
- broccoli
- Brussels sprouts
- cabbage
- cauliflower
- celery
- cucumber
- eggplant
- fiddleheads
- leafy greens, such as lettuce, arugula, kale and spinach
- marrow
- mushrooms
- okra
- onions
- green, red or orange peppers
- radishes
- summer and spaghetti squash
- tomato
- zucchini

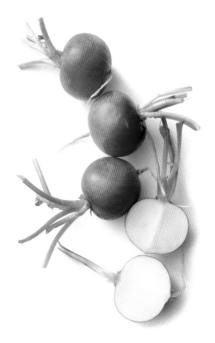

Whipped Gelatin

Makes 4 cups (1 L)

1 package (4-serving size) light gelatin of your favorite flavor

1. Make the gelatin according to the directions on the box (or use the recipe on page 117).
2. Remove the gelatin from the fridge after about 45 minutes. It should be as thick as an unbeaten egg white. Beat the gelatin with a beater until it is foamy and has doubled in size.
3. Put it back in the fridge until firm.

PER 1 CUP (250 ML)	
Calories	5
Carbohydrate	2 g
Fiber	0 g
Net carbs	2 g
Protein	0 g
Fat, total	0 g
Fat, saturated	0 g
Cholesterol	0 mg
Sodium	25 mg

Food Choices	Large Meal	Small Meal
Carbohydrate	5	4
Protein	5	3
Fat	2	1

Your Dinner Menu	Large Meal (730 calories)	Total Carbs	Net Carbs	Small Meal (550 calories)	Total Carbs	Net Carbs
Baked ham	1 thick slice (5 oz/150 g, cooked)	1	1	1 thin slice (3 oz/90 g, cooked)	1	1
Pineapple, packed in juice	2 rings, no juice	13	12	2 rings, no juice	13	12
Sweet potato	1 large	46	43	1 medium	36	31
Margarine	2 tsp (10 mL)	0	0	1 tsp (5 mL)	0	0
Cauliflower	2 cups (500 mL)	8	5	2 cups (500 mL)	8	5
Seasoned Bread Crumbs	1 tsp (5 mL)	2	2	1 tsp (5 mL)	2	2
Skim or 1% milk	1 cup (250 mL)	12	12	1 cup (250 mL)	12	12
Whipped Gelatin	1 cup (250 mL)	2	2	1 cup (250 mL)	2	2
		84 g	77 g		74 g	65 g

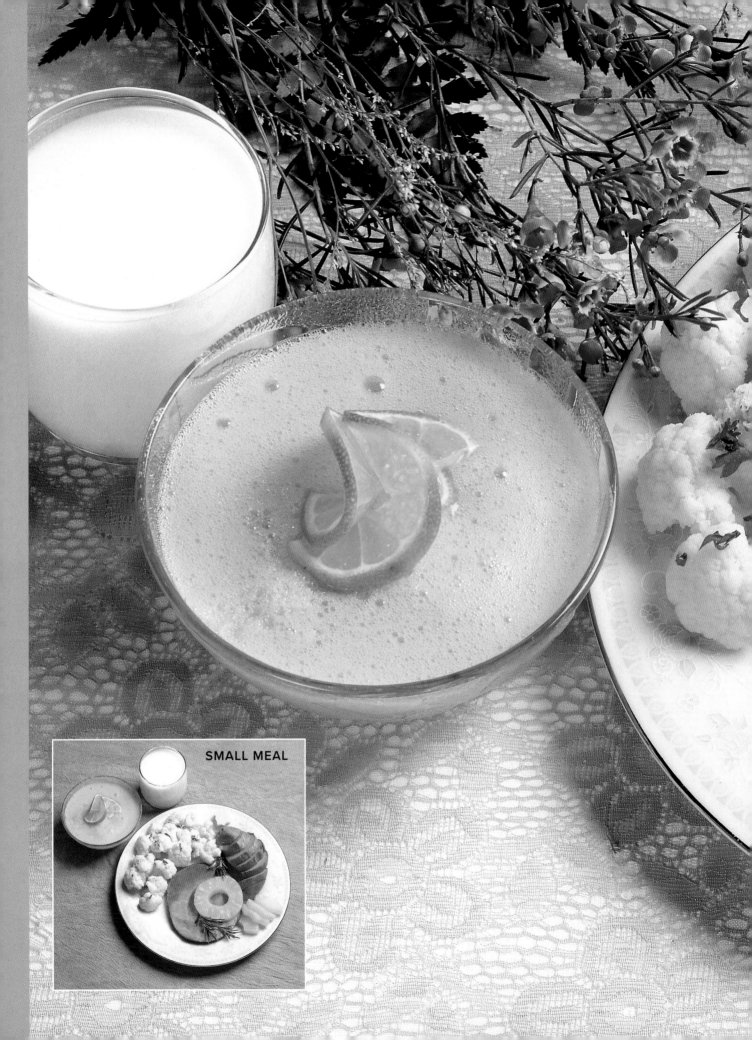

SMALL MEAL

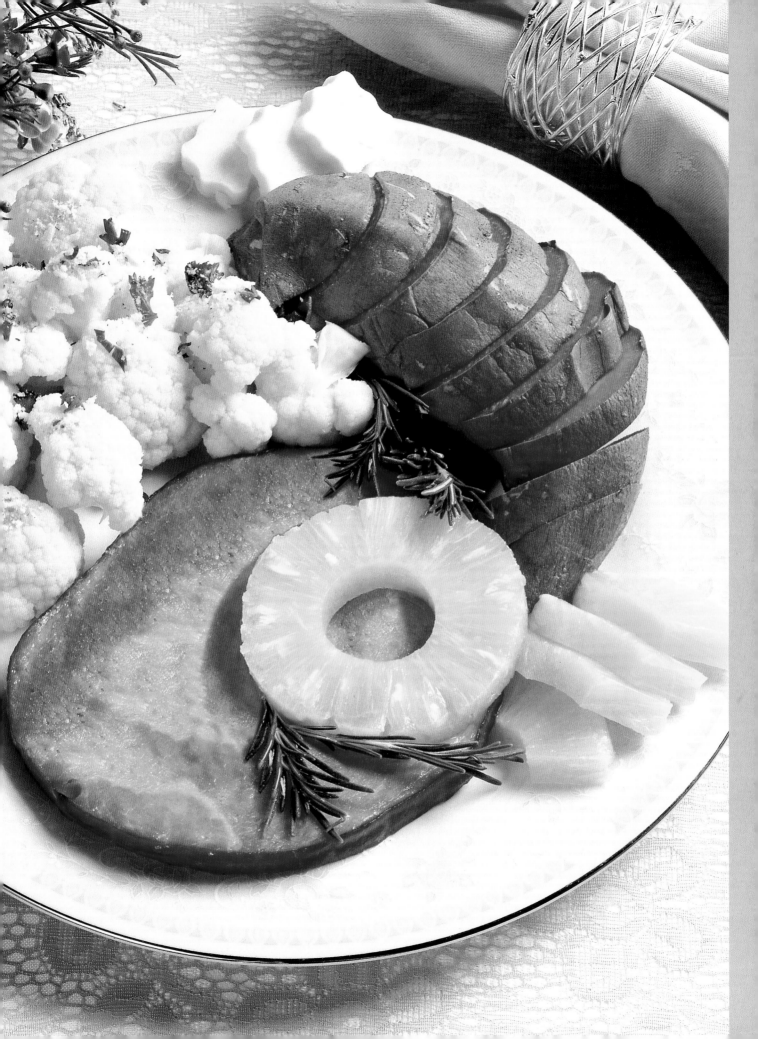

DINNER 11

Beef Stew

Beef stew served with potatoes and bread is an old favorite. Double the recipe if you want to make more to freeze for another day.

RECIPE TIP

Vegetables that go well in a stew include turnips, yellow and green beans, carrots and peas. You can use frozen mixed vegetables in this recipe in place of the fresh vegetables.

If you are in a hurry, try this:

Open a can of beef stew, put it in a pot and add some frozen or cooked vegetables. Cook until heated.

Beef Stew

Recipe makes 7 cups (1.75 L)

1 to 2 tbsp (15 to 30 mL) margarine or oil

2 medium onions, chopped

2 cloves garlic, finely chopped
(or ½ tsp/2 mL garlic powder)

1 lb (500 g) stewing beef, fat removed
and chopped into dice-size pieces

2 tbsp (30 mL) flour

1 to 2 packets (4.5 g each) reduced-salt
beef bouillon, mixed in 2 cups (500 mL) hot water

1 bay leaf (remove before serving)

2 large stalks of celery, sliced

3 medium carrots, sliced

2 cups (500 mL) other fresh vegetables
(or frozen mixed vegetables)

⅛ tsp (0.5 mL) black pepper

¼ cup (60 mL) dry wine (or wine vinegar)

PER 1 CUP (250 ML)	
Calories	164
Carbohydrate	13 g
Fiber	3 g
Net carbs	10 g
Protein	14 g
Fat, total	6 g
Fat, saturated	2 g
Cholesterol	27 mg
Sodium	179 mg

1. In a heavy pot, add margarine, onions and garlic and stir on medium heat until onions become clear. Stir often so they do not burn.
2. Add meat and stir it until it is cooked on the outside (about 5 minutes). Sprinkle flour over the onion and meat mixture, and stir until the flour disappears.
3. Take pot off the heat while you add the rest of the ingredients. Stir. Return to heat. Bring to a boil and then turn heat down to low. Cover and simmer for about an hour. Stir occasionally.
4. If you are using frozen mixed vegetables instead of fresh vegetables, add them just at the end and simmer for 10 minutes.

The beef stew is served with potatoes, a slice of bread to soak up the stew, and sliced cucumbers. For dessert, enjoy a serving of melon or other fruit.

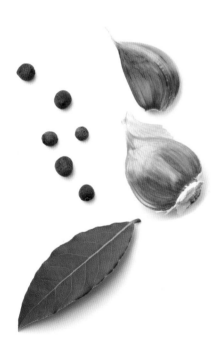

North African Stew and Couscous

For a change, you may want a spicier stew. Try a North African stew. This stew is commonly made with lamb and, for vegetables, onions, carrots, turnips, tomatoes, zucchini, pumpkin and squash. When you cook the meat, add 1 tsp (5 mL) of each of the following: turmeric, cinnamon and cumin (or try 1 tbsp/15 mL of curry powder instead), and 1 tsp (5 mL) of chili powder. Make this stew a day ahead so that the spice taste is best.

Instead of having this stew with bread and potatoes, you can serve it with couscous. Serve 1¼ cups (300 mL) couscous for the large meal and 1 cup (250 mL) for the small meal. Couscous is made from semolina wheat and can be bought in all major food stores. It looks like rice but tastes more like noodles. It is easy and quick to make because you just boil it in water. Serve the stew and couscous with mint tea.

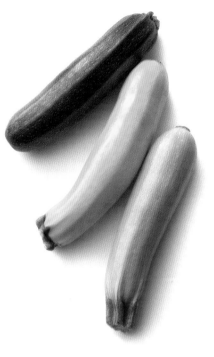

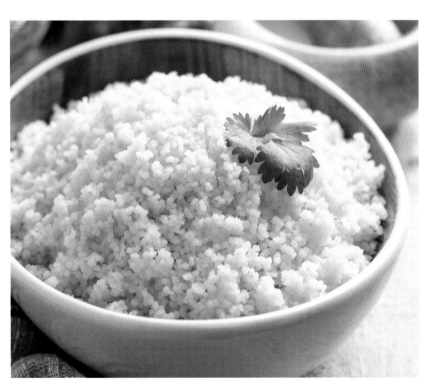

Food Choices	Large Meal	Small Meal
Carbohydrate	5	4
Protein	3½	2½
Fat	1	½

Your Dinner Menu	Large Meal (730 calories)	Total Carbs	Net Carbs	Small Meal (550 calories)	Total Carbs	Net Carbs
Beef Stew	2 cups (500 mL)	27	22	1½ cups (375 mL)	20	17
Boiled potatoes	1 large	44	41	1 medium	30	28
Bread	1 slice	17	15	1 slice	17	15
Margarine	1 tsp (5 mL)	0	0	½ tsp (2 mL)	0	0
Sliced cucumbers	½ medium cucumber	2	1	½ medium cucumber	2	1
Melon	2 slices	15	13	2 slices	15	13
		105 g	**92 g**		**84 g**	**74 g**

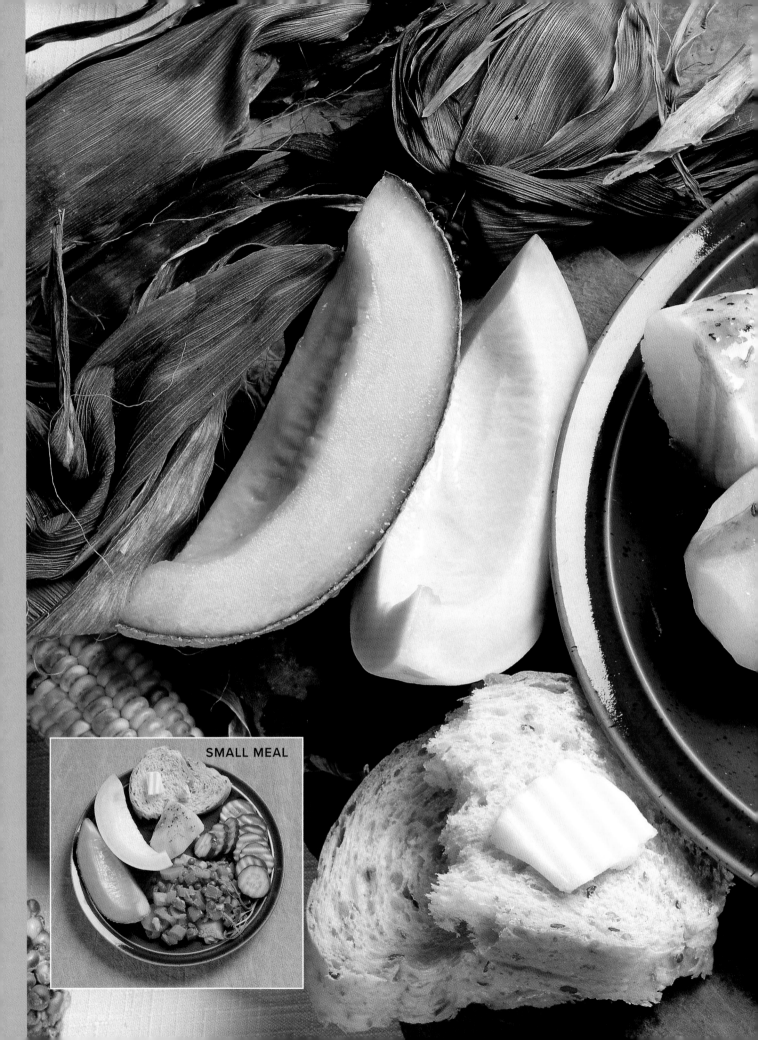

SMALL MEAL

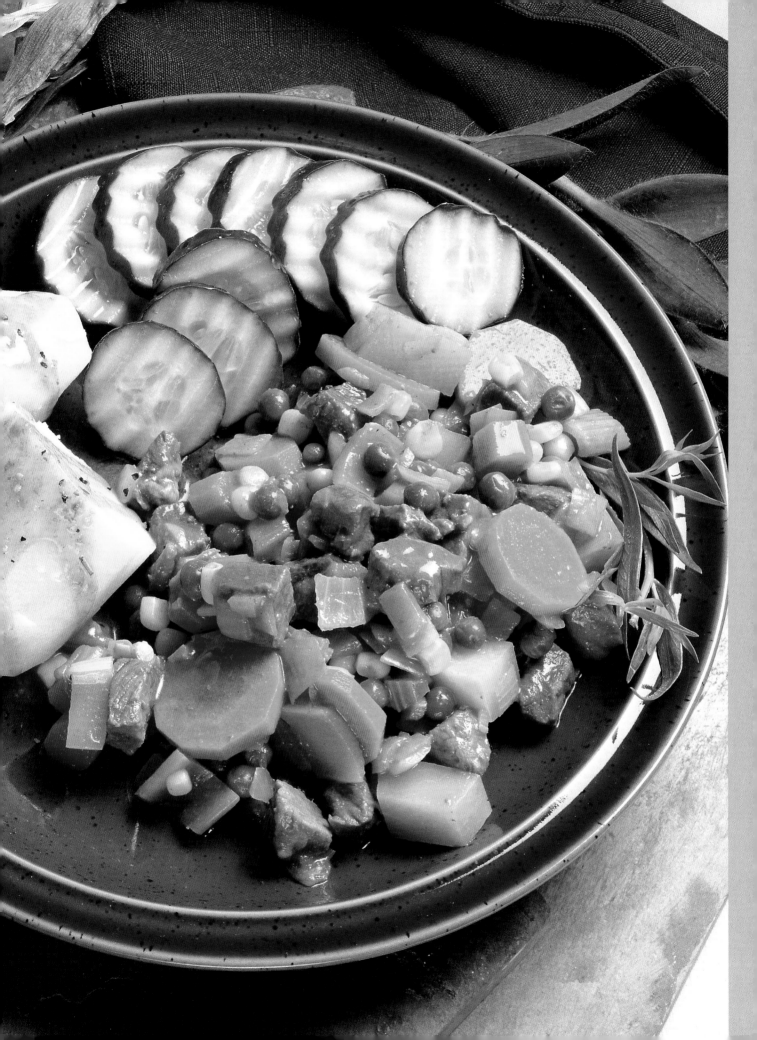

DINNER 12

Fish & Chips

This is a favorite for many, especially for those who aren't as keen on eating fish. Making a balanced meal at home is so much more nutritious than having deep fried fish with fries and a creamy coleslaw in a restaurant. Look for a brand of fish sticks that are labeled "lightly breaded." This meal includes frozen french fries but a lower fat option is Baked Low-Fat Fries (recipe below) or potato wedges tossed in oil (see page 304).

Bake the fish and fries in the oven on a cookie sheet at 450°F (230°C) for 15 minutes, or according to the package instructions.

Baked Low-Fat Fries

Makes 45 fries (15 fries for each potato)

3 medium potatoes (about 1 lb/500 g)
1 egg white
1 to 2 tsp (5 to 10 mL) packaged
   potato seasonings, or sprinkle
   on your favorite herbs or spices
   (such as curry, garlic powder, dill,
   Cajun spice or hot pepper flakes)

PER 10 FRIES	
Calories	65
Carbohydrate	14 g
Fiber	1 g
Net carbs	13 g
Protein	2 g
Fat, total	0 g
Fat, saturated	0 g
Cholesterol	0 mg
Sodium	63 mg

1. Wash and peel the potatoes.
2. Cut into fry-size pieces or chunks.
3. In a small bowl, mix the egg white and spices with a fork.
4. Dip the potato pieces into the mixture.
5. On a greased nonstick cookie sheet, bake the potato pieces at 400°F (200°C). Cook for about 30 minutes, turning them every 10 minutes.

With this meal, have one vegetable serving of squash, peas, carrots, corn, turnips or parsnips.

Here is how the squash shown in the photograph is cooked: Cut the squash in half and place the cut side down on a cookie sheet. Bake in the oven with the fish and fries. Bake for 30 minutes, or until tender.

FOOD CHARTS

See page 300, Fish, and page 304, Potatoes.

FOOD FACTS

Compare the calories of 10 french fries:

- fried in oil from a restaurant: 160 calories
- frozen fries baked in the oven: 90 calories
- Baked Low-Fat Fries: 60 calories

Squash

The orange squash shown in the photograph is an acorn squash. There are many kinds of squash. For example, you may want to try spaghetti squash, one of the less sweet squashes.

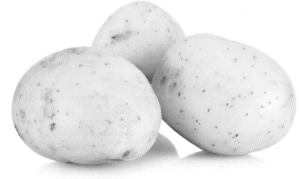

Try this Light Jellied Vegetable Salad. It is colorful and tasty and low in calories. The lime gelatin gives it a nice green color.

Light Jellied Vegetable Salad

Makes 2¹/₂ cups (625 mL) (5 servings)

1 package (4-serving size) light
    lime gelatin

1¹/₂ cups (375 mL) boiling water

2 tbsp (30 mL) lemon or lime juice

¹/₂ cup (125 mL) radish, finely chopped

¹/₂ cup (125 mL) celery, finely chopped

¹/₂ cup (125 mL) cabbage, finely chopped

1 tbsp (15 mL) fresh parsley, chopped, or
    1 tsp (5 mL) dried parsley

PER ¹/₂ CUP (125 ML)	
Calories	17
Carbohydrate	4 g
Fiber	1 g
Net carbs	3 g
Protein	1 g
Fat, total	0 g
Fat, saturated	0 g
Cholesterol	0 mg
Sodium	41 mg

RECIPE TIP

For a lightly salted and less sweet flavor in the Jellied Vegetable Salad, try this:

- add 1 packet (4.5 g) of light chicken bouillon mix, or 1 bouillon cube, to the boiling water.

1. In a medium bowl, place the gelatin powder. Add the boiling water and stir until the gelatin is mixed in. Add the lemon juice. Put this mixture in the fridge.
2. Chop all the vegetables. Once the mixture in the fridge is slightly thickened (about 45 minutes), stir in all the vegetables.
3. Chill until set (about another hour).

Jellied Vegetable Salad can be a low-calorie vegetable choice with any lunch or dinner meal — ¹/₂ cup (125 mL) has only 20 calories.

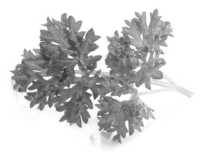

Food Choices	Large Meal	Small Meal
Carbohydrate	4	3
Protein	3	2
Fat	1	1

Your Dinner Menu	Large Meal (730 calories)	Total Carbs	Net Carbs	Small Meal (550 calories)	Total Carbs	Net Carbs
Fish sticks	6 sticks or 3 wedges	36	34	4 sticks or 2 wedges	24	23
Oven-baked frozen french fries	15	23	21	10	16	14
Ketchup	1 tbsp (15 mL)	4	4	1 tbsp	4	4
Squash	¹/₂ cup (125 mL)	15	13	¹/₂ cup (125 mL)	15	13
Light Jellied Vegetable Salad	¹/₂ cup (125 mL)	4	3	¹/₂ cup (125 mL)	4	3
Plum	1 medium	9	8	1 medium	9	8
		91 g	**83 g**		**72 g**	**65 g**

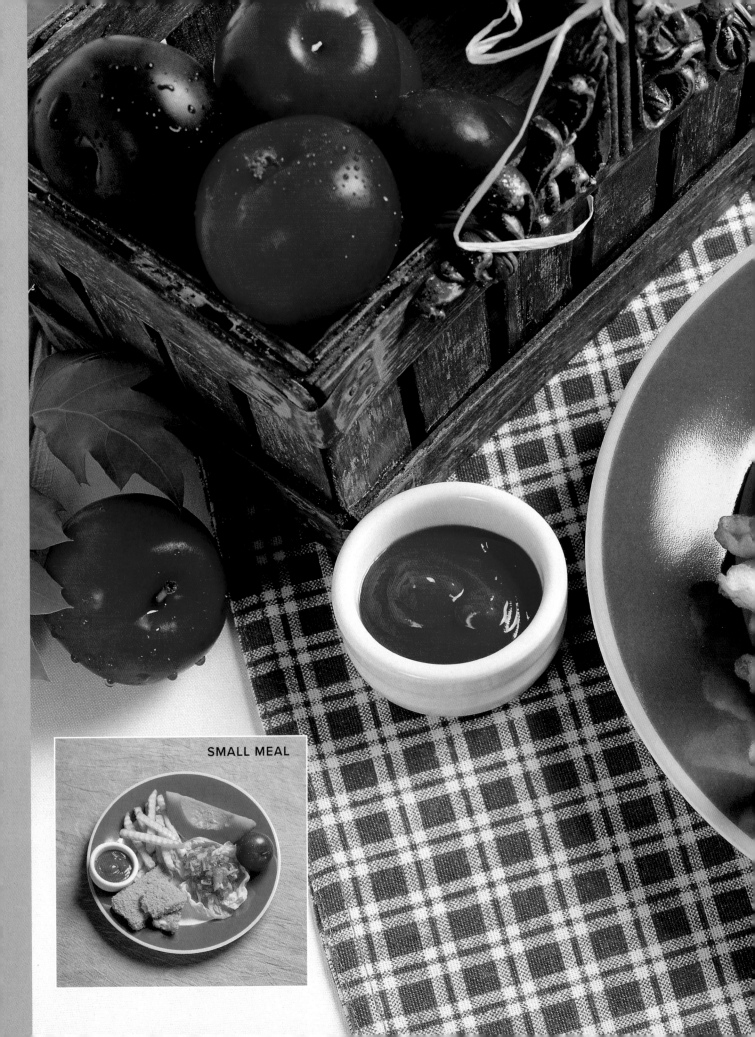

SMALL MEAL

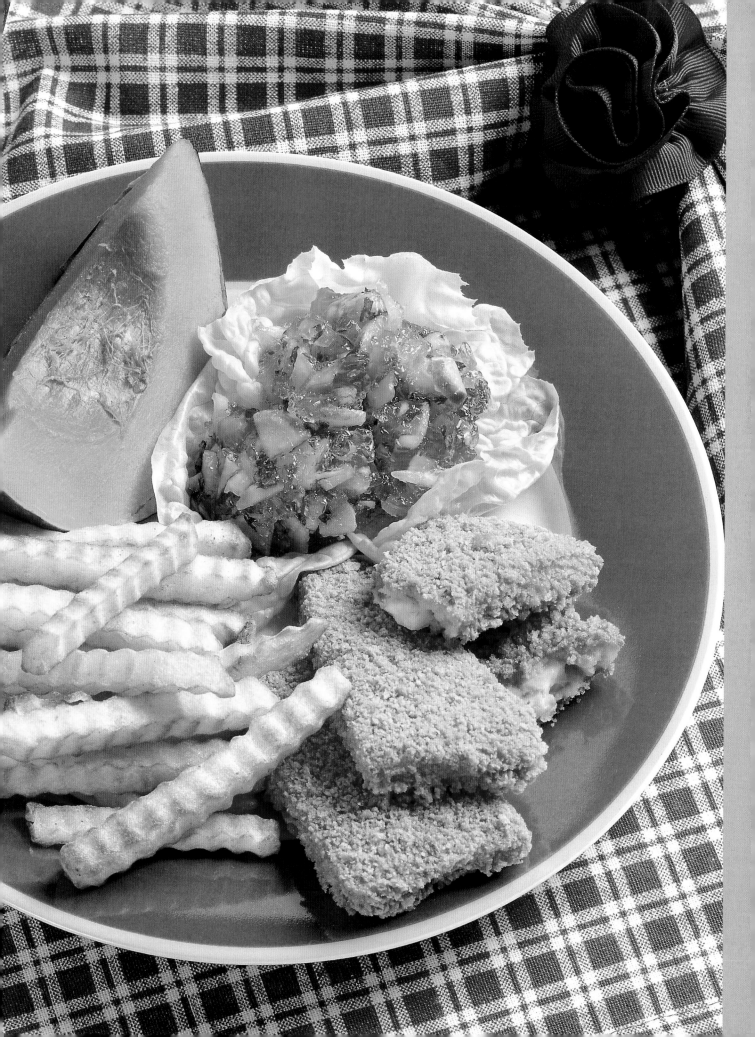

DINNER 13

Sausages & Cornbread

RECIPE TIP

Zucchini is also nice cooked in a pan with 1 tsp (5 mL) of margarine or oil and chopped onion and garlic. To this, you can add one or two other vegetables, such as:

- canned or fresh chopped tomatoes
- green pepper
- eggplant or okra

Add water to the pan, if needed. Sprinkle Parmesan cheese on top.

Here is another occasional but favorite meal. Sausages are high in fat and salt. Poke them several times so the fat can drain out, fry in a fry pan, remove from the pan and place on a paper towel to absorb the fat.

Fill up on vegetables. Zucchini is a low-calorie vegetable that is easy to prepare by slicing and steaming. If you boil zucchini, it will get soggy. Sprinkle it with Seasoned Bread Crumbs (see recipe on page 148).

Use the Coleslaw recipe in Lunch 4 on page 84.

You could replace the light ice cream bar with ½ cup (125 mL) skim milk.

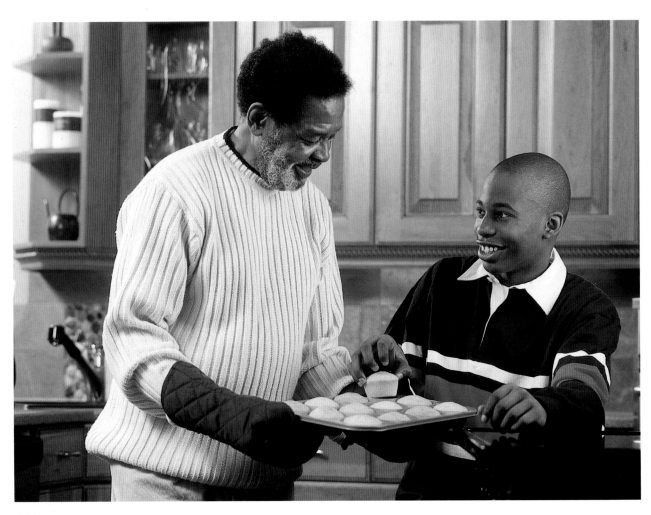

Cornbread or Corn Muffins

Makes an 8-inch (2 L) square pan (12 pieces) or 12 muffins

$^3/_4$ cup (175 mL) cornmeal

$1^1/_4$ cups (300 mL) skim milk

1 egg, slightly beaten

3 level tbsp (45 mL) oil or melted margarine, butter or shortening

1 cup (250 mL) flour

1 tbsp (15 mL) baking powder

$^1/_2$ tsp (2 mL) salt

$^1/_4$ cup (60 mL) sugar

PER PIECE ($^1/_{12}$ OF RECIPE)	
Calories	137
Carbohydrate	21 g
Fiber	1 g
Net carbs	20 g
Protein	3 g
Fat, total	4 g
Fat, saturated	0 g
Cholesterol	16 mg
Sodium	180 mg

OPTIONS

For a change, here are some starches that could take the place of one piece of cornbread:

- $^1/_2$ cup (125 mL) canned corn kernels or rice
- 1 small cob of corn

1. In a medium bowl, mix together cornmeal, milk, slightly beaten egg and oil (or melted fat).
2. In a large bowl, mix together flour, baking powder, salt and sugar.
3. Add cornmeal mixture to the flour mixture. Stir until combined. Pour into an 8-inch (2 L) square pan or muffin tin. Use a nonstick pan, or grease your pan lightly.
4. Bake in a 400°F (200°C) oven for about 20 minutes (15 minutes for muffins), or until lightly browned.
5. Cut into 12 pieces (about 3 inches by 2 inches/7.5 cm by 5 cm).

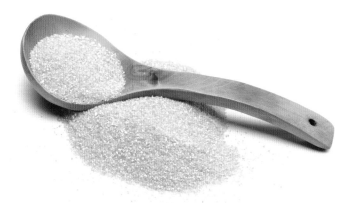

Food Choices	Large Meal	Small Meal
Carbohydrate	4	3
Protein	$1^1/_2$	1

Your Dinner Menu	Large Meal (730 calories)	Total Carbs	Net Carbs	Small Meal (550 calories)	Total Carbs	Net Carbs
Sausages	4 small links	1	1	3 small links	1	1
Cornbread	$2^1/_2$ pieces	54	52	2 pieces	43	41
Steamed zucchini	2 cups (500 mL)	14	8	2 cups (500 mL)	14	8
Seasoned Bread Crumbs	1 tbsp (15 mL)	5	5	1 tbsp (15 mL)	5	5
Coleslaw	$^1/_2$ cup (125 mL)	5	4	$^1/_2$ cup (125 mL)	5	4
Light fudge ice cream bar	1 bar	9	8	1 bar	9	8
		88 g	78 g		77 g	67 g

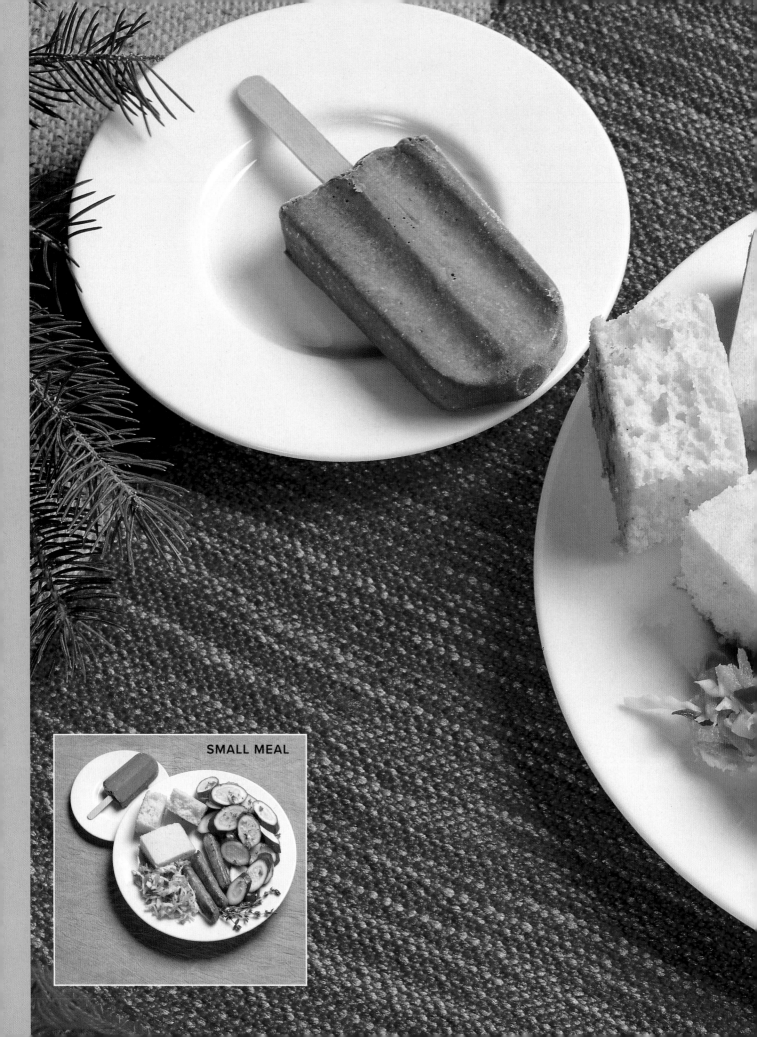

SMALL MEAL

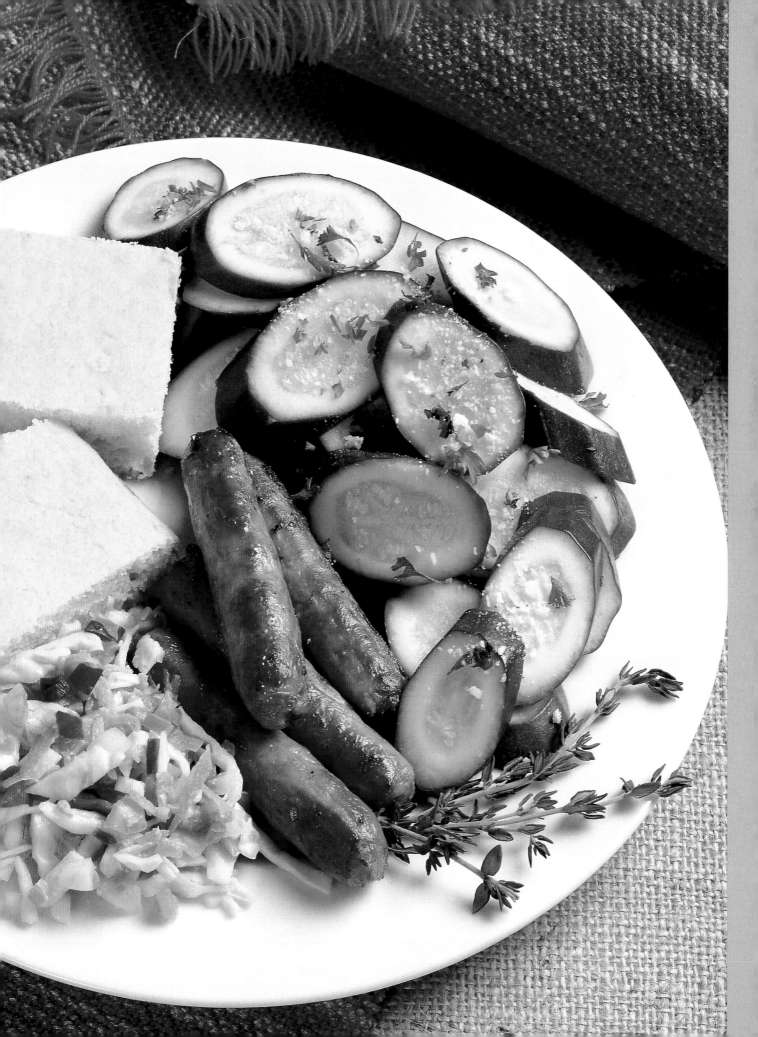

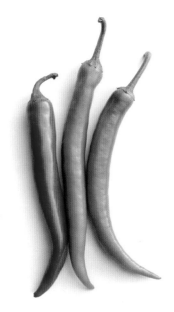

Chili Con Carne

Chili freezes well. You can easily double the recipe for freezing.

Chili Con Carne

Makes 6¼ cups (1.55 L)

1 lb (500 g) lean ground beef

2 medium onions, chopped

28-oz (796 mL) can kidney beans, drained and rinsed

10-oz (284 mL) can tomato soup

1 cup (250 mL) water

⅛ tsp (0.5 mL) black pepper

½ tsp (2 mL) chili powder

1 tbsp (15 mL) vinegar

½ tsp (2 mL) Worcestershire sauce

1 cup (250 mL) chopped vegetables, such as celery or green pepper

PER 1 CUP (250 ML)	
Calories	270
Carbohydrate	29 g
Fiber	7 g
Net carbs	22 g
Protein	21 g
Fat, total	8 g
Fat, saturated	3 g
Cholesterol	38 mg
Sodium	597 mg

1. In a large, heavy pot, brown ground beef. Drain off as much fat as you can.
2. Add all the other ingredients to the pot.
3. Cover with a lid and cook for 2 to 3 hours on low heat. Stir every now and then so the chili doesn't stick. Add extra water if it gets too thick.

Serve the meal with brown or white rice.

Add a low-calorie vegetable such as yellow beans or green beans. Carrot sticks are served on the side.

HEALTH TIP

Rinse canned beans

Drain off the liquid they are canned in and rinse them before use. This will remove about 30% of the salt.

OPTIONS

Instead of ⅓ cup (75 mL) of rice:

- 1 slice of bread
- ½ piece of bannock
- 1 small potato

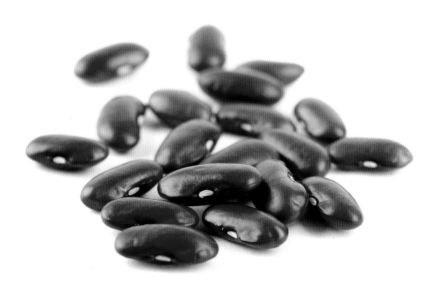

For a dessert treat, try this tasty Baked Apple or have a serving of any other kind of fruit. These baked apples have a lovely glaze because of the combination of brown sugar and butter. Margarine can be used instead, but butter makes the syrup thicker. Regular sugar is used because low-calorie sweeteners tend to make the syrup in the apple too thin.

Baked Apple

Makes 2 baked apples

2 medium apples

2 tsp (10 mL) butter or margarine

2 tsp (10 mL) brown sugar

1/4 tsp (1 mL) ground cinnamon

1/4 tsp (1 mL) lemon juice

Dash of nutmeg

1 tbsp (15 mL) raisins

PER APPLE	
Calories	150
Carbohydrate	29 g
Fiber	3 g
Net carbs	26 g
Protein	0 g
Fat, total	5 g
Fat, saturated	3 g
Cholesterol	10 mg
Sodium	43 mg

1. Remove apple core, cutting from the top of the apple. Don't cut right through to the bottom. Prick apples with a fork.
2. In a small bowl, mix together other ingredients and spoon into the apples.
3. Place apples on a dish and microwave them on High for 80 seconds, or until the apples are tender. Or place the apples in a pan with 2 tbsp (30 mL) of water and bake in a 350°F (180°C) oven for 30 minutes.

FOOD CHARTS

See page 311, Apple Dessert, for a comparison of Baked Apple to Apple Pie.

RECIPE TIP

Baked Apple in a Dish

Here's an even easier way to make this recipe! Core the apple then chop or slice it, and place the apple with the other ingredients in a microwavable bowl. Stir. Then microwave on high for about 2 minutes or until the apples are soft. Eat with a fork or spoon.

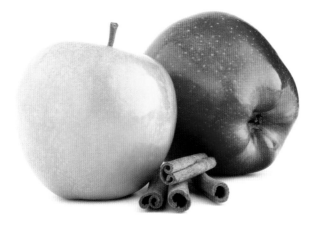

Food Choices	Large Meal	Small Meal
Carbohydrate	5½	4½
Protein	3	2

Your Dinner Menu	Large Meal (730 calories)	Total Carbs	Net Carbs	Small Meal (550 calories)	Total Carbs	Net Carbs
Chili Con Carne	1¼ cups (310 mL)	36	28	1 cup (250 mL)	29	22
Rice, long-grain, parboiled	2/3 cup (150 mL)	29	28	1/3 cup (75 mL)	14	14
Green beans	1 cup (250 mL)	10	7	1 cup (250 mL)	10	7
Carrot sticks	1 medium carrot	6	5	1 medium carrot	6	5
Baked Apple	1	29	26	1	29	26
		110 g	**94 g**		**88 g**	**74 g**

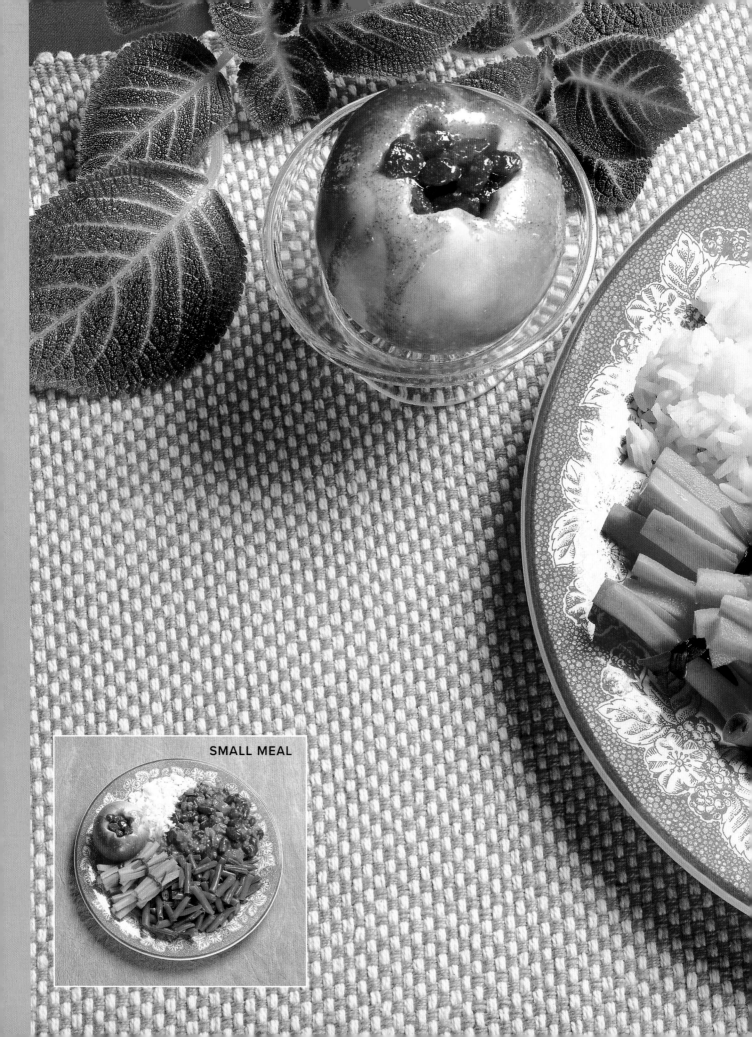

SMALL MEAL

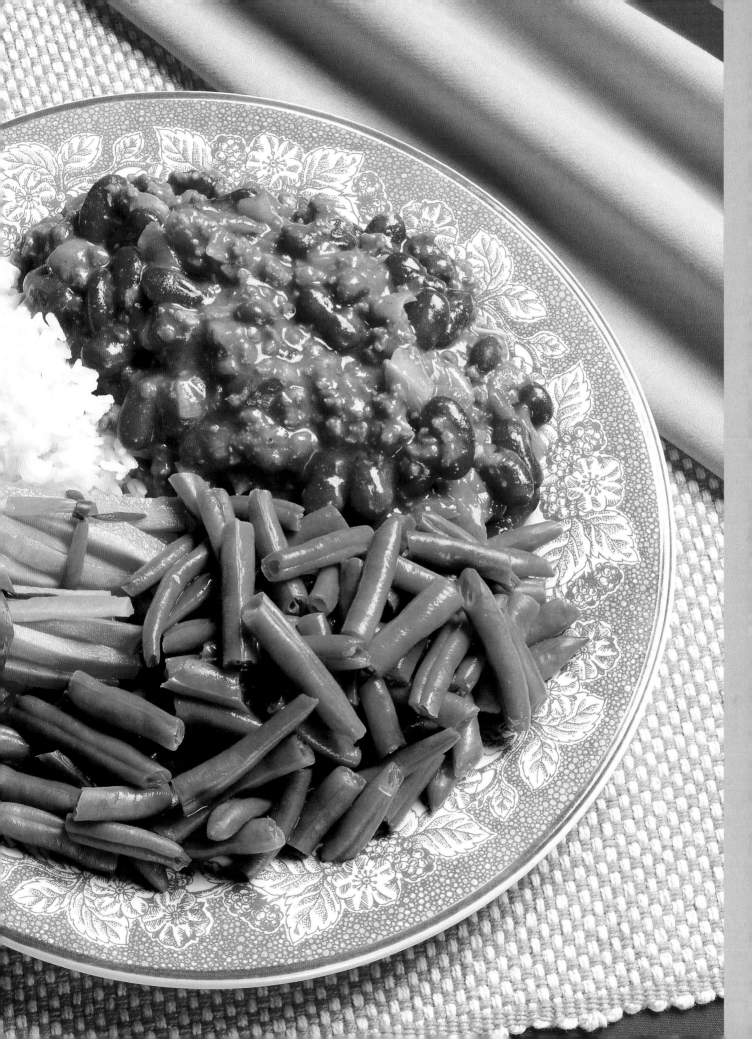

DINNER 15

Perogies

Buy frozen perogies and enjoy a fast-food meal at home. Perogies come with many fillings, such as cheese, potato and cottage cheese. The carbs in perogies can add up quickly, so be careful not to eat more than the number shown in the photograph.

First, fry onions at low heat in 2 tsp (10 mL) of butter or margarine (add water if pan gets dry). Then take the onions out of the pan so they don't get overcooked. Fry the perogies in the same pan until lightly browned. Another way to cook them is to boil them for 10 minutes.

Instead of having a 2-oz (60 g) piece of garlic sausage (kielbasa) with the large meal, you could have:

- ½ cup (125 mL) of 1% cottage cheese
- 1 small fast-fry pork chop (3 oz/85 g)
- 2 slices bologna, broiled, or fried without added fat

Sauerkraut is a low-calorie vegetable that has healthy bacteria.

A low-salt alternative to sauerkraut or a pickle would be a small salad or coleslaw.

FOOD FACTS

Perogies and sour cream go together like hugs and kisses; but go for a light hug. Enjoy 1 tbsp (15 mL) of light sour cream, or 2 tbsp (30 mL) of fat-free sour cream with your perogies. Here are the calories in a 1 tbsp (15 mL) serving:

- Fat-free sour cream: 9 calories
- Plain Greek yogurt (2%): 10 calories
- Light sour cream (7%): 16 calories
- Regular sour cream (14%): 32 calories

FOOD FACT

What is sauerkraut?

Sauerkraut is cabbage with salt added that is left to ferment (pickle). Salt is the downside of sauerkraut, but the upside is that during this fermenting process healthy bacteria grow. These are called probiotic bacteria. When you eat sauerkraut or other fermented products like Kimchi (a Korean pickled vegetable dish), these probiotic bacteria are healthy for your gut.

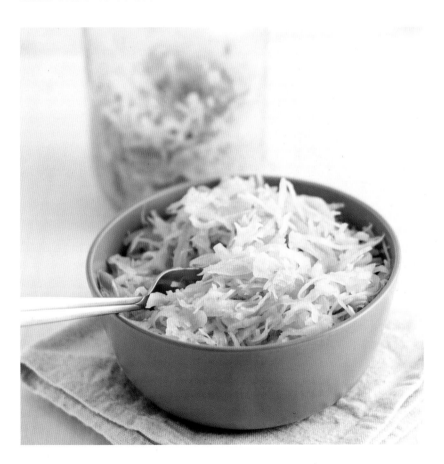

Easy Beet Soup

Makes 3½ cups (875 mL)

10-oz (284 mL) can diced beets
  (unsweetened), drained and rinsed
1½ cups (375 mL) vegetable juice
  (such as V8)
½ cup (125 mL) water
2 cups (500 mL) chopped cabbage
¼ tsp (1 mL) dried dill

PER 1 CUP (250 ML)	
Calories	46
Carbohydrate	10 g
Fiber	2 g
Net carbs	8 g
Protein	2 g
Fat, total	0 g
Fat, saturated	0 g
Cholesterol	0 mg
Sodium	363 mg

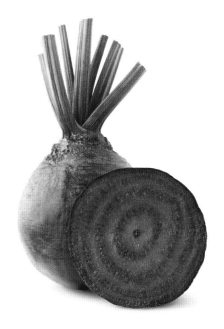

1. Place all ingredients in a pot.
2. Cover and simmer. Stir as it is cooking. It will take about 15 minutes to cook.

Serve with a dab of low-fat sour cream if desired.

Instead of the beet soup, you may want to have 1 cup (250 mL) of cooked beets. Pickled beets have added sugar, so ½ cup (125 mL) of these would equal 1 cup (250 mL) of beet soup.

For dessert, have one fresh peach. If you want canned peaches, have two halves with 2 tbsp (30 mL) of juice. Choose fruit canned in water or juice. Have one plain cookie with your fruit. Plain bought cookies include arrowroot biscuits, digestives, raisin cookies (as shown in the photograph), gingersnaps, oatmeal cookies and Graham wafers.

Food Choices	Large Meal	Small Meal
Carbohydrate	5	4
Protein	2	1
Fat	1	1

Your Dinner Menu	Large Meal (730 calories)	Total Carbs	Net Carbs	Small Meal (550 calories)	Total Carbs	Net Carbs
Perogies	6	60	54	4	40	36
Low-fat or fat-free sour cream	1 tbsp (15 mL)	2	2	1 tbsp (15 mL)	2	2
Cooked sliced onion in butter or margarine	½ small onion 2 tsp (10 mL)	3 0	2 0	½ small onion 2 tsp (10 mL)	3 0	2 0
Garlic sausage (kielbasa)	2 oz (60 g)	2	2	1 oz (30 g)	1	1
Easy Beet Soup	1 cup (250 mL)	10	8	1 cup (250 mL)	10	8
Cherry tomatoes	2, or 2 slices of tomato	1	1	2, or 2 slices of tomato	1	1
Sauerkraut	½ cup (125 mL)	3	1	½ cup (125 mL)	3	1
Peach	1 large	17	14	1 large	17	14
Plain cookie	1	6	6	1	6	6
		104 g	**90 g**		**83 g**	**71 g**

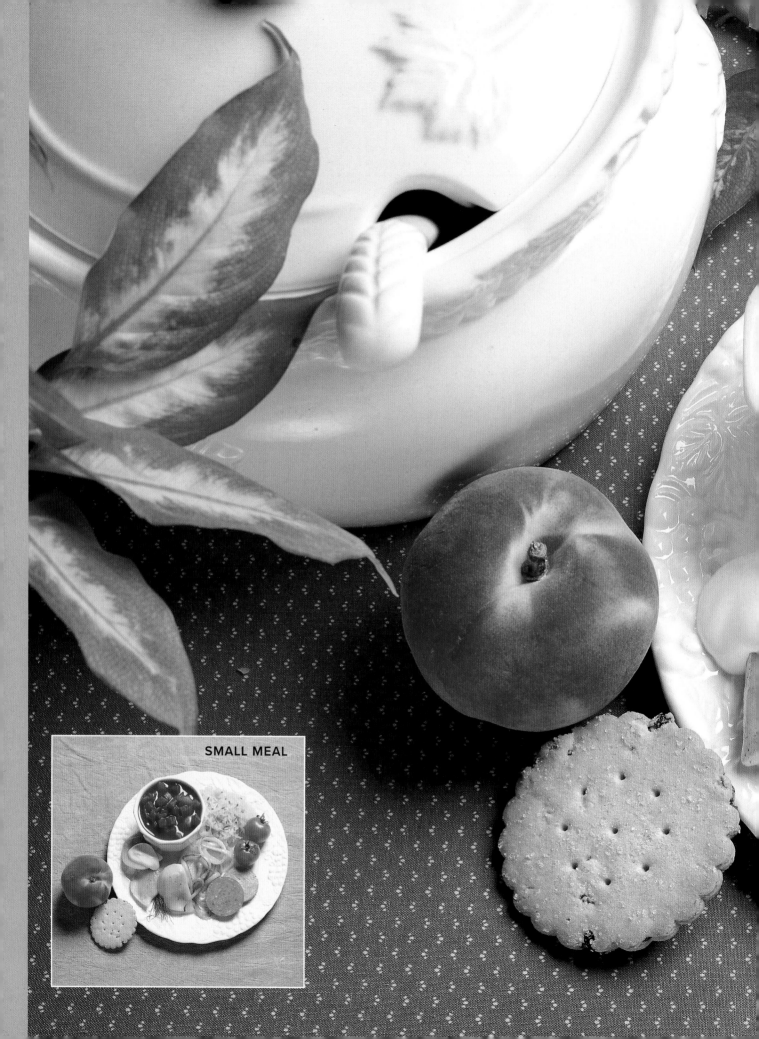

SMALL MEAL

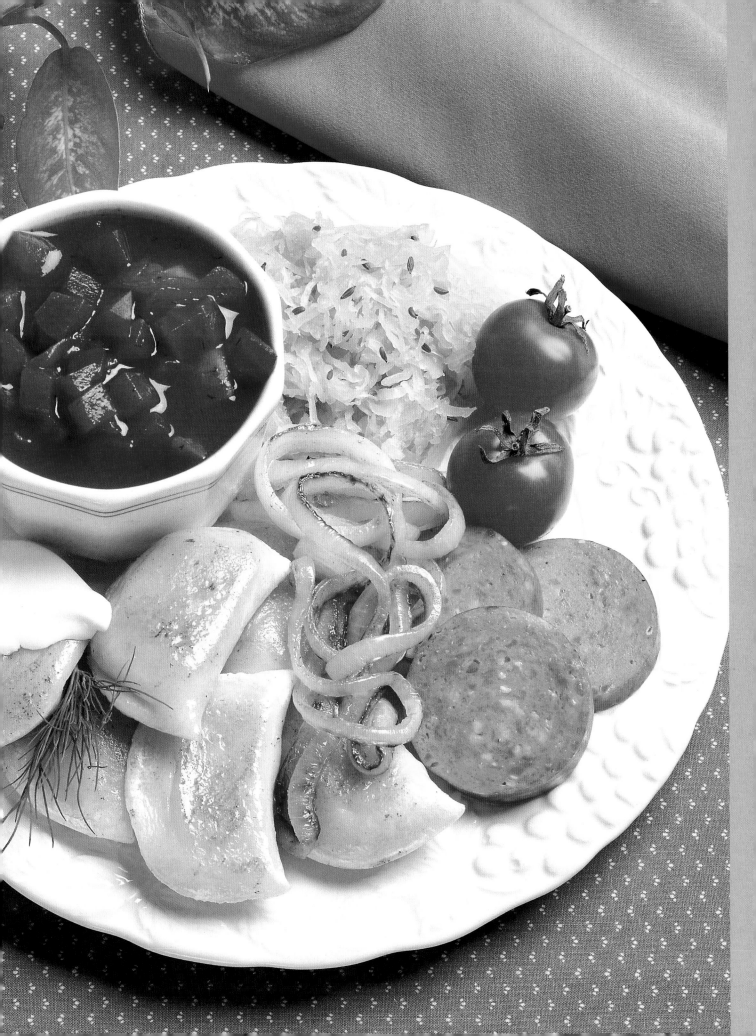

Hamburger with Potato Salad

RECIPE TIP

If you add ½ cup (125 mL) of fresh chopped mushrooms into your raw ground meat, this will keep your hamburgers moist.

CAUTION!

Hamburger safety

Cook hamburgers until well done to make sure they are safe to eat. There must be no pink showing. Refrigerate any leftovers right away.

OPTIONS

If you would like to have hot dogs (wiener in a bun with onion, ketchup and mustard) instead of hamburgers, you can have:

- instead of the cheeseburger for the large meal, two hot dogs with no cheese.

- instead of a hamburger for the small meal, one hot dog with cheese

Use lean or extra-lean ground beef when you make hamburgers. One pound (500 g) of lean ground beef will make three large or four medium cooked beef patties. For extra flavor, you can mix in 2 tsp (10 mL) of Chicken Spice Mix (page 112) or Mrs Dash type of salt-free blend into the raw beef. Options that would lightly salt your hamburger include ¼ to ½ tsp (1 to 2 mL) of Hy's Seasoning Salt or a sprinkle of dried onion soup mix.

There are several ways to cook your hamburgers:
- Grill on a barbecue.
- Place them on a rack and broil in the oven.
- Fry them in a nonstick pan, then place on a paper towel to soak up the extra fat.

Fill your hamburger bun with lots of lettuce, tomato and onion. Add 1 tsp (5 mL) of ketchup, mustard and relish or cheese spread, if you wish. For the large meal, add one slice of cheese.

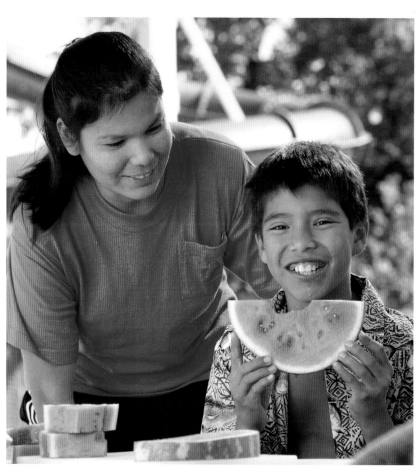

Potato Salad

Makes 4 cups (1 L) of potato salad

4 small cooked potatoes, chopped
$1/2$ green pepper, finely chopped
2 stalks celery, finely chopped
2 to 3 green onions, chopped
    (or 1 small onion, finely chopped)
5 radishes, sliced
2 tbsp (30 mL) vinegar
2 tbsp (30 mL) light mayonnaise
$1/2$ tsp (2 mL) prepared mustard
Salt and black pepper, to taste
1 hard-boiled egg, chopped
Dash of paprika to sprinkle on top

PER $1/2$ CUP (125 ML)	
Calories	85
Carbohydrate	15 g
Fiber	1 g
Net carbs	14 g
Protein	2 g
Fat, total	2 g
Fat, saturated	0 g
Cholesterol	24 mg
Sodium	52 mg

1. In a big bowl, mix together the potatoes, green pepper, celery, green onions and radishes.
2. In a small bowl, mix together the vinegar, mayonnaise, mustard, salt and pepper. Gently fold in the chopped egg. Pour this into the bowl with the potatoes, and mix gently. Sprinkle the top with paprika.

A nice drink for this meal is light iced tea. There are many kinds that you can buy. You could make your own light iced tea by mixing leftover cold tea with lemon juice and a low-calorie sweetener, to suit your taste.

Watermelon or some other fresh fruit makes a great ending to this meal.

CAUTION!

Potato salad safety
Once you've made your potato salad, keep it in your refrigerator. As soon as your meal is over, place it back in your fridge. Never leave it in the sun.

FOOD FACTS

Check the label of light iced tea packages:

- Make sure the tea you buy has fewer than 20 calories in a serving.
- It will probably say "diet," "calorie-reduced" or "light ("lite") on the label.

Food Choices	Large Meal	Small Meal
Carbohydrate	$4^{1}/_{2}$	4
Protein	5	$3^{1}/_{2}$

Your Dinner Menu	Large Meal (730 calories)	Total Carbs	Net Carbs	Small Meal (550 calories)	Total Carbs	Net Carbs
Cheeseburger/hamburger with bun and toppings	Large burger, with cheese	28	27	Medium burger	25	24
Potato Salad	$3/4$ cup (175 mL)	23	21	$1/2$ cup (125 mL)	15	14
Celery sticks	2 stalks	4	2	2 stalks	4	2
Dill pickles	2 small, or 1 medium	1	1	2 small, or 1 medium	1	1
Light iced tea	12 oz (375 mL)	1	1	12 oz (375 mL)	1	1
Watermelon	3 small slices	22	21	3 small slices	22	21
		79 g	**73 g**		**68 g**	**63 g**

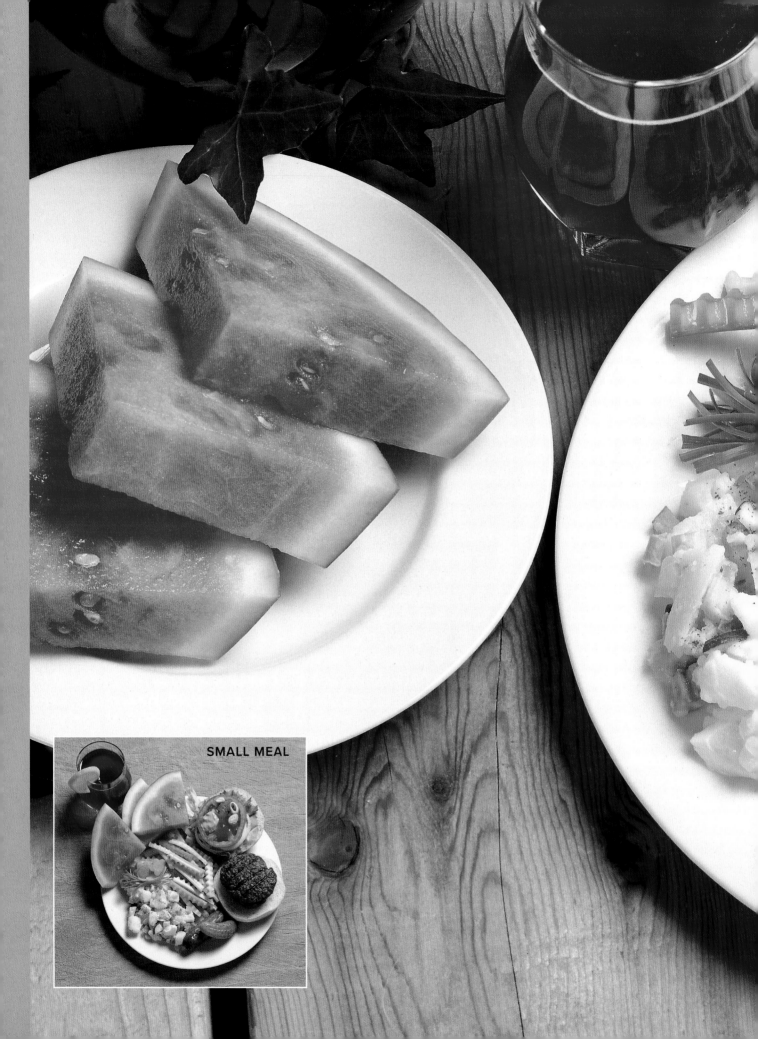

SMALL MEAL

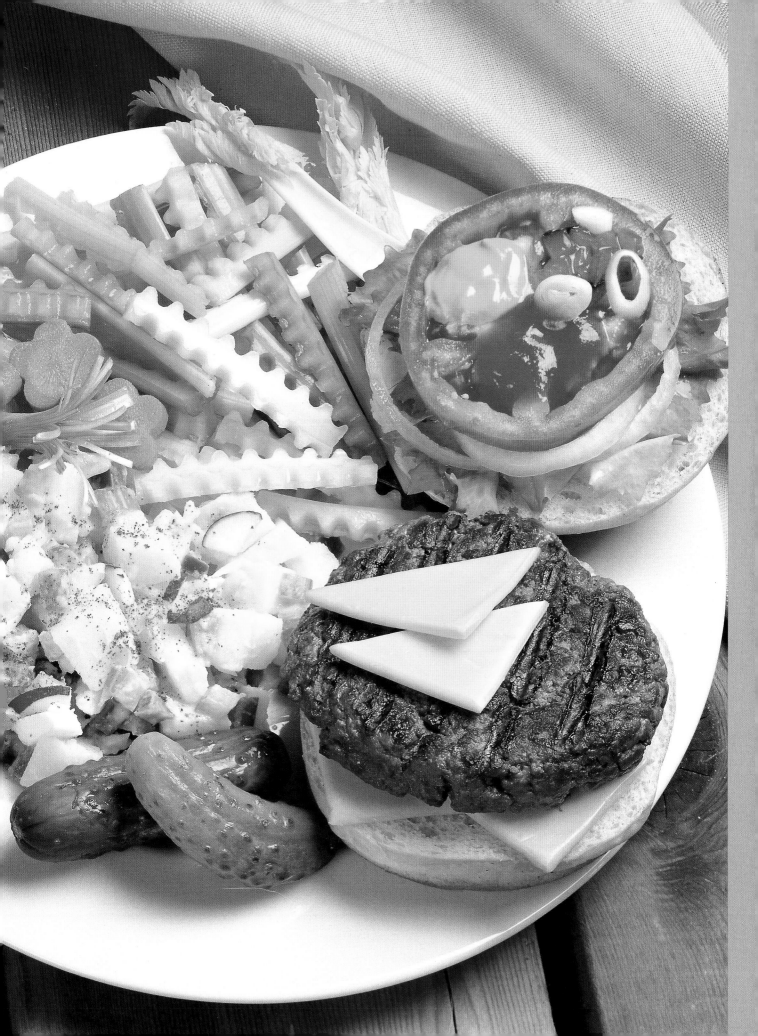

DINNER 17

Roast Turkey Dinner

Roast turkey is a great meal to have at Thanksgiving — or any time of the year! The leftovers come in so handy for sandwiches, soups and other meals.

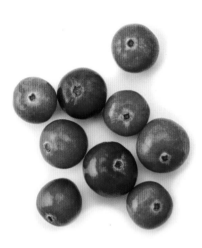

Turkey

- Place your turkey on a rack, breast side up in a covered pan. For the last 15 minutes of cooking, uncover the pan if you wish.
- Cook your turkey for about 15 minutes per pound in a 350°F (180°C) oven. Cook to 170°F (77°C) measured with a thermometer in the inner thigh. Turkey is cooked when the meat moves easily when pierced with a fork.
- Once cooked, remove most of the high-fat skin, and slice the dark and white meat. Dark meat has more fat than white meat.
- Enjoy 1 tbsp (15 mL) of canned cranberry sauce on the side.

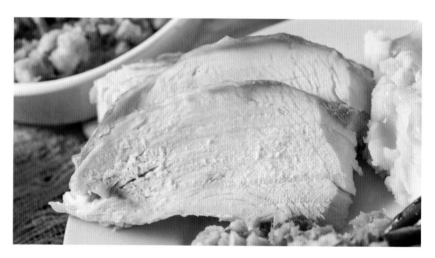

HEALTH TIP

Leave your turkey unstuffed. Bread stuffing is made with a lot of fat and soaks up more fat from the turkey. If you want to make stuffing, cook it in a greased baking dish (covered) or in foil. Eat less potato if you also want stuffing.

Potatoes and Gravy

- Use the recipes for Low-Salt Gravy (page 124) and Low-Fat Mashed Potatoes (page 141).

Vegetables

- A lot of vegetables are served with this meal, including carrots, peas, pickles, Light Jellied Vegetable Salad (see recipe on page 157) and asparagus (fresh or canned).

Beverage

In addition to your glass of water, this meal is served with a wine spritzer. A spritzer has fewer calories and alcohol than regular wine. To make a spritzer, add to a glass 2 oz (60 mL) of dry wine, and fill up the glass with diet ginger ale, diet 7-Up or soda water.

OPTIONS

If you would prefer to not have alcohol:

- Use non-alcohol wine in the spritzer.
- Drink diet soft drink, sparkling mineral water or soda water.

Dessert

This crustless pumpkin pie with whipped topping is delicious. You many not even miss the crust!

This pie is best if made the day before.

Crustless Pumpkin Pie

Makes 6 slices
(9-inch/23 cm glass pie plate)

14-oz (398 mL) can pure pumpkin
$^1/_3$ cup (125 mL) sugar
$^1/_2$ tsp (2 mL) salt
$^1/_2$ tsp (2 mL) ground ginger
1 tsp (5 mL) ground cinnamon
$^1/_4$ tsp (1 mL) ground nutmeg
$^1/_4$ tsp (1 mL) ground cloves
2 eggs, slightly beaten
13-oz (385 mL) can evaporated skim milk

PER SLICE	
Calories	146
Carbohydrate	25 g
Fiber	2 g
Net carbs	23 g
Protein	8 g
Fat, total	2 g
Fat, saturated	1 g
Cholesterol	65 mg
Sodium	298 mg

1. In a large bowl, mix pumpkin, sugar, salt and spices.
2. Stir in the 2 slightly beaten eggs and mix well.
3. Add the evaporated skim milk (shake can before opening) and stir until smooth.
4. Pour into a greased glass pie plate (this recipe works best in a glass pie plate instead of metal). Bake in a 400°F (200°C) oven for about 40 minutes, or until knife inserted near the center of the pie comes out clean.

OPTIONS

You may want to try Greek yogurt as a topping instead of whipped cream.

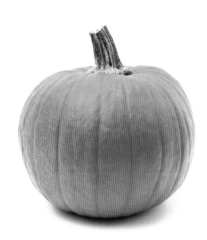

Food Choices	Large Meal	Small Meal
Carbohydrate	4	3
Protein	5	3

Your Dinner Menu	Large Meal (730 calories)	Total Carbs	Net Carbs	Small Meal (550 calories)	Total Carbs	Net Carbs
Turkey	3 oz (90 g) white meat and 2 oz (60 g) of dark meat	0	0	3 oz (90 g) white meat (or 2 oz/60 g white and 1 oz/30 g dark)	0	0
Cranberry sauce	1 tbsp (15 mL)	7	7	1 tbsp (15 mL)	7	7
Low-Fat Mashed Potatoes	1 cup (250 mL)	38	35	$^1/_2$ cup (125 mL)	19	18
Low-Fat Gravy	4 tbsp (60 mL)	4	4	2 tbsp (30 mL)	2	2
Peas and carrots	$^1/_2$ cup (125 mL)	8	6	$^1/_2$ cup (125 mL)	8	6
Asparagus	7 stalks	4	2	7 stalks	4	2
Dill pickle	1 medium	1	1	1 medium	1	1
Jellied Vegetable Salad	$^1/_2$ cup (125 mL)	4	3	$^1/_2$ cup (125 mL)	4	3
Wine spritzer	$^1/_2$ cup (125 mL)	0	0	$^1/_2$ cup (125 mL)	0	0
Crustless Pumpkin Pie	1 slice	25	23	1 slice	25	23
Whipped cream	2 tbsp (30 mL)	1	1	2 tbsp (30 mL)	1	1
		92 g	**82 g**		**71 g**	**63 g**

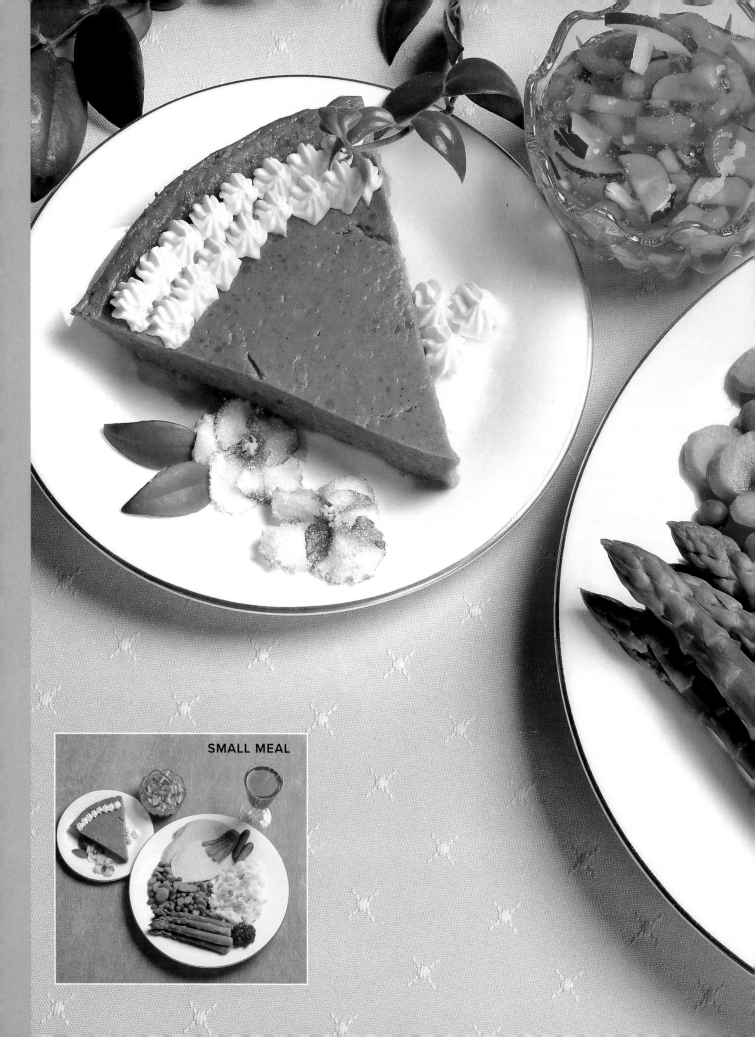

SMALL MEAL

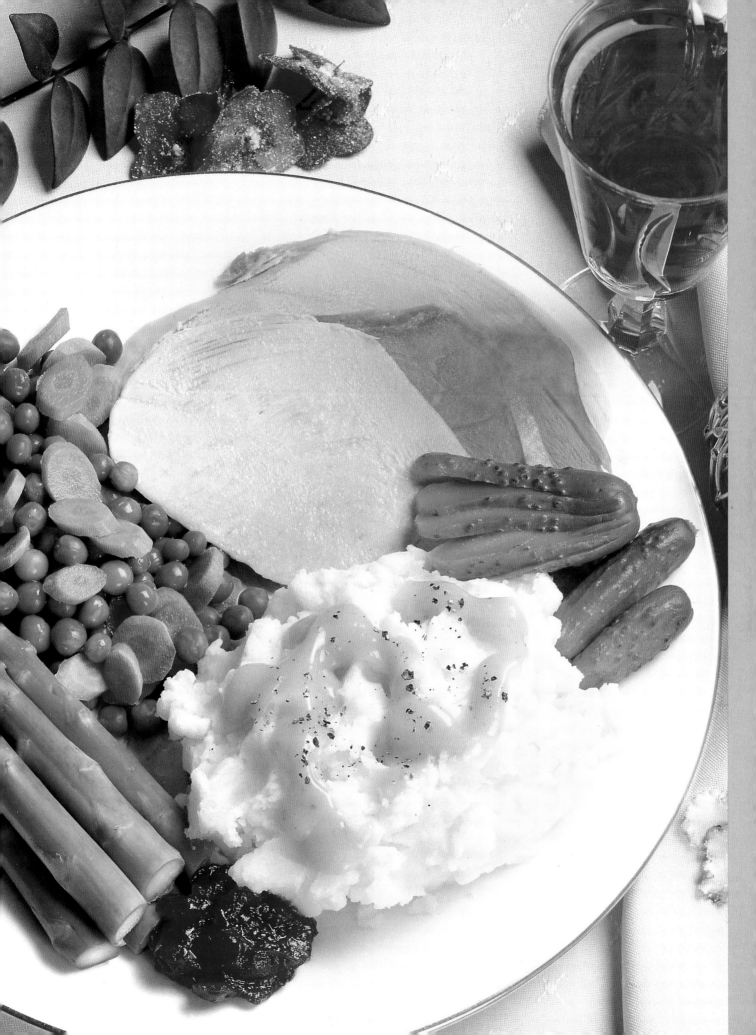

DINNER 18

Baked Macaroni & Cheese

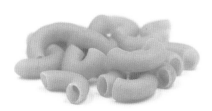

Baked Macaroni and Cheese

Makes about 5½ cups (1.375 L)

1¾ cups (425 mL) dry macaroni

2 tbsp (30 mL) skim milk

2 eggs, beaten with a fork

½ of a 10-oz (284 mL) can tomato soup

1 cup (250 mL) loosely packed, shredded Cheddar cheese (regular)

2 tbsp (30 mL) Seasoned Bread Crumbs (see page 148) (optional)

PER 1 CUP (250 ML)	
Calories	264
Carbohydrate	31 g
Fiber	1 g
Net carbs	30 g
Protein	13 g
Fat, total	10 g
Fat, saturated	5 g
Cholesterol	100 mg
Sodium	365 mg

1. Fill a heavy pot with water and bring to a boil. Add the macaroni and boil for 10 minutes. Drain.
2. Add the milk, then the eggs, to the macaroni and stir quickly on low heat until the eggs are cooked. Add the tomato soup and cheese and stir some more. It should be ready in 2 minutes.
3. It is ready to eat now if you want. If you want it baked (as in the picture), place it in a baking dish and sprinkle Seasoned Bread Crumbs on top. Bake in a 375°F (190°C) oven for 30 minutes.

Vegetables

- Cut broccoli in pieces and steam or lightly boil. For other low-calorie vegetable choices, see page 149.
- Try raw pieces of rutabaga or turnip. For a change, cook turnip with carrots, and mash together once cooked.

RECIPE TIP

Macaroni and cheese is a high-carbohydrate dish, so an option to boost protein is to add 1 cup (250 mL) of chopped leftover meat, chicken or canned drained tuna to the recipe and omit the dessert.

OPTIONS

For extra flavor, add one of these to the Baked Macaroni & Cheese recipe:

- few dashes of hot pepper sauce
- few tablespoons of salsa
- ¼ tsp (1 mL) each of oregano and garlic powder

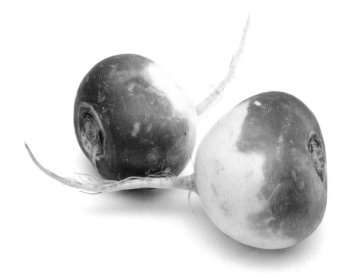

For dessert, try this easy and delicious treat made with bananas, pineapple, pudding and Graham wafers. It looks as good as it tastes.

Pineapple Surprise

Makes 6 servings

1½ cups (375 mL) skim milk

1 package (4-serving size) light vanilla instant pudding mix

1 cup (250 mL) frozen whipped topping (regular or light), thawed

8-oz (227 mL) can crushed pineapple, drained

2 small bananas, sliced thinly

¼ cup (60 mL) Graham cracker crumbs (equal to about 4 Graham crackers)

1. In a medium bowl, pour skim milk and add the pudding mix.
2. Beat with a whisk or an electric mixer until thickened (about 2 minutes).
3. Fold in frozen whipped topping and pineapple until well blended.
4. Add sliced bananas and Graham cracker crumbs to the pudding mixture. Save some bananas and crumbs for the top. If you want, you can layer the pudding mixture, bananas and crumbs.
5. Put in the fridge until ready to serve.

PER SERVING	
Calories	141
Carbohydrate	25 g
Fiber	1 g
Net carbs	24 g
Protein	3 g
Fat, total	4 g
Fat, saturated	3 g
Cholesterol	1 mg
Sodium	283 mg

OPTIONS

If you make Pineapple Surprise with regular pudding instead of light, you will add an extra 2½ tsp (10 g) of sugar to each serving.

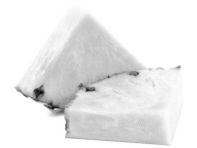

Food Choices	Large Meal	Small Meal
Carbohydrate	5½	4
Protein	2	1

Your Dinner Menu	Large Meal (730 calories)	Total Carbs	Net Carbs	Small Meal (550 calories)	Total Carbs	Net Carbs
Baked Macaroni & Cheese	2 cups (500 mL)	62	60	1¼ cups (300 mL)	39	37
Broccoli	1½ cups (375 mL)	8	5	1½ cups (375 mL)	8	5
Rutabaga or turnip sticks	½ cup (125 mL)	6	4	½ cup (125 mL)	6	4
Bread & butter pickles	4 slices	6	6	4 slices	6	6
Pineapple Surprise	1 serving	25	24	1 serving	25	24
		107 g	**99 g**		**84 g**	**76 g**

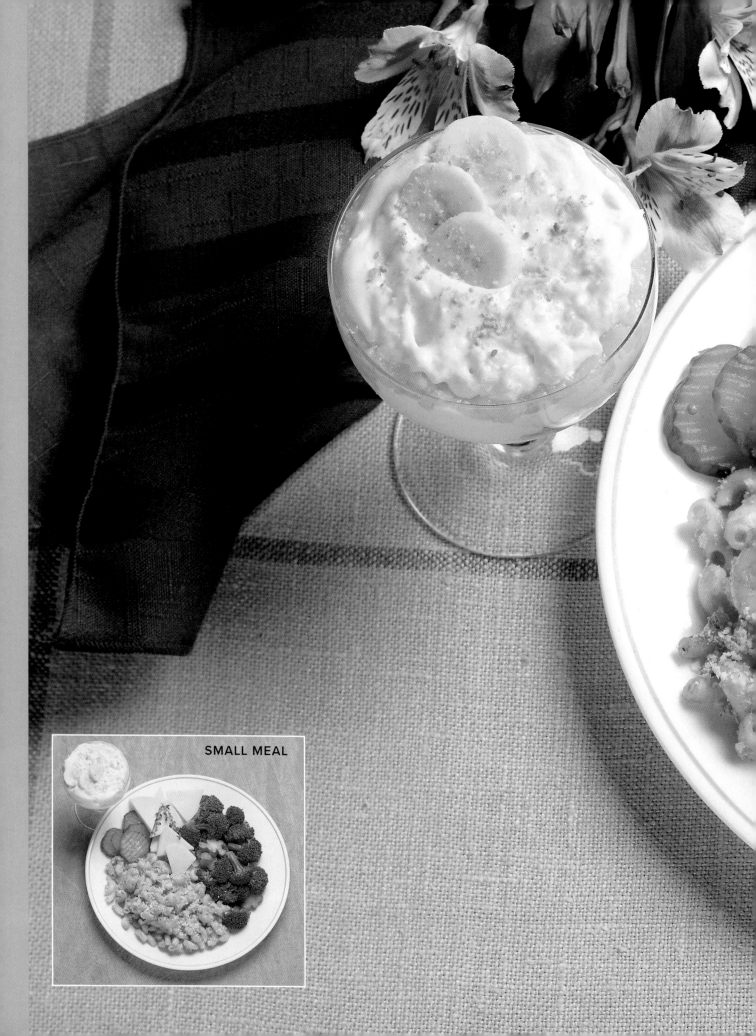

SMALL MEAL

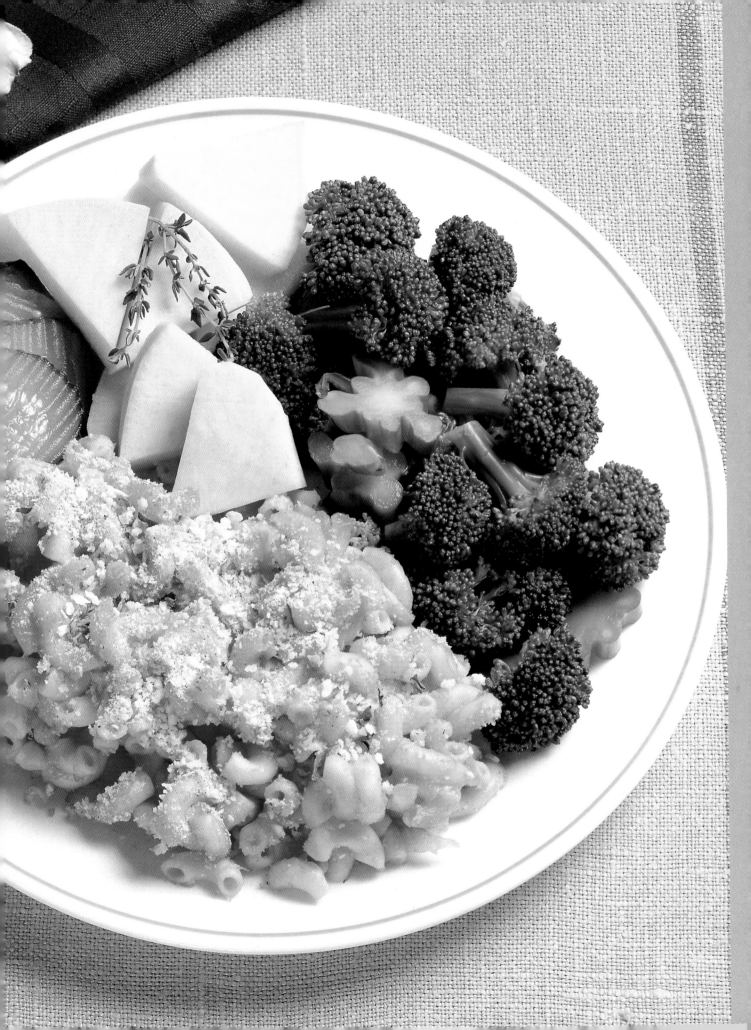

DINNER 19

Pork Chop & Applesauce

RECIPE TIP

You can place a rack over a pan and broil the meat in the oven. The fat will drip into the pan.

HEALTH TIP

Here are some lower-fat cuts of pork:

- loin or tenderloin
- leg, inside round

Pork does not have to be a rich meal. Trim the fat and barbecue or broil small pork chops. Or cook without fat in a nonstick pan. Pork goes nicely with boiled potatoes sprinkled with fresh or dried parsley.

A small dish of applesauce is served with the pork chop. Instead of applesauce, you could slice an apple and an onion and cook them with the pork.

For another nice change, try a lamb chop with mint sauce, instead of pork chop with applesauce.

This meal is served with an easy-to-make German Bean Salad. This salad will keep in the fridge for a week. This German Bean Salad has a tangy bite; it's not sweet at all. Try making it with a flavored vinegar.

German Bean Salad

Makes 4 cups (1 L)

4 cups (1 L) fresh yellow or green beans, cooked, or two 14-oz (398 mL) cans of cut beans (drained and rinsed)

$1/2$ medium onion, thinly sliced

2 tbsp (30 mL) vinegar or flavored vinaigrette

$1/4$ tsp (1 mL) salt (no salt if using canned beans)

PER 1 CUP (250 ML)	
Calories	40
Carbohydrate	9 g
Fiber	3 g
Net carbs	6 g
Protein	2 g
Fat, total	0 g
Fat, saturated	0 g
Cholesterol	0 mg
Sodium	149 mg

1. Cut the beans into 1-inch (2.5 cm) pieces and place in a salad bowl. If you are using canned beans, drain them and place them in the bowl.
2. Mix with the other ingredients.
3. Leave to stand for 30 minutes. Serve.

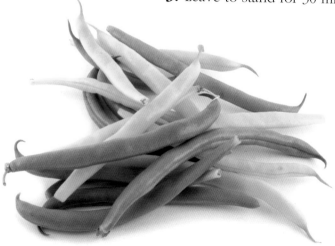

Tapioca pudding is easy to make and healthy.

Tapioca Pudding

Makes 4 servings

1 egg, separated

2 tbsp (30 mL) sugar

2 cups (500 mL) skim milk

3 tbsp (45 mL) quick-cooking tapioca

3 tbsp (45 mL) sugar

Dash of salt

1/2 tsp (2 mL) vanilla

PER SERVING	
Calories	149
Carbohydrate	28 g
Fiber	0 g
Net carbs	28 g
Protein	6 g
Fat, total	1 g
Fat, saturated	1 g
Cholesterol	49 mg
Sodium	79 mg

OPTIONS

Instead of Tapioca Pudding, you may choose a boxed light pudding, or one of the dessert choices from the other meals, or 1 cup (250 mL) of milk with a plain cookie.

1. Place the egg white in a bowl and the egg yolk in a small pot. Beat the egg white with a beater until foamy. Gradually add 2 tbsp (30 mL) of sugar until mixture forms soft peaks.
2. In the pot, beat yolk with a fork. Add milk to the yolk. Stir in tapioca, then add 3 tbsp (45 mL) of sugar and salt.
3. Cook this yolk mixture to a rolling boil, stirring. Take off heat.
4. Pour a small amount of the tapioca mixture over the beaten egg white and blend. Fold the rest of the tapioca mixture into the egg white. Cool on the counter.
5. Stir tapioca after 15 minutes. Add vanilla and chill.
6. Before serving, put 1 tsp (5 mL) of diet jam or a small piece of fruit on top of each serving, if you want.

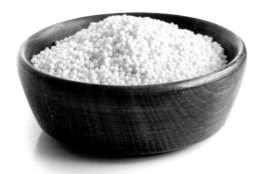

Tapioca "pearls" are made from the flour from the root of a tropical plant called cassava.

Food Choices	Large Meal	Small Meal
Carbohydrate	5½	4½
Protein	5	3

Your Dinner Menu	Large Meal (730 calories)	Total Carbs	Net Carbs	Small Meal (550 calories)	Total Carbs	Net Carbs
Pork chop	1 medium (5 oz/150 g, cooked)	0	0	1 small (3 oz/90 g, cooked)	0	0
Applesauce	¼ cup (60 mL)	7	6	¼ cup (60 mL)	7	6
Boiled potatoes with parsley	8 mini or 1½ medium	50	46	6 mini or 1 medium	38	35
German Bean Salad	1 cup (250 mL)	9	6	1 cup (250 mL)	9	6
Tapioca Pudding	1 serving	28	28	1 serving	28	28
Coffee	1 cup (250 mL)	1	1	1 cup (250 mL)	1	1
		95 g	87 g		83 g	76 g

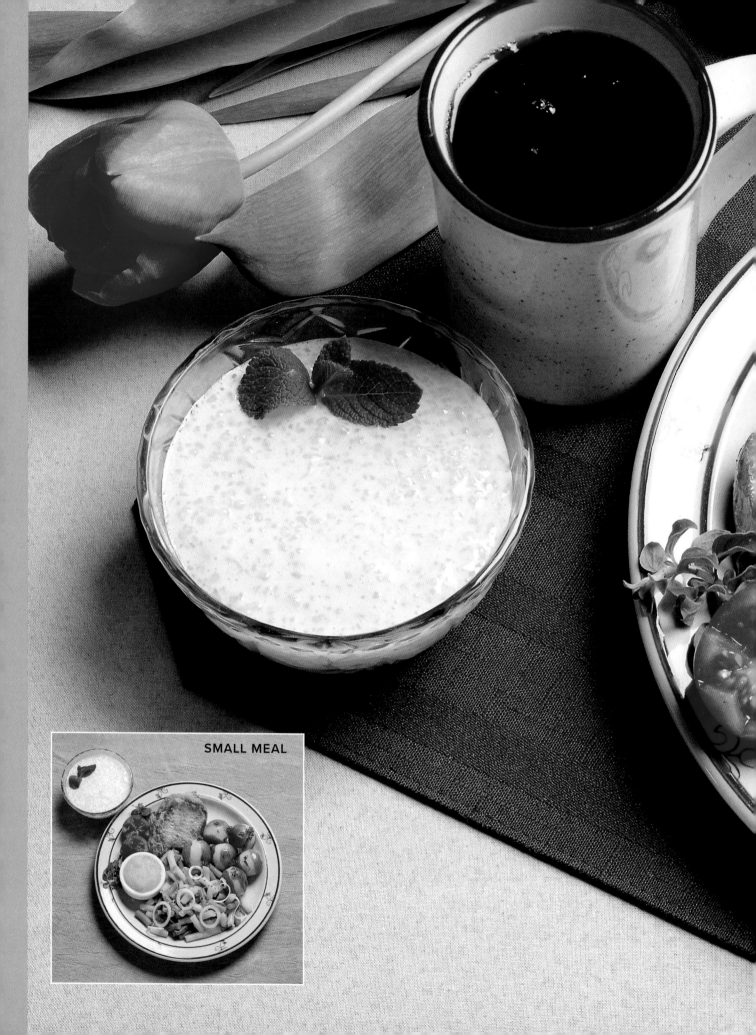

SMALL MEAL

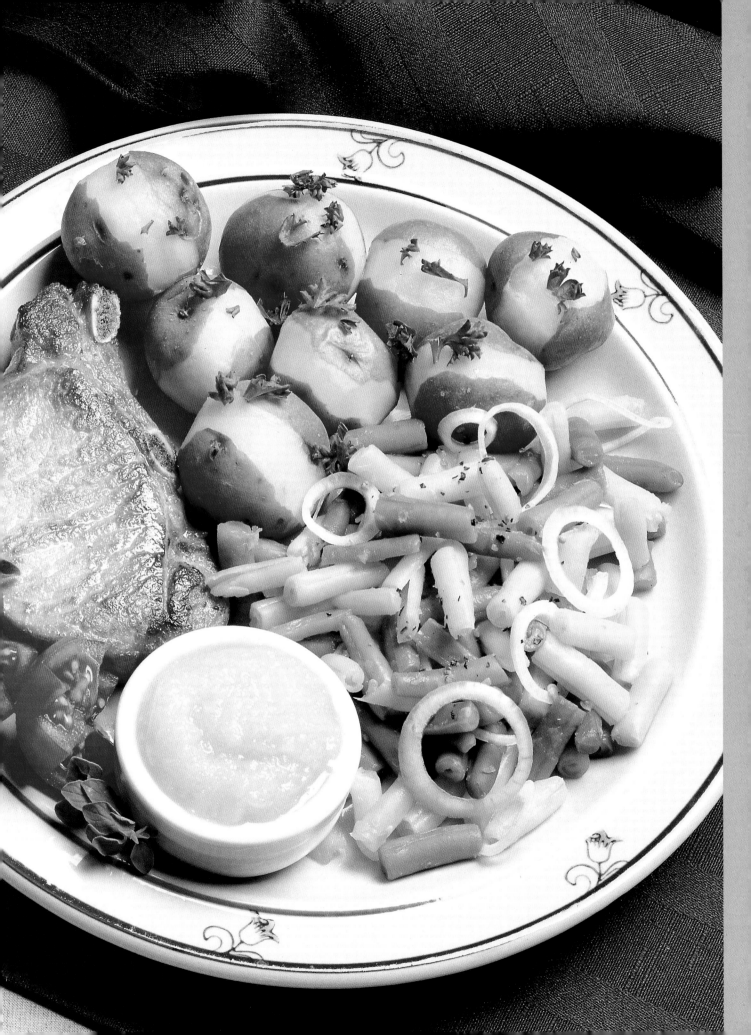

Tacos

You can make tacos using the Bean and Meat Filling below, or using leftover spaghetti sauce, chili con carne or chopped turkey or meat. Tacos are so easy and kids love to help (even if it does get a bit messy making them — and eating them). For a change, you can make burritos by using a soft flour tortilla shell instead of a hard taco shell.

RECIPE TIP

Here are some low-calorie vegetables that taste good in tacos:

- bean sprouts
- chopped tomatoes
- chopped green, red or yellow peppers
- celery
- shredded lettuce
- salsa
- cilantro

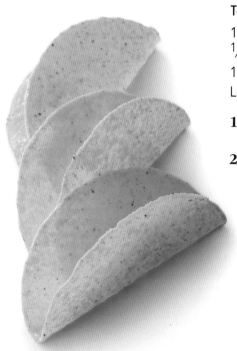

Bean and Meat Filling

Makes 5 cups (1.25 L) (enough for 20 tacos)

1 lb (500 g) lean ground beef
1 cup (250 mL) water
1 tsp (5 mL) each cumin, oregano, paprika and garlic powder
2 tsp (10 mL) chili powder
1/2 tsp (2 mL) black pepper
28 oz (796 mL) can kidney beans or white beans, drained and rinsed

PER 1/4 CUP (60 ML)	
Calories	70
Carbohydrate	6 g
Fiber	2 g
Net carbs	4 g
Protein	6 g
Fat, total	2 g
Fat, saturated	1 g
Cholesterol	12 mg
Sodium	146 mg

1. In a medium pot, brown ground beef. Drain off as much fat as you can.
2. Stir in the water and spice mix. Cook on medium heat for 10 minutes. Add the beans and cook for another 5 minutes. Add extra water if needed to keep moist.

Tacos

To make each taco you will need:

1 taco shell
1/4 cup (60 mL) Bean and Meat Filling
1 1/2 tbsp (22 mL) shredded cheese
Lots of vegetables

PER TACO	
Calories	174
Carbohydrate	16 g
Fiber	3 g
Net carbs	13 g
Protein	10 g
Fat, total	8 g
Fat, saturated	4 g
Cholesterol	23 mg
Sodium	256 mg

1. Heat the taco shells in the oven at 350°F (180°C) for 5 minutes.
2. Into each hot taco shell, put the meat and bean mixture, cheese and vegetables.

Since you eat burritos or tacos with your hands, it's nice to serve other finger foods, too. Try fresh vegetables with this dip.

Vegetable Dip

Makes 1½ cups (375 mL)

1 cup (250 mL) plain skim milk yogurt
½ cup (125 mL) low-fat sour cream
2 tbsp (30 mL) dried onion soup mix
Green onion tops or parsley, chopped

1. Mix the first three ingredients together.
2. Put the green onions or parsley on top.

PER 2 TBSP (30 ML)	
Calories	26
Carbohydrate	4 g
Fiber	0 g
Net carbs	4 g
Protein	1 g
Fat, total	1 g
Fat, saturated	0 g
Cholesterol	3 mg
Sodium	152 mg

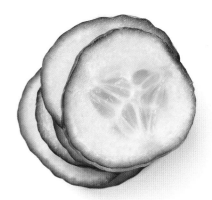

If you are looking for a low-salt vegetable dip, try this alternative recipe, which has similar calories. It has a tangy, sweet taste and is sure to be popular.

Garlic Vegetable Dip

Makes ¼ cup (60 mL)

¼ cup (60 mL) fat-free sour cream
1 tsp (5 mL) fat-free mayonnaise
1 tsp (5 mL) white vinegar
⅛ tsp (0.5 mL) no-salt-added garlic and
    herb seasoning, or garlic powder
½ tsp (2 mL) low-calorie sweetener
    (1 package)

1. Combine all ingredients.

PER 2 TBSP (30 ML)	
Calories	28
Carbohydrate	6 g
Fiber	0 g
Net carbs	6 g
Protein	1 g
Fat, total	0 g
Fat, saturated	0 g
Cholesterol	0 mg
Sodium	66 mg

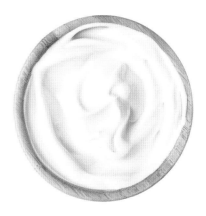

For dessert, make an angel food cake from a mix, or buy one from a bakery. Angel food cake has the lowest amount of fat of any cake. Serve the angel food cake with fruit, such as strawberries (either fresh or unsweetened frozen), and a spoonful of Greek yogurt or non-dairy whipped topping.

Food Choices	Large Meal	Small Meal
Carbohydrate	4	3
Protein	2½	2

Your Dinner Menu	Large Meal (730 calories)	Total Carbs	Net Carbs	Small Meal (550 calories)	Total Carbs	Net Carbs
Bean & Meat Tacos	3	44	35	2	29	23
Fresh vegetables on the side	2 cups (500 mL)	8	6	2 cups (500 mL)	8	6
Garlic Vegetable Dip	2 tbsp (30 mL)	6	6	2 tbsp (30 mL)	6	6
Angel food cake	⅒ of a 10-inch (25 cm) cake	20	19	⅒ of a 10-inch (25 cm) cake	20	19
Strawberries	½ cup (125 mL)	5	3	½ cup (125 mL)	5	3
Greek yogurt (0 to 2%), or non-dairy whipped topping	2 tbsp (30 mL)	0	0	2 tbsp (30 mL)	0	0
		83 g	**69 g**		**68 g**	**57 g**

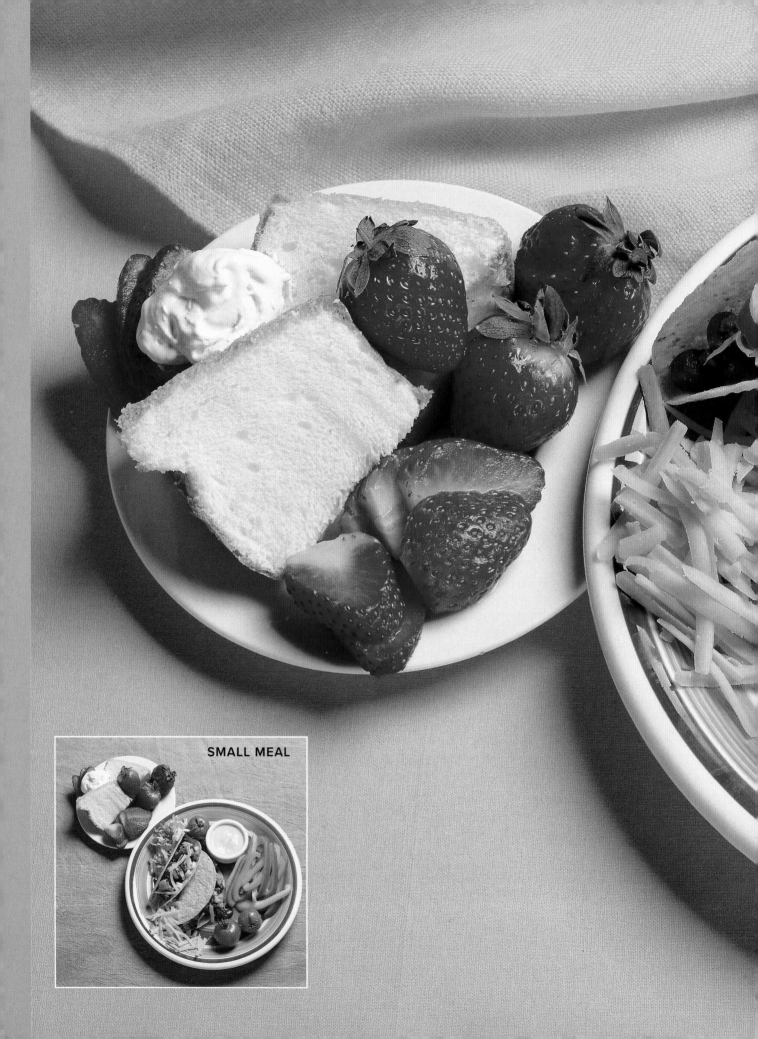

SMALL MEAL

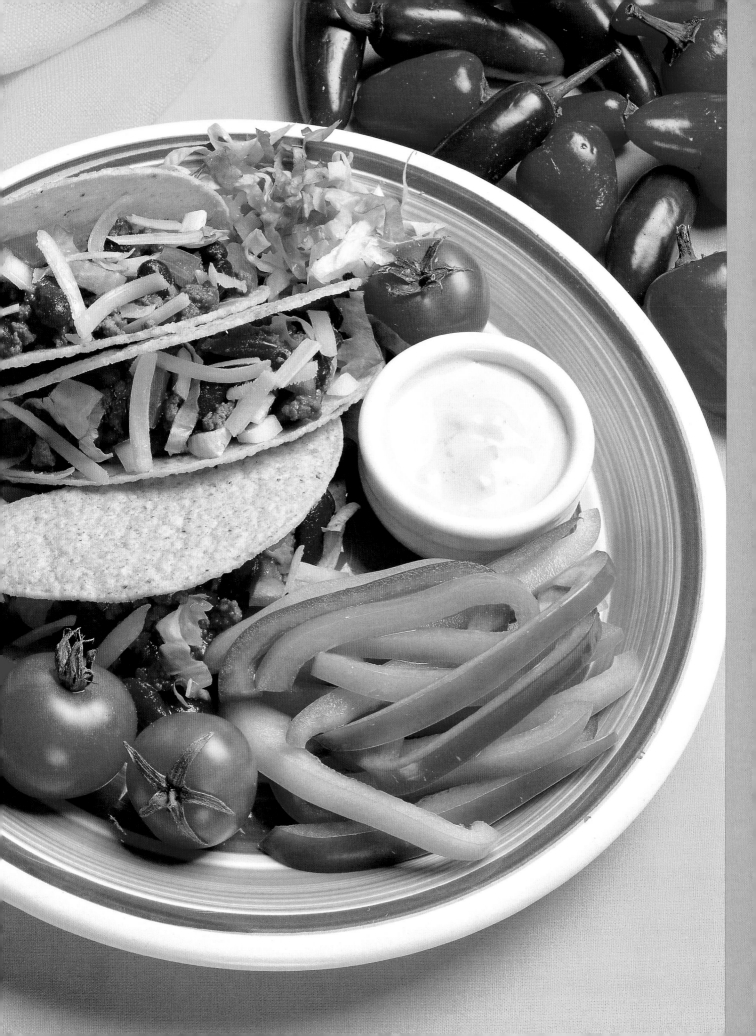

DINNER 21

Caribbean Chicken Roti

Rotis, originally from Trinidad, are a popular Caribbean food. It is a curry stew folded within a special flatbread, like a tortilla, but different! These flatbreads are tender and soft, fragrant and include a middle layer of dried yellow split pea. The curry stew that fills the roti is rich in spices and commonly made with potatoes and a meat such as chicken, goat, beef or shrimp, or vegetarian with chickpeas. Make your curry stew several hours ahead or the day before, so the spices have a chance to infuse, then the curry and roti shell can be reheated later for a fast dinner. The completed filled rotis can also be frozen and reheated for another day.

Caribbean Chicken Roti

Chicken Curry Stew

Makes 6 cups: four 1½-cup large servings *or* six 1-cup small servings

2 tbsp (30 mL) canola oil
1 medium onion, chopped
3 cloves of garlic, minced
    or finely chopped
1 tbsp (15 mL) curry powder
1 tbsp (15 mL) garam masala
1 tsp (5 mL) cumin
½ tsp (2 mL) salt
¼ tsp (1 mL) black pepper
Dash of hot pepper sauce, optional
1 package chicken bouillon, reduced salt
1½ cups (375 mL) water
1 lbs (454 g) boneless skinless chicken thighs or breasts,
    cut in 1-inch (2.5 cm) pieces
2 medium (about 3-inch/7.5 cm round) potatoes, raw,
    peeled and diced
2 cups raw cauliflower, roughly chopped

PER 1 CUP (250 ML)	
Calories	190
Carbohydrate	17
Fiber	3
Net carbs	14
Protein	17
Fat, total	6
Fat, saturated	1
Cholesterol	44
Sodium	340

1. Prepare your ingredients.
2. In a large heavy pot, heat oil over medium heat. Add onion and garlic and sauté for 5 minutes or until softened. Add spices, salt and pepper, and hot sauce. Add 1 to 2 tbsp (15 to 30 mL) water if dry. Continue to stir for another minute.
3. Add bouillon and water, chicken, potatoes and cauliflower and bring to a boil. Let simmer uncovered until the chicken, potato and cauliflower are cooked and the sauce is thickened, about 30 minutes. Stir occasionally. Cool and put in the fridge overnight.

FOOD FACTS

Where to get the roti flatbread?

The flatbread used to make Caribbean rotis may be called Trinidadian dhalpourie or roti shells or wraps. It is different than typical roti in Indian cuisine. They can be bought at Caribbean food stores or restaurants.

If you can't find Caribbean roti flatbread:

You could also use another flatbread sold in your supermarket.

Compare the net carbs to a 13-inch/33 cm (98 g) roti dahlpourie roti shell at 46 g net carb:

- 13-inch/33 cm (105 g) extra-large soft flour tortilla (Mexican) — 50 g
- 10-inch/25 cm (65 g) soft flour tortilla (Mexican) — 32 g
- 8-inch/20 cm (50 g) thin roti or chapatti (Indian) — 18 g

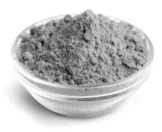

Roti Shells

4 Caribbean roti shells, 13-inch (33 cm) each
   (not included in nutrition calculation)

The next day, reheat the filling and place a serving of Chicken Curry Stew in the middle of each roti shell. Fold one side over the mixture, then the other. Gently fold ends toward the center to make a neat package. Turn it over on the plate so the folds are underneath. Microwave on High for 3 minutes. Let sit for a few minutes so the curry stew inside is not boiling.

Tropical Green Salad

Serves 4

4 to 6 cups (1 to 1.5 L) torn salad greens,
   such as Boston lettuce
¾ cup (175 mL) fresh pineapple chunks
2 tbsp (30 mL) dried unsweetened
   medium coconut, plain or toasted
3 tbsp (45 mL) light coleslaw dressing
Squirt of fresh lime, optional

PER SERVING	
Calories	69
Carbohydrate	8
Fiber	2
Net carbs	6
Protein	1
Fat, total	3
Fat, saturated	2
Cholesterol	4
Sodium	125

1. In a large bowl, combine salad greens, pineapple and/or other fruit and coconut.
2. Toss with the salad dressing, or place on side with lime (optional).
3. Sprinkle with sesame seeds in the amount shown in menu box (not included in nutrition calculation).

OPTIONS

There are many wonderful tropical fruits you can put in your salad, such as thinly sliced papaya or mango, or orange sections.

OPTIONS

Vegetarian Roti

Instead of chicken, roti can be made with chickpeas. This vegetarian version will have 16 grams more net carbs per roti.

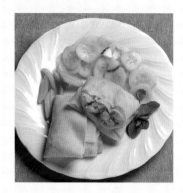

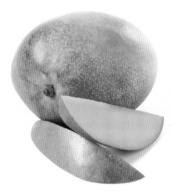

Food Choices	Large Meal	Small Meal
Carbohydrate	4½	4
Protein	3	2
Fat	1	–

Your Dinner Menu	Large Meal (730 calories)	Total Carbs	Net Carbs	Small Meal (550 calories)	Total Carbs	Net Carbs
Chicken Roti						
• Chicken Curry Stew	1½ cups (375 mL)	25	21	1 cup (250 mL)	17	14
• Caribbean roti shell (98 g)	one 13-inch (33 cm)	50	46	one 13-inch (33 cm)	50	46
Tropical Green Salad	1 serving	8	6	1 serving	8	6
Sesame seeds, toasted	1½ tbsp (22 mL)	13	11	1 tsp (5 mL) sprinkle	3	2
		96 g	**84 g**		**78 g**	**68 g**

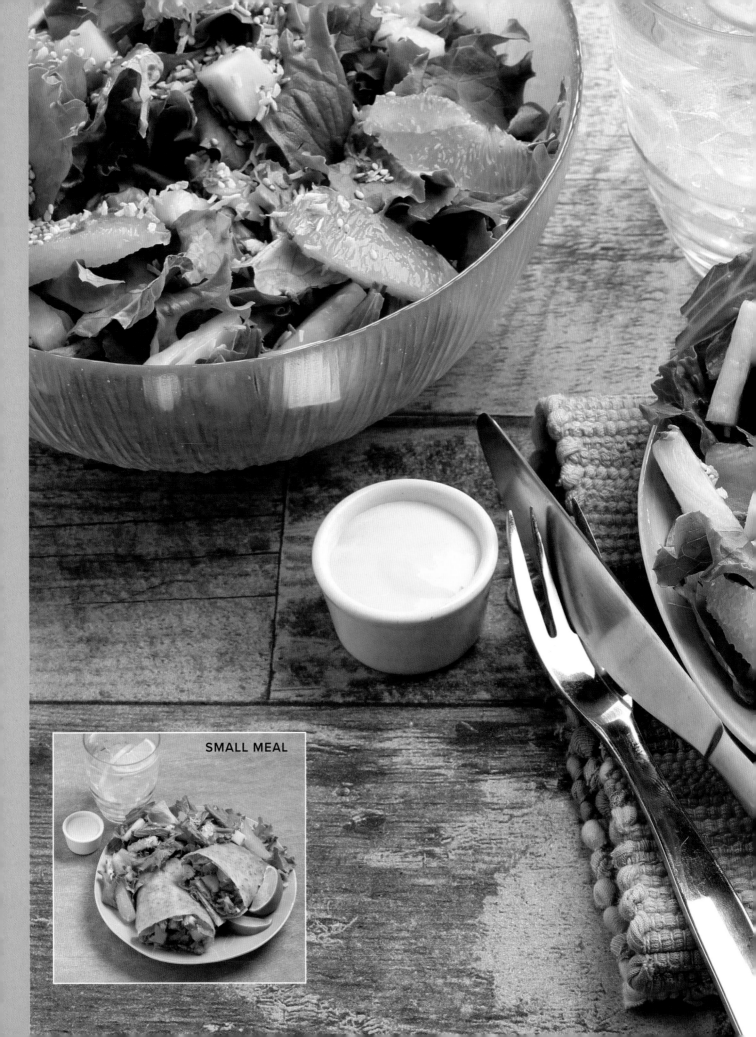

SMALL MEAL

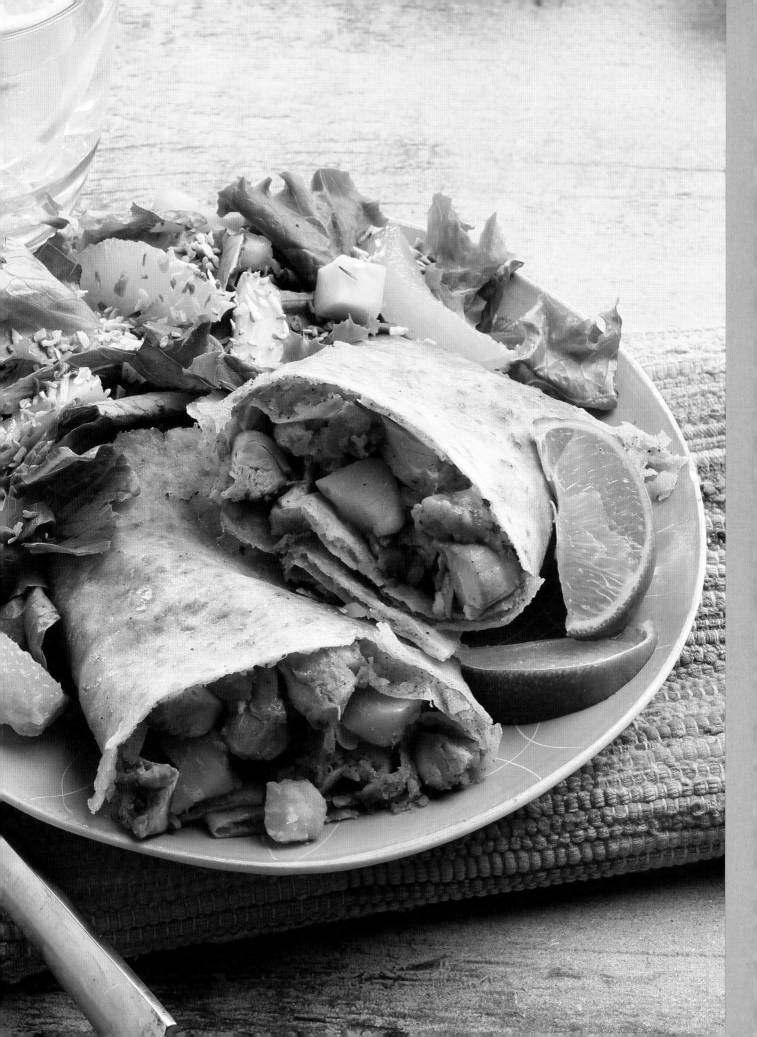

DINNER 22

Liver & Onions

Do you love liver? Then you'll enjoy this meal. Organ meats such as liver, kidney, gizzards and heart are all rich in iron and other nutrients. But they are also high in cholesterol, so eat the large or small serving portion as shown, and choose no more than once a month.

FOOD FACT

Calf liver is the tastiest and most tender, but it costs more than beef liver. Pork liver is a bit stronger-tasting than beef liver.

OPTIONS

Chicken liver is cheap, tender and tasty. Six chicken livers are equal to about one large serving of beef liver.

You can cook an equal portion of beef kidney as a change from beef liver.

RECIPE TIP

Boil chicken gizzards in a bit of chicken broth for at least an hour until they are tender. About 5 oz (140 g) raw chicken gizzards is an equal portion to the large serving of beef liver.

Liver and Onions

Makes 3 large or 4 small servings

3 small to medium onions,
   thinly sliced, lightly pounded
2 tbsp (30 mL) butter
1 lb (500 g) beef liver
1/2 cup (125 mL) beef broth, made
   from 1/2 cup (125 mL) water
   plus 1/2 packet (2 g) reduced-salt
   beef bouillon mix
1/4 cup (60 mL) dry wine or wine vinegar

PER SMALL SERVING	
Calories	222
Carbohydrate	8 g
Fiber	1 g
Net carbs	7 g
Protein	24 g
Fat, total	10 g
Fat, saturated	5 g
Cholesterol	344 mg
Sodium	170 mg

1. In a nonstick or cast-iron pan, over low heat, cook onion slices in the butter until soft. Take onions out of the pan, and set to the side.
2. Place liver in pan and sear it on high heat for a minute or two on each side.
3. Return onions to the pan, along with the broth and wine, and simmer for a minute or two until liver is cooked through but not overcooked. Overcooking makes liver tough.
4. At the table, pour the broth from the pan over your liver and rice, if desired.

Liver is also easy and tasty cooked on the barbecue. On a hot barbecue the liver will cook quickly — be careful it doesn't overcook.

HEALTH TIP

Iron is needed for healthy blood. Organ meats are one of the best sources of iron. Other good sources of iron include beef, pork and chicken, eggs, oysters, kidney beans, whole wheat bread, cereals, spinach and dark greens, and dried fruit such as raisins.

For your starch, have rice, as shown, or potatoes. Two-thirds of a cup (150 mL) of rice equals 1 cup (250 mL) of potatoes.

The vegetables for this meal are carrots and tomatoes. Choose either canned tomatoes or fresh sliced tomatoes.

For dessert, there is fruit salad served with two small vanilla wafers (or one plain cookie, such as an arrowroot biscuit). To make your fruit salad, mix together any of your favorite fresh or frozen fruits.

FOOD CHARTS
See page 309: Cookies.

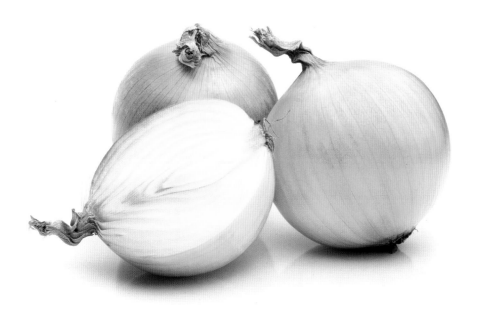

Food Choices	Large Meal	Small Meal
Carbohydrate	5	3½
Protein	4	3
Fat	3	2

Your Dinner Menu	Large Meal (730 calories)	Total Carbs	Net Carbs	Small Meal (550 calories)	Total Carbs	Net Carbs
Liver and Onions	1 large serving	10	8	1 small serving	8	7
Rice, long-grain, parboiled	1¼ cups (300 mL)	55	54	⅔ cup (150 mL)	29	28
Carrots	½ cup (125 mL)	8	6	½ cup (125 mL)	8	6
Canned tomatoes	1 cup (250 mL)	10	8	1 cup (250 mL)	10	8
Fresh fruit salad	¾ cup (175 mL)	19	17	¾ cup (175 mL)	19	17
Vanilla wafers	2 small	6	6	2 small	6	6
		108 g	**99 g**		**80 g**	**72 g**

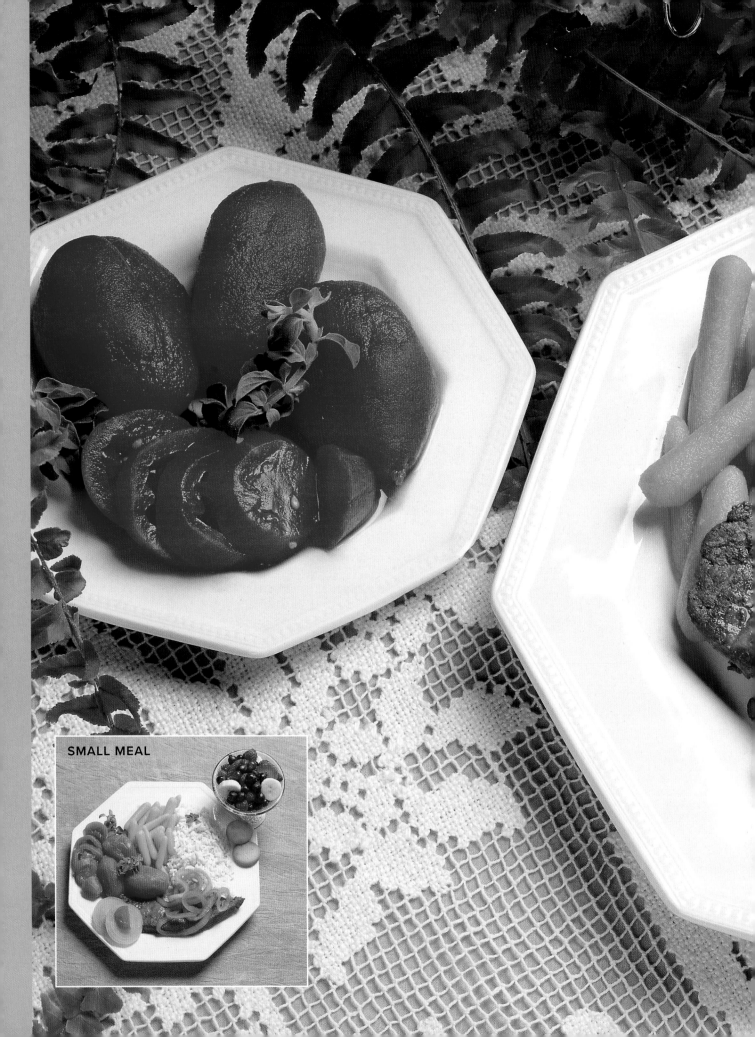

SMALL MEAL

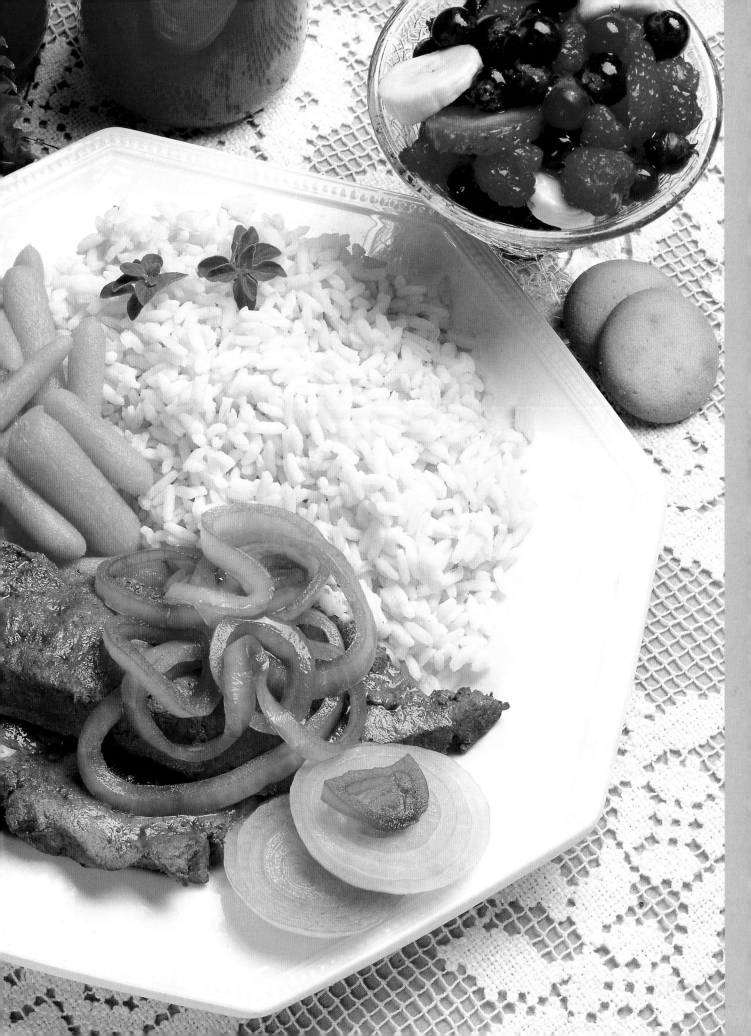

DINNER 23

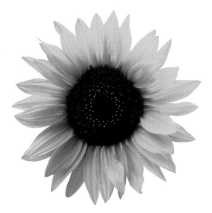

Sun Burger

These meatless burgers are delicious when served on a bagel or hamburger bun. Add to your bagel lots of vegetables, such as lettuce, tomatoes, onions and cucumbers.

Sun Burgers

Makes 12 burgers

1½ cups (375 mL) cooked rice
    (brown or white), or cooked quinoa
19-oz (540 mL) can romano beans,
    drained (or other beans, such as
    pinto or kidney)
⅓ cup (75 mL) sesame seeds
⅓ cup (75 mL) sunflower seeds
2 tbsp (30 mL) wheat germ or ground flaxseed
¼ tsp (1 mL) dried basil
¼ tsp (1 mL) black pepper
½ tsp (2 mL) garlic powder
1 tsp (5 mL) dried parsley
1 tsp (5 mL) of dried dillweed
1 to 2 eggs
1 cup (250 mL) loosely packed mozzarella cheese

PER BURGER PATTY	
Calories	143
Carbohydrate	15 g
Fiber	4 g
Net carbs	11 g
Protein	8 g
Fat, total	6 g
Fat, saturated	2 g
Cholesterol	22 mg
Sodium	113 mg

1. Cook rice or use cold rice from the night before.
2. In a large bowl, put drained beans and mash them with a fork or a masher.
3. Add all the other ingredients. Mix with a large spoon or fork, or use your hands.
4. Form mixture into patties. Cook until nicely browned in a nonstick frying pan or heavy frying pan (lightly greased).

Add a shake of dried dill to the mayonnaise you spread on your burger.

OPTIONS

Bagels come in many sizes, and some are very large. A 3-inch (7.5 cm) bagel (used in this meal) is equivalent to two slices of bread. A 4-inch (10 cm) bagel is equivalent to four slices.

For a lower-carb option, you could choose a small whole-grain bun instead of a bagel.

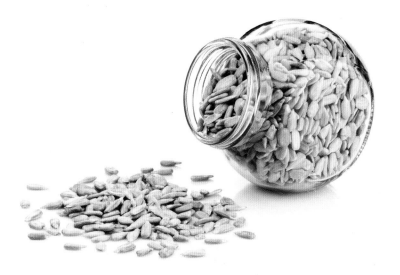

Kale and Orange Salad

Makes 1 serving

$^3/_4$ cup (175 mL) stemmed kale leaves,
    chopped into pieces

$^1/_3$ cup (75 mL) sliced bok choy

$^1/_3$ cup (75 mL) chopped broccoli

$^1/_2$ orange, broken into segments

3 strawberries, sliced

Sprinkle of sesame seeds, ground
    flaxseed or walnuts (optional)

PER SERVING	
Calories	64
Carbohydrate	14 g
Fiber	4 g
Net carbs	10 g
Protein	3 g
Fat, total	1 g
Fat, saturated	0 g
Cholesterol	0 mg
Sodium	47 mg

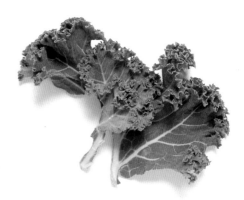

1. Combine all ingredients.

2. Add your favorite light salad dressing.

Dream Delight

Makes four 1-cup (250 mL) servings

1 package (4-serving size) unflavored
    gelatin

1 package (4-serving size) light gelatin,
    raspberry or any other flavor

1$^1/_4$ cups (300 mL) boiling water

1$^1/_4$ cups (300 mL) cold water

1 package dessert topping mix
    (enough to make 2 cups/500 mL)

PER CUP (250 ML)	
Calories	73
Carbohydrate	8 g
Fiber	0 g
Net carbs	8 g
Protein	2 g
Fat, total	4 g
Fat, saturated	4 g
Cholesterol	0 mg
Sodium	43 mg

OPTIONS

You may want to make
this dessert with regular
gelatin instead of light.
By doing so, you will
add an extra 4 tsp (20 mL)
of sugar to each serving.

1. Place the unflavored gelatin and the light gelatin in a bowl.

2. Stir in boiling water until the gelatin is mixed in. Then stir in
    cold water. Refrigerate.

3. Remove the gelatin from the fridge after about 45 minutes.
    It should be as thick as an unbeaten egg white. Do not
    allow it to get too firm.

4. Mix the topping mix as directed on the box.

5. Blend topping with a beater into gelatin mixture until
    well mixed.

6. Pour into four dessert bowls. Refrigerate to set.

This dessert is easy to make and has a nice light flavor.

Food Choices	Large Meal	Small Meal
Carbohydrate	4	3
Protein	2	1
Fat	2	2

Your Dinner Menu	Large Meal (730 calories)	Total Carbs	Net Carbs	Small Meal (550 calories)	Total Carbs	Net Carbs
Sun Burgers	2	31	22	1	15	11
Bagel	1 (3-inch/7.5 cm)	31	30	1 (3-inch/7.5 cm)	31	30
Light mayonnaise	1 tbsp (15 mL)	1	1	1 tbsp (15 mL)	1	1
Kale and Orange Salad	1 serving	14	10	1 serving	14	10
Citrus Vinaigrette (page 137)	2 tbsp (30 mL)	5	5	2 tbsp (30 mL)	5	5
Dream Delight	1 cup (250 mL)	8	8	1 cup (250 mL)	8	8
		90 g	**76 g**		**74 g**	**65 g**

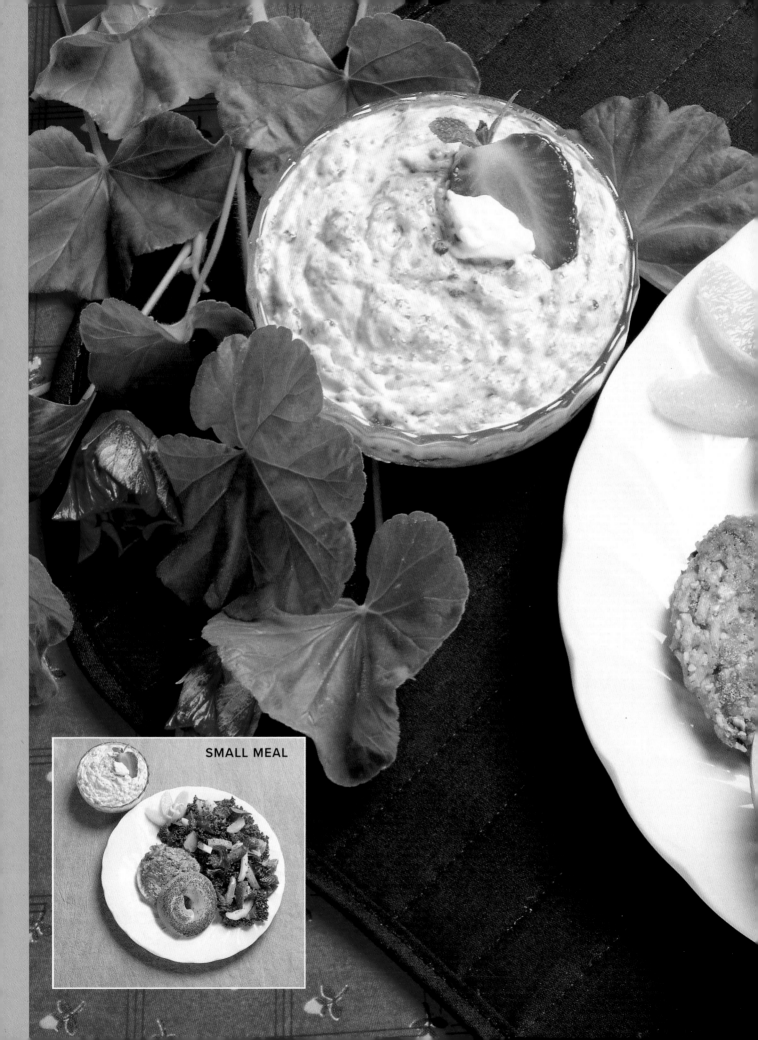

SMALL MEAL

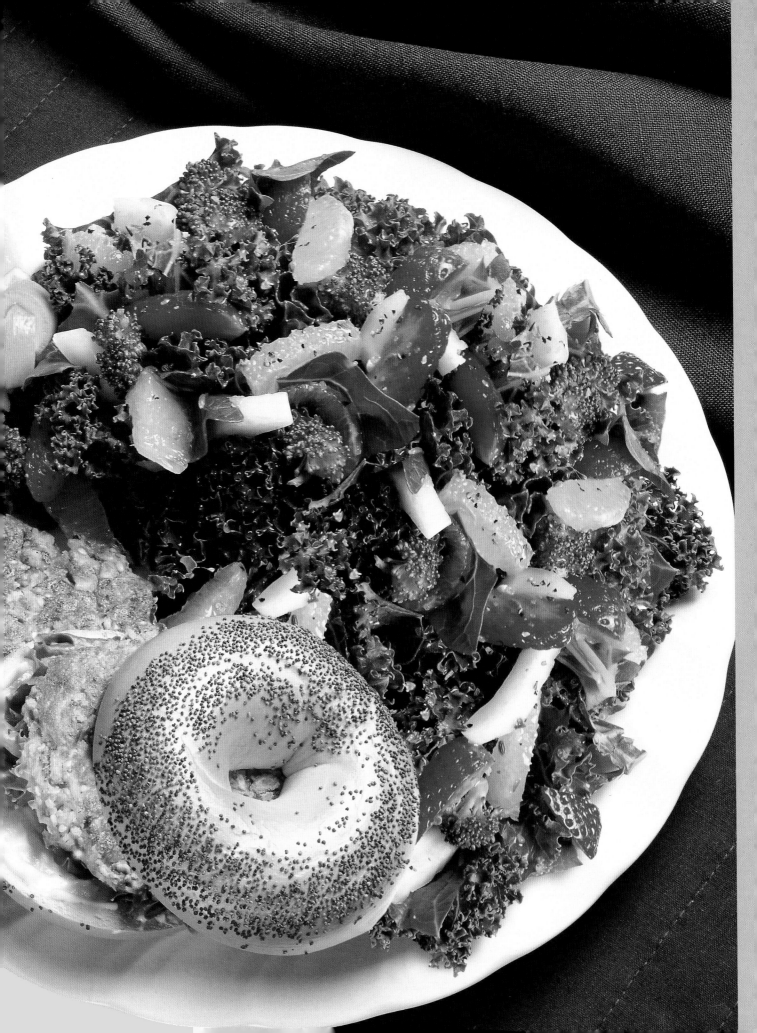

Salmon & Potato Dish

This meal can be made with canned salmon or tuna, or any kind of leftover fish. This three-ingredient dish is the perfect combination of flavors.

OPTIONS

No-salt-added canned salmon contains about 85% less sodium than the regular variety. If it's available, you can use it in this Salmon & Potato Dish to reduce the sodium per serving to about 400 mg.

Salmon and Potato Dish

**Makes one small baking dish
(2 large or 3 small servings)**

1 can (7½ oz/213 g) pink or
    red salmon, drained
Pinch of black pepper
1 cup (250 mL) loosely packed,
    shredded Cheddar cheese
2 cups (500 mL) mashed potato
    (leftover or fresh)

PER LARGE SERVING	
Calories	519
Carbohydrate	39 g
Fiber	3 g
Net carbs	36 g
Protein	39 g
Fat, total	23 g
Fat, saturated	13 g
Cholesterol	133 mg
Sodium	731 mg

1. Mash the salmon with the bones. Put the salmon on the bottom of a small baking dish. Sprinkle with pepper and half the shredded cheese.
2. Spread the mashed potato on top of the salmon and cheese.
3. Sprinkle the rest of the cheese on top.
4. Bake in a 350°F (180°C) oven for 30 minutes, or microwave for 8 minutes.

For a change, this dish can also be made into patties. Add your favorite herbs and fry in a nonstick pan with a small amount of oil or other fat.

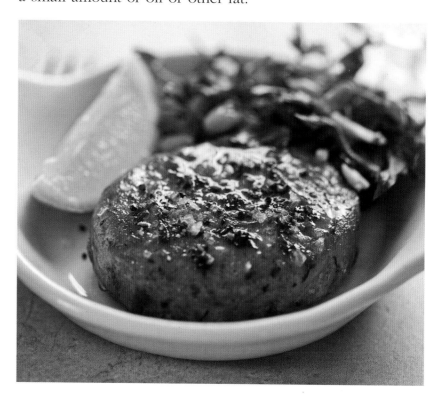

Corn is the sweet vegetable with this meal, and spinach and tomato juice are the low-calorie vegetables.

You can buy spinach fresh or frozen.

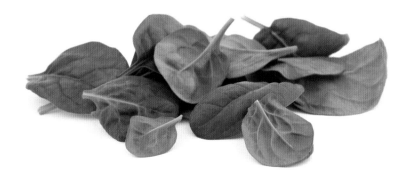

HEALTH TIP

Spinach is rich in iron and folic acid.

The dessert is light gelatin with fruit.

Light Gelatin with Fruit

Makes three 1-cup (250 mL) servings

1 package (4-serving size) light gelatin
1 cup (250 mL) boiling water
1/4 cup (60 mL) cold water
14-oz (398 mL) can fruit cocktail, with juice

1. Put the gelatin in a medium bowl (not plastic).
2. Add the boiling water. Stir until gelatin is all mixed in.
3. Add the cold water and fruit cocktail and stir.
4. Pour into three dessert bowls. Refrigerate to set.

PER 1 CUP (250 ML)	
Calories	68
Carbohydrate	18 g
Fiber	1 g
Net carbs	17 g
Protein	1 g
Fat, total	0 g
Fat, saturated	0 g
Cholesterol	0 mg
Sodium	37 mg

OPTIONS

Instead of fruit cocktail, you can use a can of other fruit, such as peaches. Chop the fruit into pieces.

Food Choices	Large Meal	Small Meal
Carbohydrate	5	3½
Protein	4½	3

Your Dinner Menu	Large Meal (730 calories)	Total Carbs	Net Carbs	Small Meal (550 calories)	Total Carbs	Net Carbs
Salmon & Potato Dish	½ the recipe	39	36	⅓ the recipe	26	24
Corn	¾ cup (175 mL)	24	22	½ cup (125 mL)	16	14
Spinach	½ cup (125 mL)	3	1	½ cup (125 mL)	3	1
Tomato juice	½ cup (125 mL)	5	4	½ cup (125 mL)	5	4
Celery	¼ stalk (in tomato juice)	1	1	1¼ stalks	3	2
Light Gelatin with Fruit	1 cup (250 mL)	18	17	1 cup (250 mL)	18	17
		90 g	**81 g**		**71 g**	**62 g**

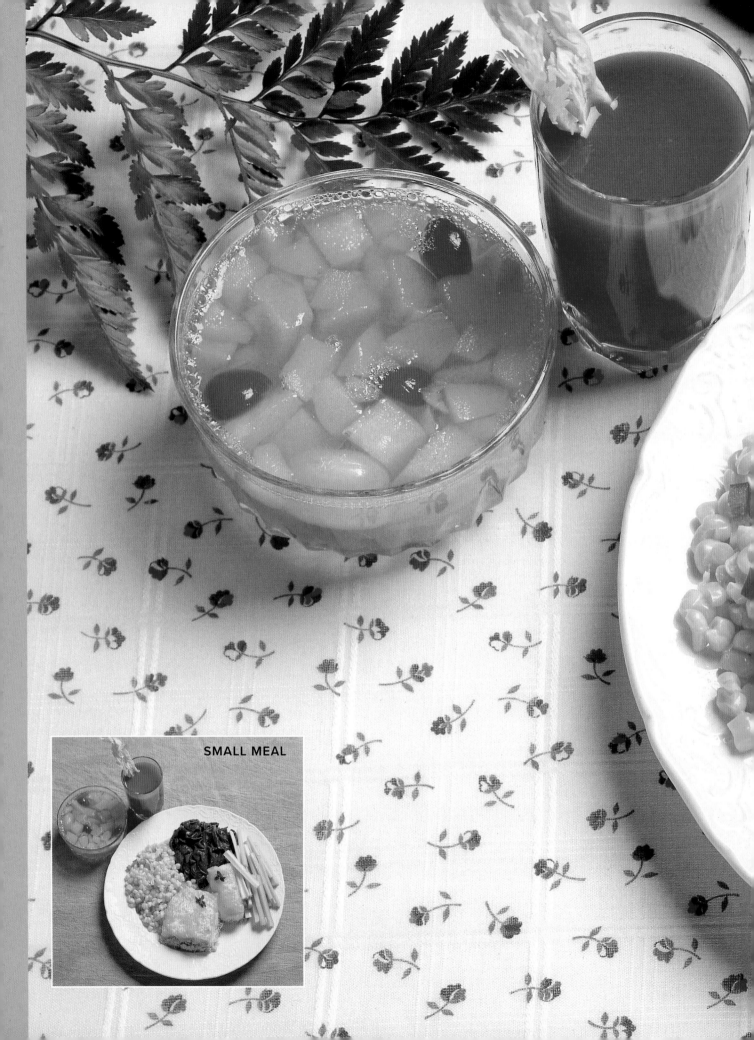

SMALL MEAL

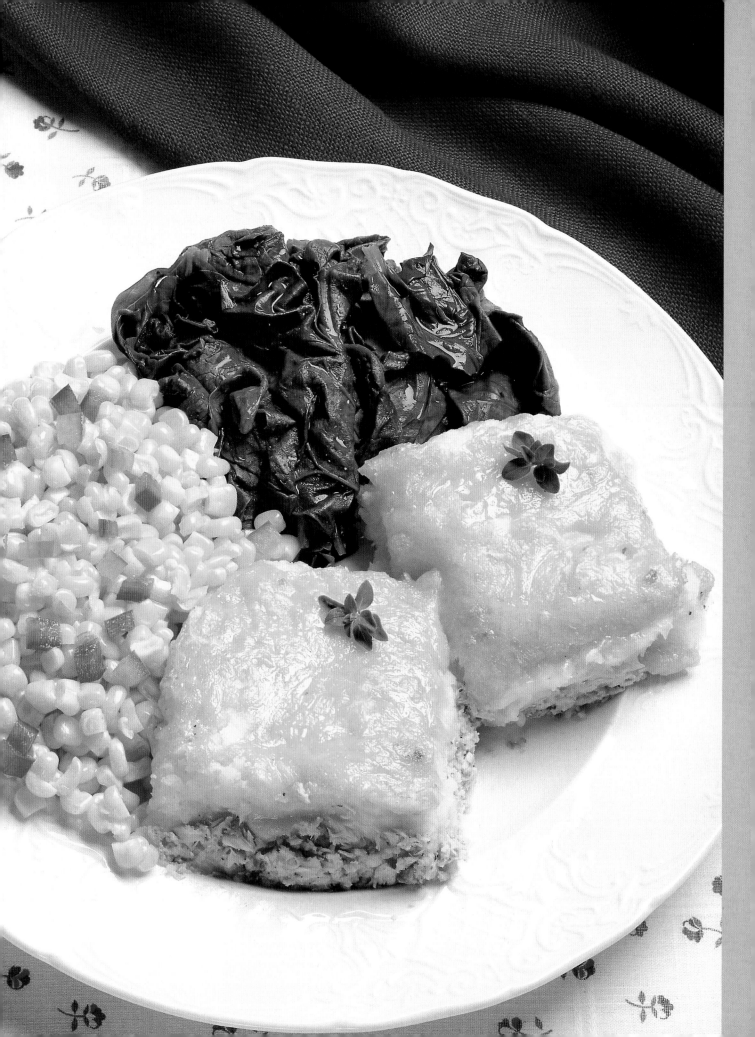

DINNER 25

Hamburger Noodle Dish

Most packages of noodles and sauce mix (hamburger "helper") added to ground beef are high in fat. This recipe is lower in fat.

Hamburger Noodle Dish

Makes 7⅓ cups (1.825 L)
(about 4 large or 6 small servings)

1 lb (500 g) lean ground beef

1 large onion, chopped

¼ tsp (1 mL) black pepper

10-oz (284 mL) can tomato soup

10-oz (284 mL) can mushroom pieces (drained)

1 cup (250 mL) skim milk

1 tsp (5 mL) Worcestershire sauce

4 cups (1 L) dry corkscrew noodles (or 2½ cups/625 mL dry macaroni)

PER 1 CUP (250 ML)	
Calories	293
Carbohydrate	38 g
Fiber	3 g
Net carbs	35 g
Protein	18 g
Fat, total	7 g
Fat, saturated	3 g
Cholesterol	33 mg
Sodium	382 mg

1. In a large, heavy pan, brown ground beef. Drain off the fat.
2. Add chopped onion to the beef and cook until the onions are soft. Add water if too dry. Add all other ingredients except the noodles. Cook for 15 minutes.
3. While the beef and onions are cooking, add noodles to a pot of boiling water and cook as directed on package. Drain the cooked noodles.
4. Add cooked noodles to the hamburger mixture. Cook for 5 more minutes.

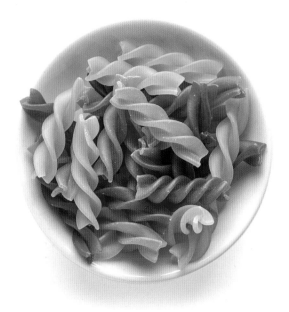

This meal is served with mixed vegetables and steamed cabbage. You could dab 1 tbsp (15 mL) of light cheese spread on your cabbage, instead of the butter or margarine.

Enjoy a serving of fresh fruit for dessert.

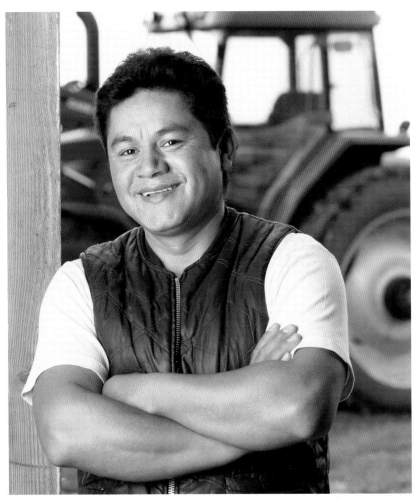

"Healthy meals and snacks give me the energy
I need to do my work."

Food Choices	Large Meal	Small Meal
Carbohydrate	5	4
Protein	2½	1½
Fat	1	½

Your Dinner Menu	Large Meal (730 calories)	Total Carbs	Net Carbs	Small Meal (550 calories)	Total Carbs	Net Carbs
Hamburger Noodle Dish	1½ cups (375 mL)	57	53	1 cup (250 mL)	38	35
Mixed vegetables	¾ cup (175 mL)	18	14	½ cup (125 mL)	12	9
Cabbage	1 cup (250 mL)	8	4	1 cup (250 mL)	8	4
Margarine or butter	1 tsp (5 mL)	0	0	½ tsp (2 mL)	0	0
Grapes	1 cup (250 mL)	27	25	1 cup (250 mL)	27	25
		110 g	96 g		85 g	73 g

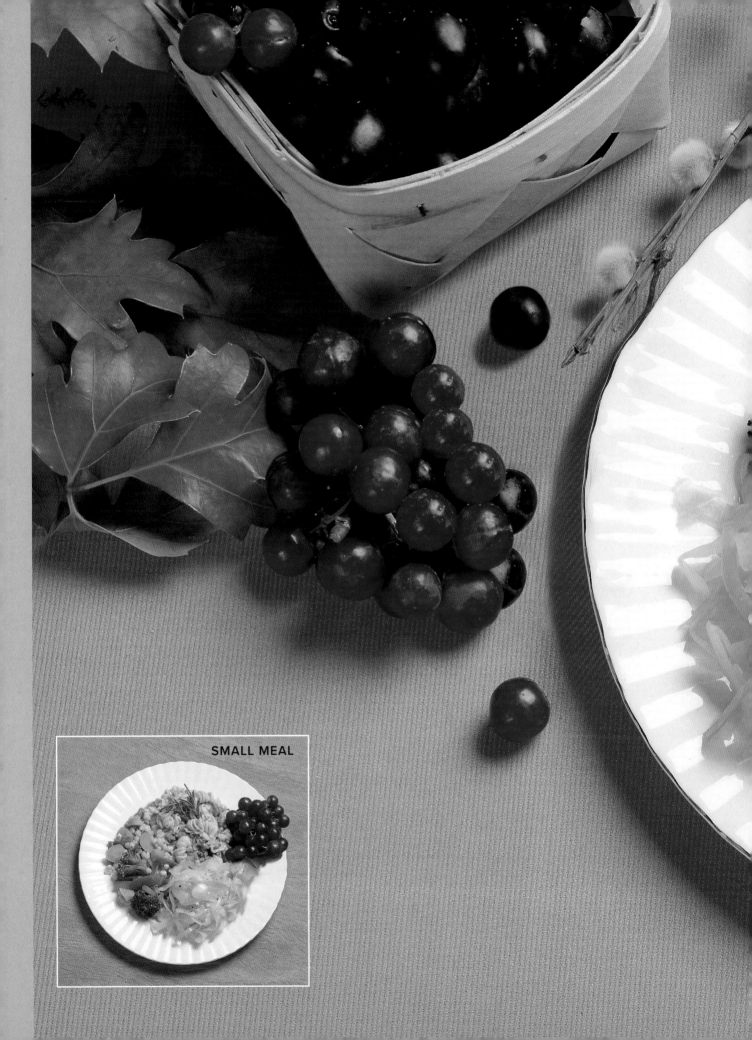

SMALL MEAL

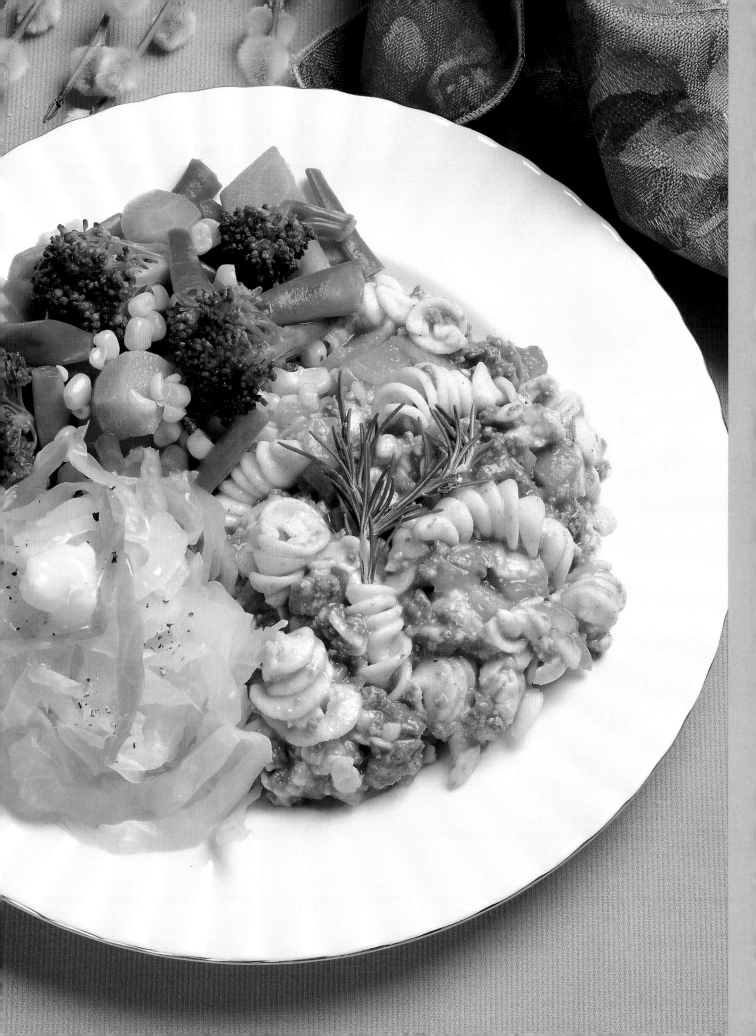

DINNER 26

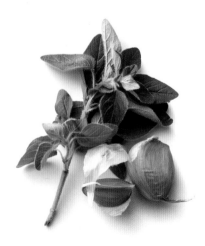

Pizza

This homemade thick crust pizza has lots of vegetables, and less cheese and meat compared to a restaurant pizza. Therefore, it has half the calories and sodium of a typical restaurant pizza (as shown on page 302). You can reduce the sodium further by using roasted chicken pieces instead of the ham, sausage or pepperoni.

Homemade Pizza

Makes one 12-inch (30 cm) pizza (6 large or 8 medium slices)

Pizza shell (ready-made, 12-inch/30 cm)
1/2 cup (125 mL) Pizza Sauce (see below)
Vegetables, such as mushrooms, peppers, onions, tomatoes, broccoli, zucchini, or eggplant
3/4 cup (175 mL) pineapple chunks
2 oz (60 g) sliced ham, sausage or pepperoni
1 cup (250 mL) loosely packed shredded cheese

PER LARGE SLICE (1/6 OF PIZZA)	
Calories	293
Carbohydrate	41 g
Fiber	3 g
Net carbs	38 g
Protein	13 g
Fat, total	9 g
Fat, saturated	4 g
Cholesterol	18 mg
Sodium	570 mg

1. Spread pizza sauce on the pizza shell.
2. Add vegetables, pineapple and meat. Top with cheese.
3. Place on your oven rack or use a pizza pan, if you have one. Bake in a 350°F (180°C) oven for 15 minutes, until the cheese bubbles.

Pizza Sauce

Makes about 1²/₃ cups (400 mL)

14-oz (398 mL) can tomato sauce
1/2 tsp (2 mL) oregano
1/2 tsp (2 mL) garlic powder or 1 garlic clove, finely chopped
Any of the following are optional for extra flavoring: 1 finely chopped small onion, 1/2 stalk finely chopped celery or a pinch of cinnamon or cloves

PER 2 TBSP (30 ML)	
Calories	10
Carbohydrate	2 g
Fiber	0 g
Net carbs	0 g
Protein	0 g
Fat, total	0 g
Fat, saturated	0 g
Cholesterol	0 mg
Sodium	157 mg

1. Combine all ingredients.

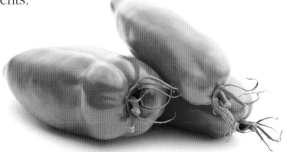

When you have a salad with your pizza, it helps fill you up so you are less likely to reach for another piece of pizza.

With your meal, enjoy a diet soft drink (as shown) or a small glass of tomato juice. Also have water to drink.

Have a fruit for dessert.

If you eat out in a restaurant:

- Eat a fruit or a fresh vegetable snack before you go to a restaurant so you won't be so hungry and overeat.
- It may help if you decide what you'll order before you go. Or better still, decide what you won't order.
- Start with a salad, and ask for low-fat salad dressings on the side.
- Don't be shy about asking for foods to be made to your liking. For example, you can request a plain roll instead of garlic bread.
- If your meal is bigger than your portions should be, ask the waiter to package your leftovers so you can take them home.

HEALTH TIP

Drinking regular soft drinks, sweetened beverages and even unsweetened juices will give you extra sugar you don't need. Remember, water is what your body needs when you are thirsty (see page 21).

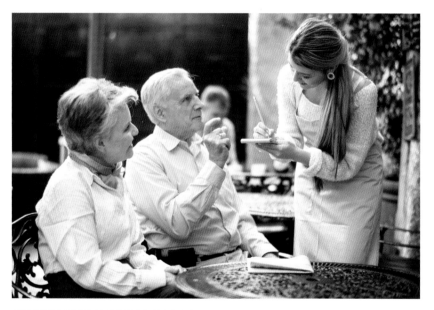

Food Choices	Large Meal	Small Meal
Carbohydrate	5	4
Protein	2	1½

Your Dinner Menu	Large Meal (730 calories)	Total Carbs	Net Carbs	Small Meal (550 calories)	Total Carbs	Net Carbs
12-inch (30 cm) Pizza, thick crust	2 large slices (⅓ pizza)	82	76	2 medium slices (¼ pizza)	61	56
Tossed salad	Large	6	5	Large	6	5
Oil-free Italian salad dressing	1 tbsp (15 mL)	2	2	1 tbsp (15 mL)	2	2
Diet soft drink	Large	1	1	Large	1	1
Nectarine	1 large	16	13	1 large	16	13
		107 g	**97 g**		**86 g**	**77 g**

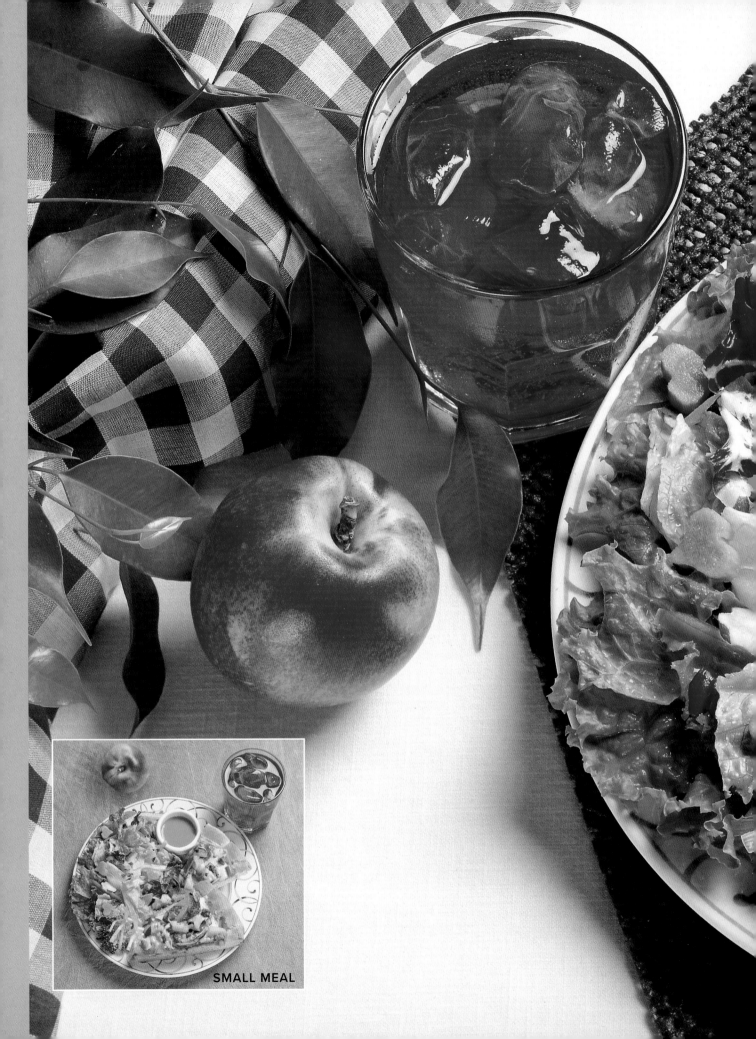

SMALL MEAL

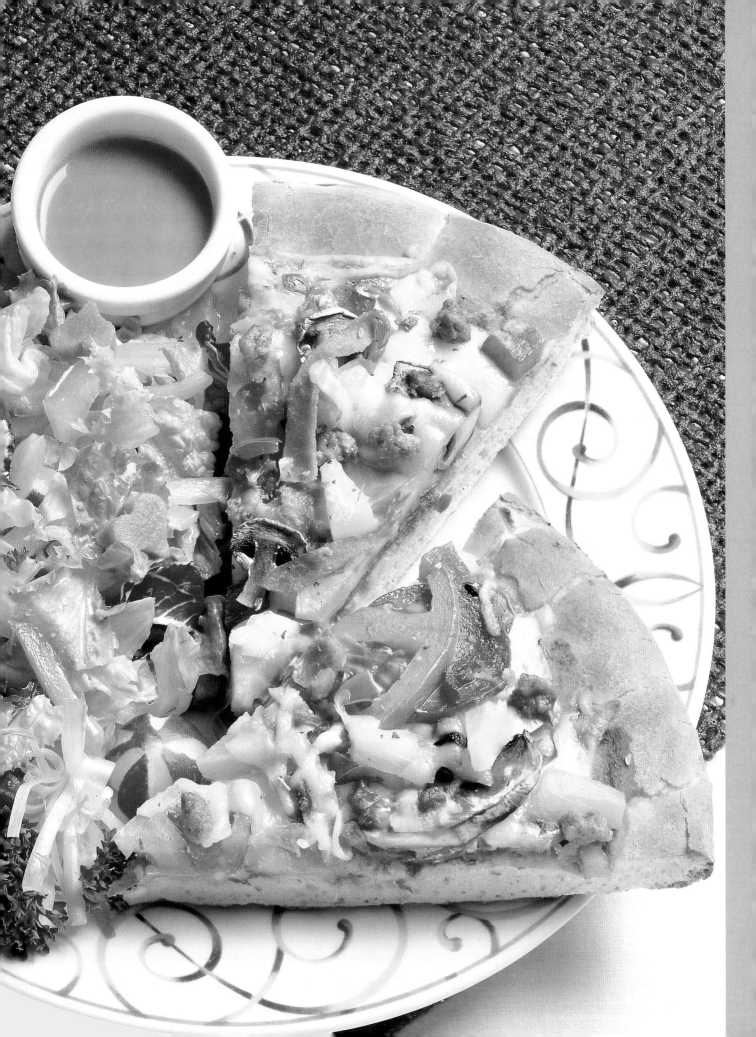

DINNER 27

Fast-Food Dinner

FOOD CHARTS

See page 301: Fast-Food Burger with All the Toppings.

OPTIONS

If you decide to make this meal at home, make Baked Low-Fat Fries (page 156), baked frozen french fries or a baked potato.

You can also try the meatless Sun Burger on page 200.

Yes, you may still eat out at fast-food restaurants — occasionally. Most foods in restaurants are high in fat and sodium and the portions are too often large or supersize. These may be called "deluxe."

Since fries are the most common food ordered in restaurants, they are included in this meal; but choose a small order.

Burger/Sandwich Options (for large meal)

Instead of a grilled chicken breast on a bun (as shown in the photograph), you could order:

- a small serving of 6 chicken nuggets with sauce
- a single fish burger
- a cheeseburger
- a veggie burger

Veggie Burgers/Sandwiches

These are made from plants rather than meat. Often the base is soya beans or pea protein. Specialty restaurants may make veggie burgers from high-protein grains like quinoa. Then other vegetables and fats and oils may be added to mimic the taste and texture of meat. Veggie burgers are a way to reduce your meat intake, but keep in mind that restaurant veggie burgers are not usually low in calories. Typically they have 400 to 500 calories, with "deluxe" or "gourmet" versions having 600 or more calories. To boost flavor, more salt is often added to veggie burgers compared to, for example, a cheeseburger.

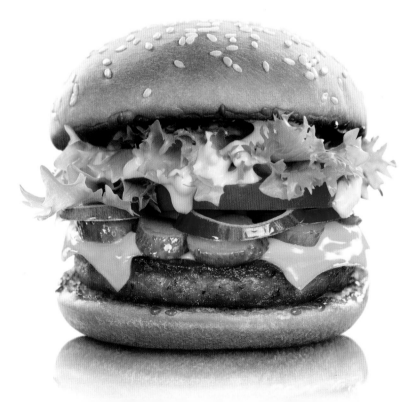

Salad with a light vinaigrette dressing and a diet drink are included with this meal.

Nutrition Information at Fast-Food Restaurants

- **Calories on the order boards.** This is a last minute check that might convince you to avoid the deluxe and higher calorie options, or the "extras."

- **Printed nutrition information sheet.** You can ask for one of these at the order desk. Most restaurants have a printed sheet, but may be reluctant to give it out; don't be surprised if they tell you they are "out of stock."

- **Get nutrition information online or with a nutrition app.** Go online to the website of the restaurant chain and search "nutrition information." Nutrients listed will include calories, carbohydrates, sugar, protein, fat and sodium. Some companies have a clear list of all their food items. Other companies make it awkward, and you have to choose item by item. There are also some great food apps that make it easy to look up fast foods. Make sure these apps get updated regularly, as restaurants change their products, plus bring in new products.

- **Get the nutrition for** *all* **the items you are ordering.** When using online apps and websites, make sure the item you choose includes the extras or condiments. For example, a salad and the salad dressing will usually be listed separately even though they are sold together. Ketchup will be listed separately from the fries; if you are going to eat both, then count the nutrients of both.

FOOD FACTS

Salad dressings

- Some of the "light" salad dressings in restaurants are still high in calories. They can have up to 100 calories in one package. Check the label.

- The regular salad dressings in restaurants may have 200 calories in one package.

- Most restaurant salad dressings are also high in salt.

FOOD CHARTS

See page 306: Caesar Salad. A restaurant Caesar salad has the same calories as a larger burger (page 301).

Food Choices	Large Meal	Small Meal
Carbohydrate	5	3
Protein	3½	2
Fat	3	3

Your Dinner Menu	Large Meal (730 calories)	Total Carbs	Net Carbs	Small Meal (550 calories)	Total Carbs	Net Carbs
Grilled burger on a bun (chicken, veggie, beef or fish)	1 burger (450–500 calories)	49	46	6 chicken nuggets (250–300 calories)	15	15
Barbecue dipping sauce	–	–	–	1 package	11	11
French fries	1 small order	31	28	1 small order	31	28
Ketchup	½ tbsp (7 mL)	1	1	½ tbsp (7 mL)	1	1
Side salad	1 small	1	1	1 small	1	1
Light vinaigrette salad dressing	½ package	2	2	½ package	2	2
Diet soft drink	Large	1	1	Large	1	1
		85 g	**79 g**		**62 g**	**59 g**

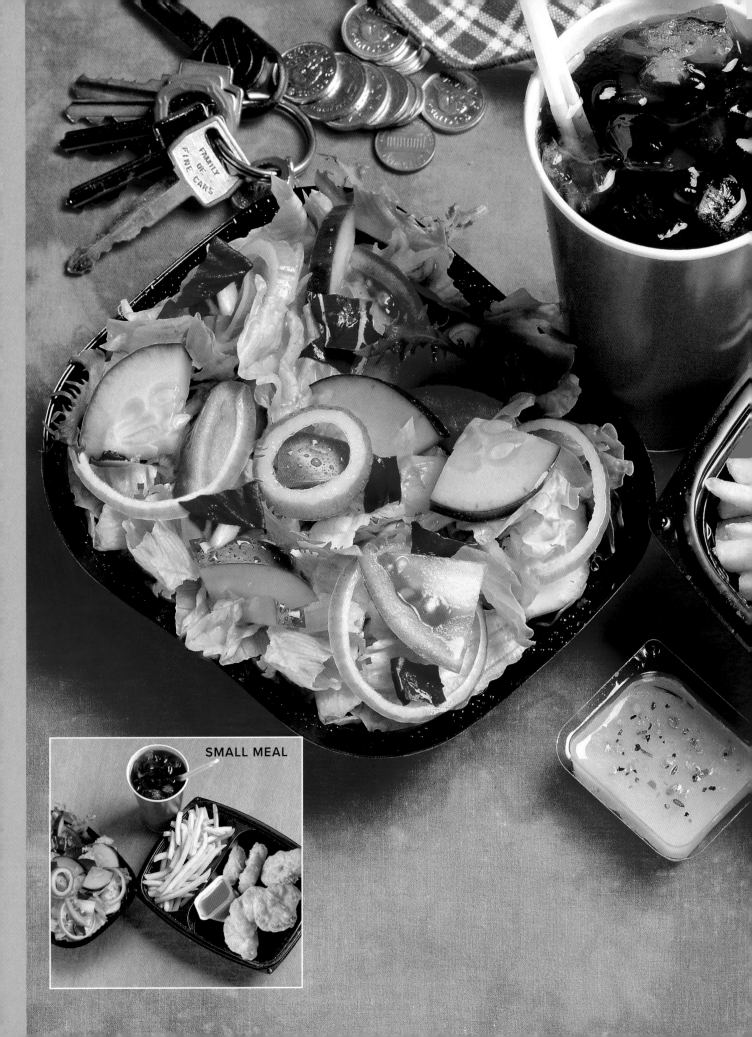

SMALL MEAL

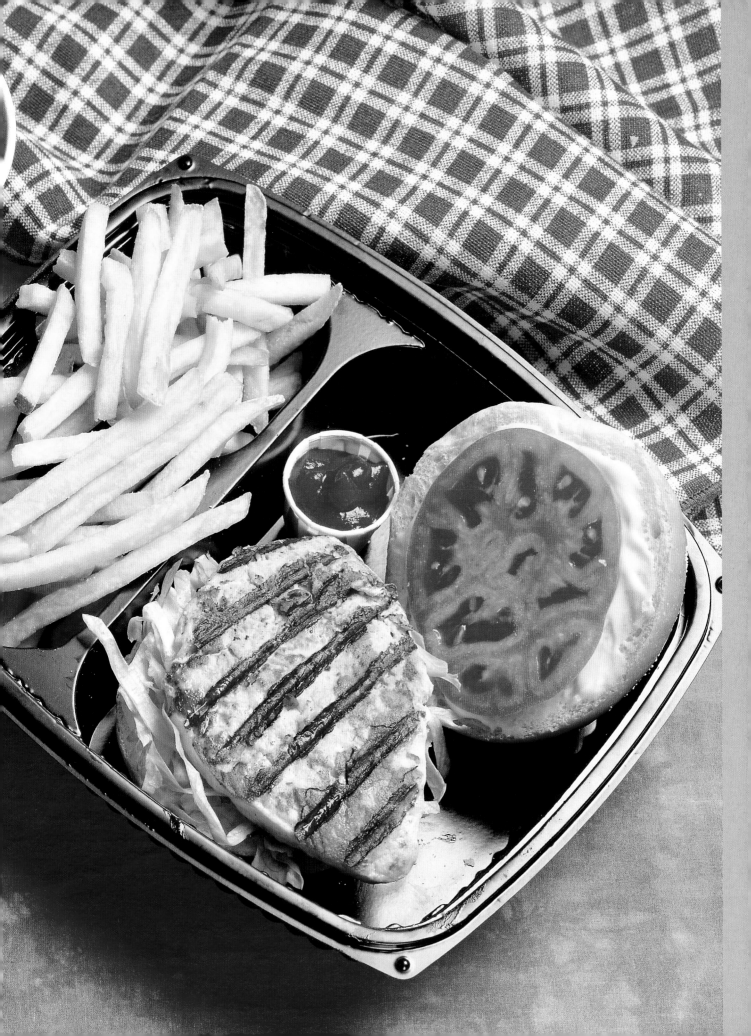

Stir-Fry

Put your rice on to cook before you start making the stir-fry.

Stir-Fry

Makes 4 cups (1 L)
(2 large meal servings)

1 small onion, sliced

1 tbsp (15 mL) vegetable oil

1 to 2 cloves garlic, finely chopped

4 to 6 cups (1 to 1.5 L) loosely packed vegetable pieces

1 packet (4.5 g) reduced-salt chicken or beef bouillon mix

¾ cup/175 mL (or 6 oz/175 g) raw lean red meat, chicken or fish, thinly sliced

2 tsp (10 mL) cornstarch

¼ cup (60 mL) cold water

1 tbsp (15 mL) reduced-sodium soy sauce

1 tsp (1 mL) ground ginger

PER 1 CUP (250 ML)	
Calories	111
Carbohydrate	13 g
Fiber	3 g
Net carbs	10 g
Protein	12 g
Fat, total	2 g
Fat, saturated	0 g
Cholesterol	18 mg
Sodium	293 mg

1. Prepare your vegetables. Place the onions and garlic in one bowl. Then put the vegetables that need the most cooking, such as carrots and broccoli in another bowl. In a third bowl, put the vegetables that need less cooking, such as bean sprouts. Set the bowls of vegetables to the side.

2. In a wok or large frying pan, heat oil over medium heat. Add onion and garlic and sauté for 5 to 10 minutes until softened. Add bouillon and raw meat (or other protein choice) and cook until partially cooked. If you are using cooked leftover meat instead of raw meat, it doesn't need to be cooked first.

3. Now add vegetables, adding the ones needing more cooking first. Stir at high heat for 5 to 10 minutes, until both vegetables and meat are cooked.

4. In a small bowl, mix together cornstarch, water, soy sauce and ginger. Add this to wok. Cook for another minute or two.

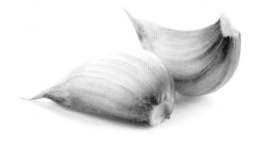

Fresh vegetables are best in a stir-fry, but you can also use frozen or canned vegetables. Try any of these vegetables:

- bamboo shoots (canned)
- bean sprouts
- bok choy (sliced)
- broccoli (pieces)
- cabbage (shredded)
- carrots or celery (sliced)
- cauliflower (pieces)
- baby corn (canned)
- mushrooms (sliced)
- green onions (chopped)
- frozen peas or whole fresh snow peas
- green pepper (strips)

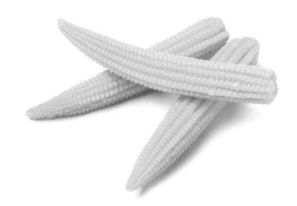

For dessert, a fortune cookie is a good low-calorie choice. Good luck!

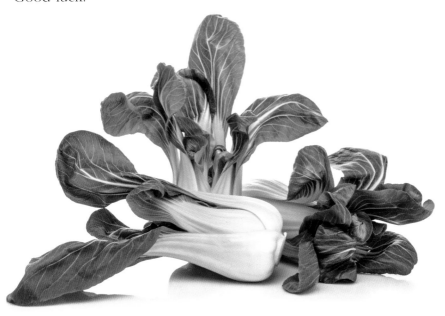

Food Choices	Large Meal	Small Meal
Carbohydrate	5	4
Protein	2½	2

Your Dinner Menu	Large Meal (730 calories)	Total Carbs	Net Carbs	Small Meal (550 calories)	Total Carbs	Net Carbs
Stir-Fry	2 cups (500 mL)	26	21	1½ cups (375 mL)	19	15
White or brown rice	1 cup (250 mL)	43	42	⅔ cup (150 mL)	29	28
Soy beverage	¾ cup (175 mL)	3	2	¾ cup (175 mL)	3	2
Pear	1 medium	25	20	1 medium	25	20
Fortune cookies	2	13	13	1	7	7
Green Tea	1 cup (250 mL)	0	0	1 cup (250 mL)	0	0
		110 g	**98 g**		**83 g**	**72 g**

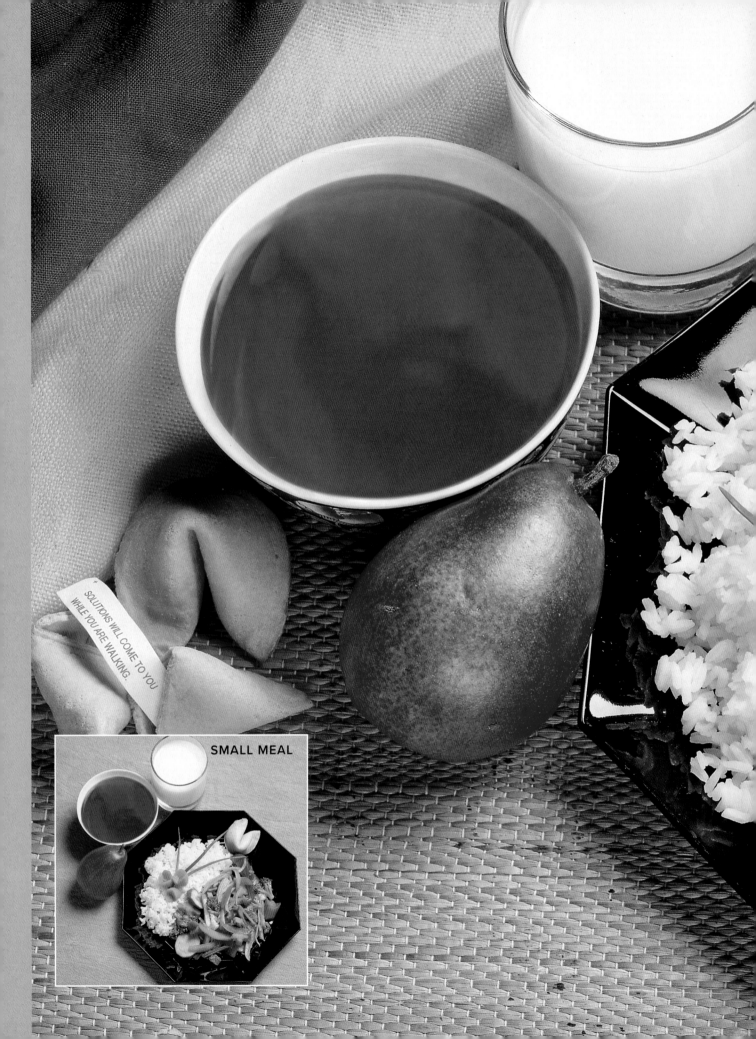

SOLUTIONS WILL COME TO YOU WHILE YOU ARE WALKING.

SMALL MEAL

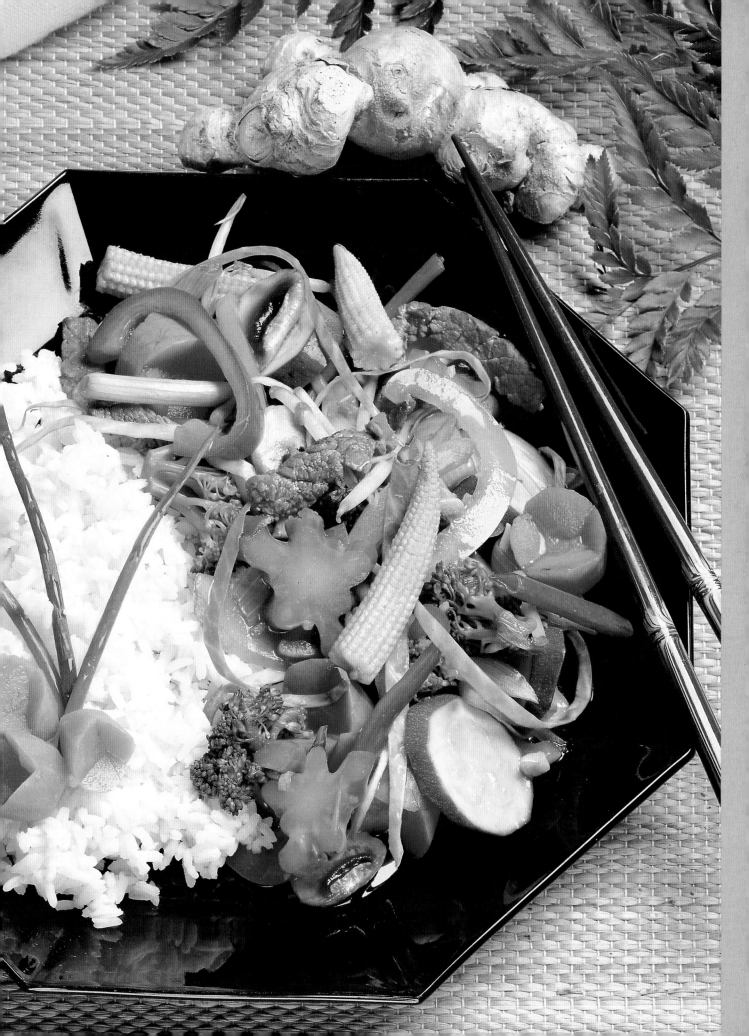

Denver Sandwich & Soup

OPTIONS

These cracker servings have about the same calories and carbs:

- 1 bread stick
- 2 soda crackers
- 1 snackbread cracker
- 2 melba toasts
- 1 Ritz-type party cracker

A sandwich and soup is a light choice for dinner in a restaurant. The sandwich could be a Denver, a Western, a clubhouse or a bacon, lettuce and tomato sandwich. Ask for your bread or toast to be spread with little or no butter or mayonnaise. Also ask the waiter to hold the french fries. If you want to make a Denver sandwich at home, here's the recipe.

Denver Sandwich

Makes 1 sandwich

1 slice bacon or 1 oz (30 g) ham, chopped

2 eggs

1 tbsp (15 mL) parsley, green onion tops, onion or chives, chopped

Black pepper to taste

2 slices toast, each spread with
$\frac{1}{2}$ tsp (2 mL) margarine or butter,
or 1 tsp (5 mL) light mayonnaise

Lettuce

PER SANDWICH	
Calories	363
Carbohydrate	27 g
Fiber	4 g
Net carbs	23 g
Protein	21 g
Fat, total	20 g
Fat, saturated	5 g
Cholesterol	381 mg
Sodium	661 mg

1. In a nonstick pan, fry chopped bacon. Drain off the fat. If you are using chopped ham instead of bacon, you don't need to cook it first.
2. In a small bowl, beat eggs with a fork. Add bacon or ham and the parsley or onion tops.
3. Cook in the nonstick pan. Stir on and off.
4. Place egg mixture on piece of toast.
5. Add lettuce or other vegetables to the sandwich.

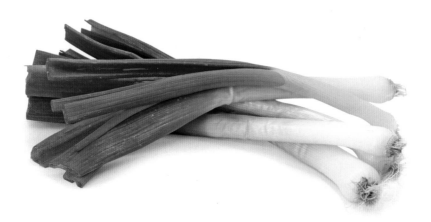

There is no dessert with this meal. If you would like to have a small fruit, then omit the bread sticks. Or choose a light gelatin or a store-bought sugar-free popsicle.

Walking after a meal makes you feel better and helps to bring down your blood sugar.

Your blood sugar goes up after a meal, and a short walk about an hour or so after eating will help you bring it down. If you can manage a half-hour or full-hour walk, this is best, but even a shorter walk of 10 to 15 minutes can help bring down your blood sugar and blood pressure after you've eaten.

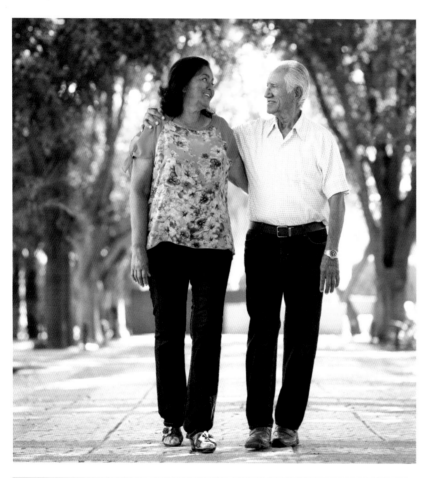

Food Choices	Large Meal	Small Meal
Carbohydrate	4½	3½
Protein	3	2
Fat	3	2

Your Dinner Menu	Large Meal (730 calories)	Total Carbs	Net Carbs	Small Meal (550 calories)	Total Carbs	Net Carbs
Tomato soup (made with water)	1 cup (250 mL)	17	16	1 cup (250 mL)	17	16
Bread sticks	1½	7	7	1½	7	7
Denver Sandwich	1½ sandwiches	40	34	1 sandwich	27	23
Salad	Large	6	5	Large	6	5
Fat-free ranch salad dressing	1 tbsp (15 mL)	4	3	1 tbsp (15 mL)	4	3
		74 g	**65 g**		**61 g**	**54 g**

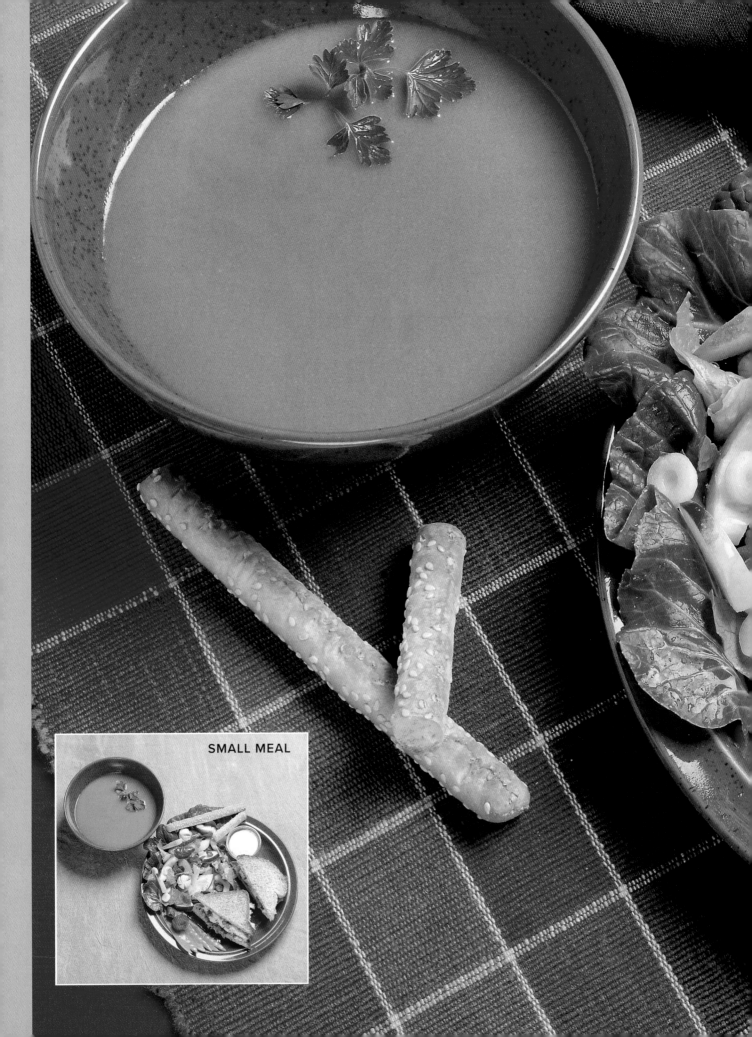

SMALL MEAL

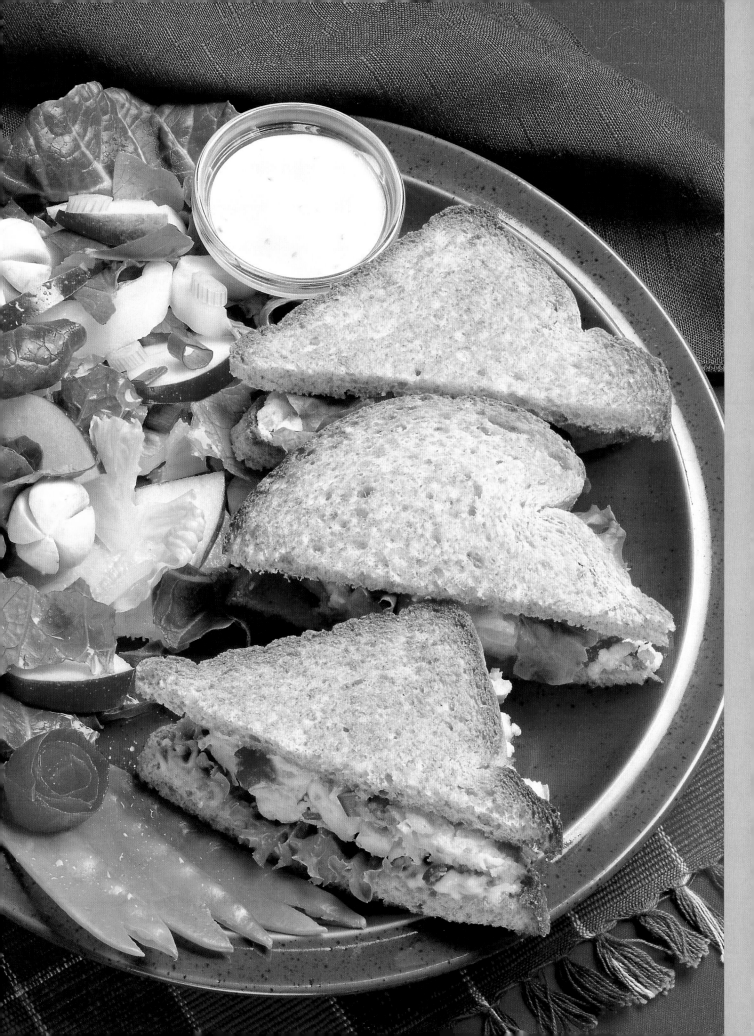

Shish Kebabs

Shish kebabs can be one of the lowest-fat meal choices in a Greek or Middle Eastern restaurant. Try this delicious low-fat marinade for your meat, or lightly baste your meat with olive oil and oregano.

FOOD FACT

A traditional Greek shish kebab is called souvlaki and is made only with meat.

Shish Kebab Marinade

Makes enough for 2 shish kebabs

1 to 2 tbsp (30 mL) reduced-sodium
   soy sauce
2 tbsp (30 mL) onion, finely chopped
1 clove garlic, crushed or finely chopped
   (or 1/2 tsp/2 mL garlic powder)
1 tbsp (15 mL) minced gingerroot
   (or 1 tsp/5 mL ground ginger)
2 tbsp (30 mL) dry wine (or wine vinegar)

PER 1 TBSP (15 ML)	
Calories	9
Carbohydrate	1 g
Fiber	0 g
Net carbs	1 g
Protein	0 g
Fat, total	0 g
Fat, saturated	0 g
Cholesterol	0 mg
Sodium	100 mg

1. Mix the marinade ingredients together in a dish. Place the meat in the marinade and let it sit in the fridge for a couple of hours.

Shish Kebabs

To make each shish kebab you will need:

Meat

1½-inch/4 cm cubes of lean lamb or beef
For large meal: 4 cubes (6 oz/175 g, raw)
For small meal: 3 cubes (4 oz/125 g, raw)

Vegetables

Cherry tomatoes, whole fresh mushrooms, cubes of green pepper, whole small onions (or chunks of onion), zucchini, eggplant, or any other vegetables you like

1. Put meat and vegetables on skewers, as shown in the picture. Brush with the marinade. If you want your meat well done, broil or barbecue it for 5 minutes before adding the vegetables.
2. Broil or barbecue for 5 to 10 minutes or until cooked.

Greek Salad

Makes 2 servings

2 large tomatoes, cut into wedges
$\frac{1}{2}$ medium red onion, sliced
$\frac{1}{2}$ green pepper, cut into chunks
$\frac{1}{2}$ small cucumber, cut into chunks
12 small black olives (or 4 large)
$\frac{1}{4}$ cup (60 mL) feta cheese,
    crumbled or chunks
1 tbsp (15 mL) olive oil
1 tbsp (15 mL) red wine vinegar
1 tsp (5 mL) dried oregano

PER SERVING	
Calories	205
Carbohydrate	17 g
Fiber	2 g
Net carbs	15 g
Protein	5 g
Fat, total	15 g
Fat, saturated	4 g
Cholesterol	17 mg
Sodium	478 mg

HEALTH TIP

If you are having this meal in a restaurant, remember to ask for the salad dressing on the side so you can control the amount.

1. In a large bowl, combine tomatoes, onions, green pepper, cucumber, olives and feta cheese.

2. In a small bowl, whisk together oil, vinegar and oregano. Pour over salad and toss to coat.

This meal ends with a low-fat dessert: apple sprinkled with a touch of cinnamon and icing sugar. Instead of apple, you could have an orange or $\frac{1}{2}$ cup (125 mL) of cantaloupe, melon or grapes.

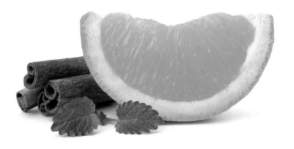

Food Choices	Large Meal	Small Meal
Carbohydrate	$4\frac{1}{2}$	$2\frac{1}{2}$
Protein	4	$2\frac{1}{2}$
Fat	3	2

Your Dinner Menu	Large Meal (730 calories)	Total Carbs	Net Carbs	Small Meal (550 calories)	Total Carbs	Net Carbs
Shish Kebab	1 made with 4 cubes of beef	6	5	1 made with 3 cubes of beef	6	5
White or brown rice	$\frac{2}{3}$ cup (150 mL)	29	28	$\frac{2}{3}$ cup (150 mL)	29	28
Greek Salad with dressing	1 serving	16	12	1 serving	16	12
Crusty white bun	1	15	14	–	–	–
Butter or margarine	1 tsp (5 mL)	0	0	–	–	–
Cinnamon apple rings	$\frac{1}{2}$ medium apple with $\frac{1}{2}$ tsp (2 mL) icing sugar plus cinnamon	12	11	$\frac{1}{2}$ medium apple with $\frac{1}{2}$ tsp (2 mL) icing sugar plus cinnamon	12	11
		78 g	**70 g**		**63 g**	**56 g**

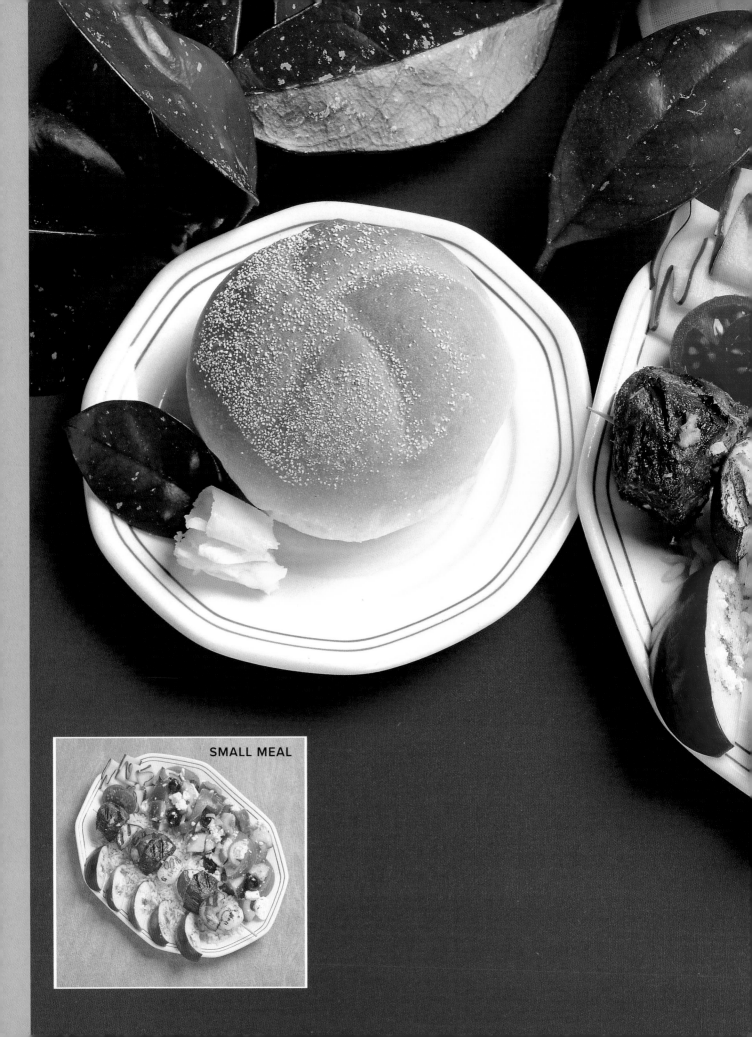

SMALL MEAL

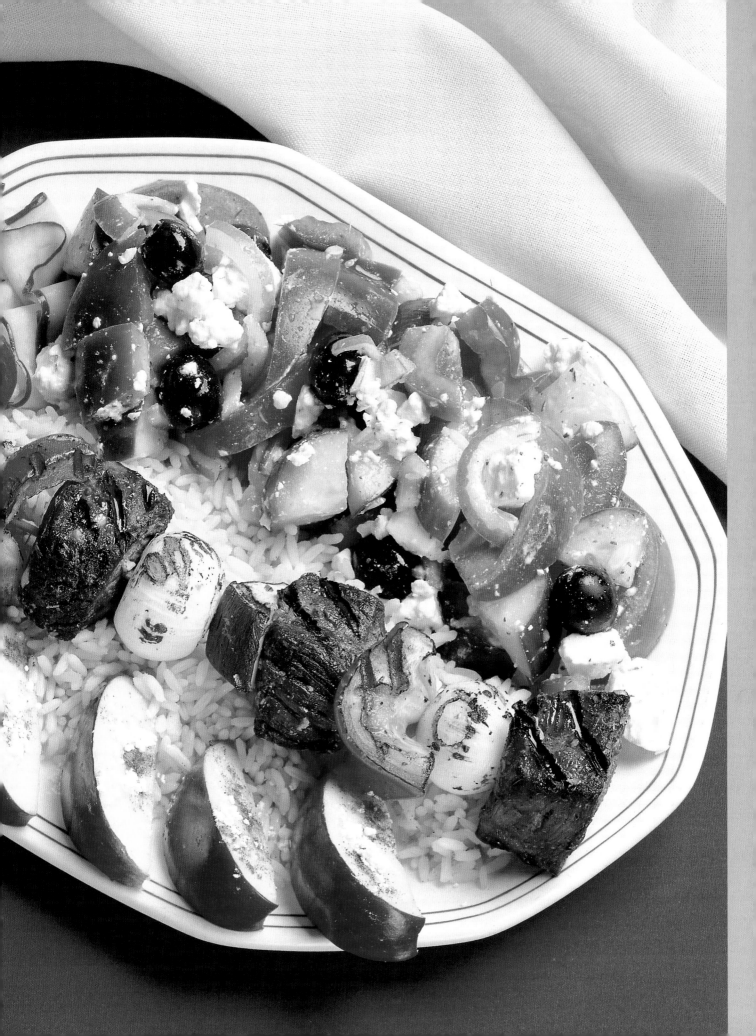

Tandoori Chicken & Rice

Karen fell in love with tandoori chicken when she lived in Kenya. This delicious meal is spicy but not hot. The chicken is coated in a tasty low-fat coating and then broiled or barbecued.

Tandoori Chicken and Sauce

Makes 5 large or 8 small servings

Sauce

1½ cups (375 mL) low-fat plain yogurt

1½ tbsp (22 mL) store-bought tandoori spice mix

1½ tbsp (22 mL) vinegar

1½ tbsp (22 mL) lemon juice

2½ lbs (1 kg) chicken pieces (weight with bones and skin), skin removed

PER 1 TBSP (15 ML) SAUCE	
Calories	7
Carbohydrate	1 g
Fiber	0 g
Net carbs	1 g
Protein	1 g
Fat, total	0 g
Fat, saturated	0 g
Cholesterol	0 mg
Sodium	9 mg

1. In a large bowl or pot, mix all the ingredients for the sauce.
2. Make some small cuts in each chicken piece so the yogurt sauce can flavor the meat. Add the chicken to the bowl or pot, making sure that it is covered with sauce. Cover and place in the fridge for at least 4 hours or overnight.
3. Gently shake any extra sauce from the chicken. Then barbecue or place on a rack in a pan and grill in the oven (about 5 in/12.5 cm from the grill). Cook for 10 to 15 minutes on each side, until well done.
4. Put the leftover sauce in a small, heavy pan and boil for 5 minutes. Give each person a small dish of this sauce for dunking their chicken and putting on their rice.

OPTIONS

Tandoori chicken can be served with either:

- basmati rice, as shown in the photograph
- chapati or naan bread (East Indian breads)

This recipe is also delicious when made with curry powder instead of the tandoori mix. If you use curry powder, the sauce will be a golden curry color. The tandoori mix makes the sauce reddish.

CAUTION!

It is important to boil the marinade sauce for 5 minutes. Raw chicken has a lot of bacteria, and boiling will make the sauce safe to eat.

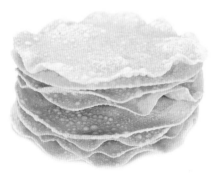

Poppadoms

If you've never had poppadoms, you don't know what you're missing! They can be bought in large food stores and in specialty food stores. They are 5 to 7 inches (12.5 to 17.5 cm) round and come in mild or hot (spicy). All you need to do is place them under a hot broiler and in 1 or 2 minutes they will bubble and turn a golden brown. Broil both sides. Or run them quickly under tap water to wet them and then pop them in the microwave on High for about 40 seconds. These crunchy treats are great with a curry meal or can be eaten as a snack.

A nice finish to this meal is a small piece of tropical fruit, such as mango or papaya.

Indian Spiced Tea

Makes 5 cups (1.25 L)

1 tea bag
3 cardamom pods
1 2-inch (5 cm) stick cinnamon
$\frac{1}{2}$ tsp (2 mL) lemon juice
$2\frac{1}{2}$ cups (625 mL) boiling water
$2\frac{1}{2}$ cups (625 mL) hot skim or 1% milk

PER 1 CUP (250 ML)	
Calories	44
Carbohydrate	6 g
Fiber	0 g
Protein	4 g
Net carbs	6 g
Fat, total	0 g
Fat, saturated	0 g
Cholesterol	2 mg
Sodium	67 mg

RECIPE TIP

Serve this meal with chai tea. For an alternative to the commercial chai tea in a bag, try this homemade version.

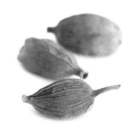

1. Place tea, cardamom, cinnamon and lemon juice in your teapot. Add boiling water and let steep for 4 minutes. Remove bag, cardamom and cinnamon from the pot.
2. Serve the tea with an equal part of hot milk and, if you want, 1 tsp (5 mL) of sugar, honey or low-calorie sweetener.

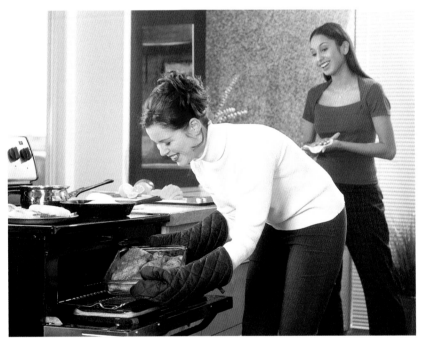

Food Choices	Large Meal	Small Meal
Carbohydrate	5	4
Protein	5	3

Your Dinner Menu	Large Meal (730 calories)	Total Carbs	Net Carbs	Small Meal (550 calories)	Total Carbs	Net Carbs
Tandoori Chicken	1 large leg	0	0	1 small leg	0	0
Tandoori Sauce	4 tbsp (60 mL)	4	4	2 tbsp (30 mL)	2	2
Rice (basmati)	1 cup (250 mL)	46	45	$\frac{2}{3}$ cup (150 mL)	31	30
Sliced raw vegetables	As desired	2	1	As desired	2	1
Poppadoms	2	10	8	2	10	8
Mango	$\frac{1}{2}$ medium	17	15	$\frac{1}{2}$ medium	17	15
Indian Spiced Tea	1 cup (250 mL)	6	6	1 cup (250 mL)	6	6
		85 g	**79 g**		**68 g**	**62 g**

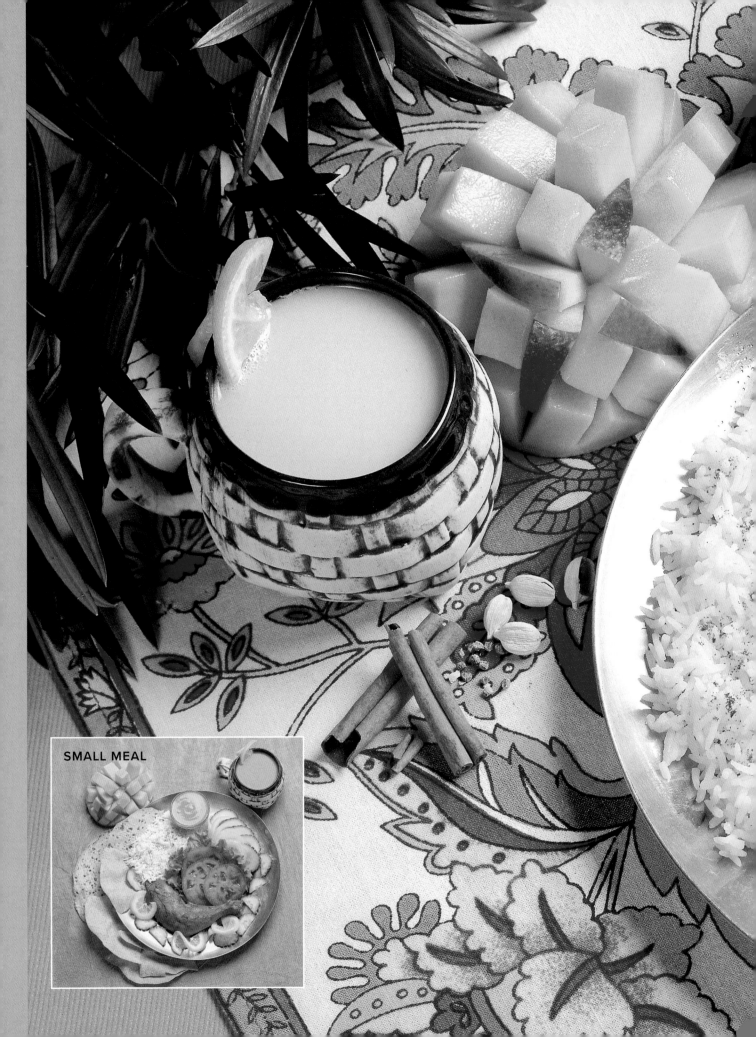

SMALL MEAL

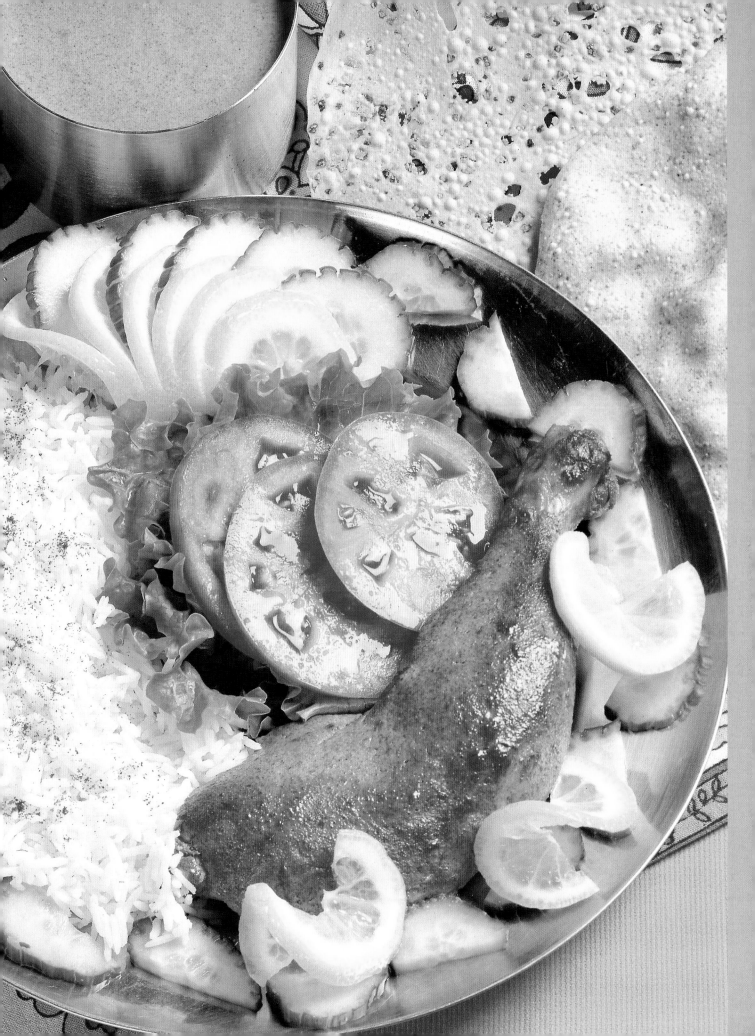

Swiss Steak

Karen adapted this recipe from her mother-in-law's Swiss Steak by reducing the butter and using a dry wine instead of a sweet wine. It is so tender and gets rave reviews!

Grandma's Swiss Steak

Makes 6 large or 8 small servings

3 lbs (1.5 kg) sirloin tip steaks

1 tsp (5 mL) Hy's Seasoning Salt

¼ tsp (1 mL) black pepper

2 tbsp (30 mL) butter

1 large onion, chopped or sliced

5 cups (1.25 L) washed and sliced fresh mushrooms

1 tbsp (15 mL) butter

¼ cup (60 mL) dry red or white wine

¾ cup (175 mL) water

PER LARGE SERVING (⅙ OF RECIPE)	
Calories	324
Carbohydrate	5 g
Fiber	1 g
Net carbs	4 g
Protein	47 g
Fat, total	11 g
Fat, saturated	6 g
Cholesterol	122 mg
Sodium	363 mg

1. Pound the steak on both sides with a meat pounder. If you don't have a meat pounder, use the edge of a small plate to flatten the meat. Trim off visible fat. Poke holes in the meat with a fork. Cut the meat into pieces the size of a deck of cards or smaller. Place meat on a large cookie sheet.
2. Sprinkle Hy's Seasoning Salt and pepper on both sides of the meat, and rub it in with the back of a spoon.
3. In a large, heavy pan or nonstick frying pan, fry onions and mushrooms in the 2 tbsp (30 mL) of butter until the onions are soft. Set aside in a bowl.
4. Add 1 tbsp (15 mL) of butter to the pan, and fry the seasoned meat at medium heat. Brown the outside of the meat on both sides.
5. Move the meat to a casserole dish (or roasting pan) and cover with wine, cooked onions and mushrooms.
6. Add the water to the frying pan to stir up any brown bits and seasoning, then add this meat juice to the casserole.
7. Put the lid on the casserole and cook the steak for 2 hours at 325°F (160°C), or longer, until it is fork-tender. Add a small amount of water as necessary to keep the meat cooking in juice.

RECIPE TIP

Tenderizing steak

This recipe is made with sirloin tip steak, which is the less expensive cut of the "best steak." It will need some tenderizing to break down the tough muscle fibers. In this recipe, the meat is tenderized by pounding, marinated with store-bought tenderizer, and slow-cooked. Each bite is succulent and tender.

FOOD FACT

Seasoning for steak

One important ingredient in this recipe is the Hy's Seasoning Salt. This is such a great Canadian seasoning that there are websites devoted to it! It also adds great flavor to steaks and hamburgers.

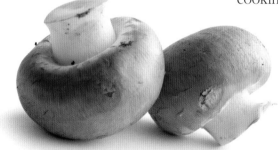

Serve the Swiss Steak with boiled potatoes, peas and carrots, and red pepper strips, either fresh or roasted.

Roasted Pepper Strips

Place halved peppers under your oven grill (or on a barbecue), with the skin side to the grill, until the surface is blackened, about 5 to 8 minutes. Remove from the oven (or barbecue) and place in a closed paper bag (or wrap in paper towel) for a few minutes. Then take them out of the bag, pull off the blackened skin and cut the peppers into strips.

This dessert is a winning finish to the meal.

Lemon Pear-fection

Makes 1 serving

3 small (or 2 medium) canned pear halves, with 3 tbsp (45 mL) of Lemon Sauce

Lemon Sauce

$^3/_4$ cup (175 mL) pear juice (the usual amount of juice in a 14-oz/398 mL can)

1 tbsp (15 mL) cornstarch

1 tsp (5 mL) lemon zest and 1 tbsp (15 mL) lemon juice (from $^1/_2$ lemon)

1 tbsp (15 mL) sugar

PER SERVING	
Calories	88
Carbohydrate	23 g
Fiber	2 g
Net carbs	21 g
Protein	0 g
Fat, total	0 g
Fat, saturated	0 g
Cholesterol	0 mg
Sodium	6 mg

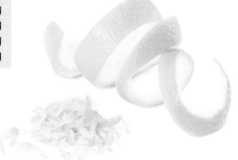

1. Place 2 pear halves in a dessert dish.
2. In a small pot, pour the pear juice. Add the cornstarch and blend well with a whisk so there are no lumps. Add the lemon zest, lemon juice and sugar, and mix.
3. With the pot on medium heat, stir constantly until the lemon sauce has thickened and the color has lightened.
4. Pour 3 tbsp (45 mL) of the warm Lemon Sauce over the pears, and serve immediately.

Food Choices	Large Meal	Small Meal
Carbohydrate	5½	4
Protein	4	3

Your Dinner Menu	Large Meal (730 calories)	Total Carbs	Net Carbs	Small Meal (550 calories)	Total Carbs	Net Carbs
Swiss Steak	4-oz (125 g) piece of steak, plus sauce (⅙ of recipe)	5	4	3-oz (90 g) piece of steak, plus sauce (⅛ of recipe)	3	2
Boiled potatoes	7 mini	44	40	5 mini	30	28
Peas and carrots	¾ cup (175 mL)	12	8	¾ cup (175 mL)	12	8
Red pepper, roasted or fresh	6 strips	2	2	3 strips	1	1
Skim or 1% milk	1 cup (250 mL)	12	12	½ cup (125 mL)	6	6
Lemon Pear-fection	3 small pear halves + 3 tbsp (45 mL) sauce	22	20	3 small pear halves + 3 tbsp (45 mL) sauce	22	20
		97 g	86 g		74 g	65 g

237

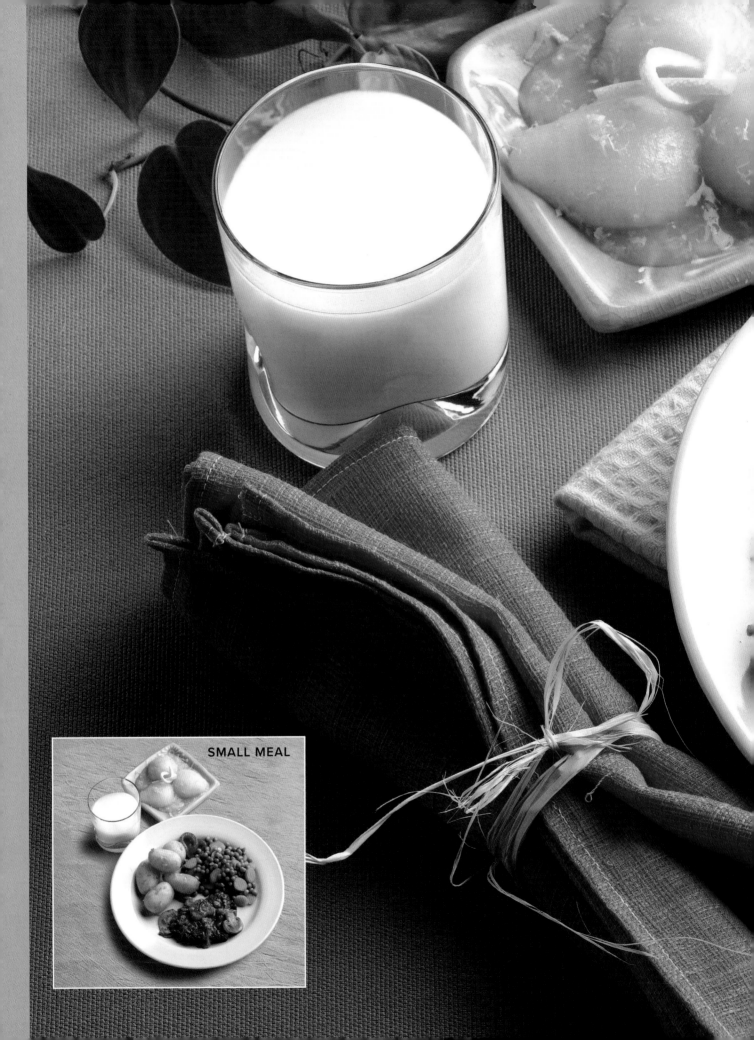

SMALL MEAL

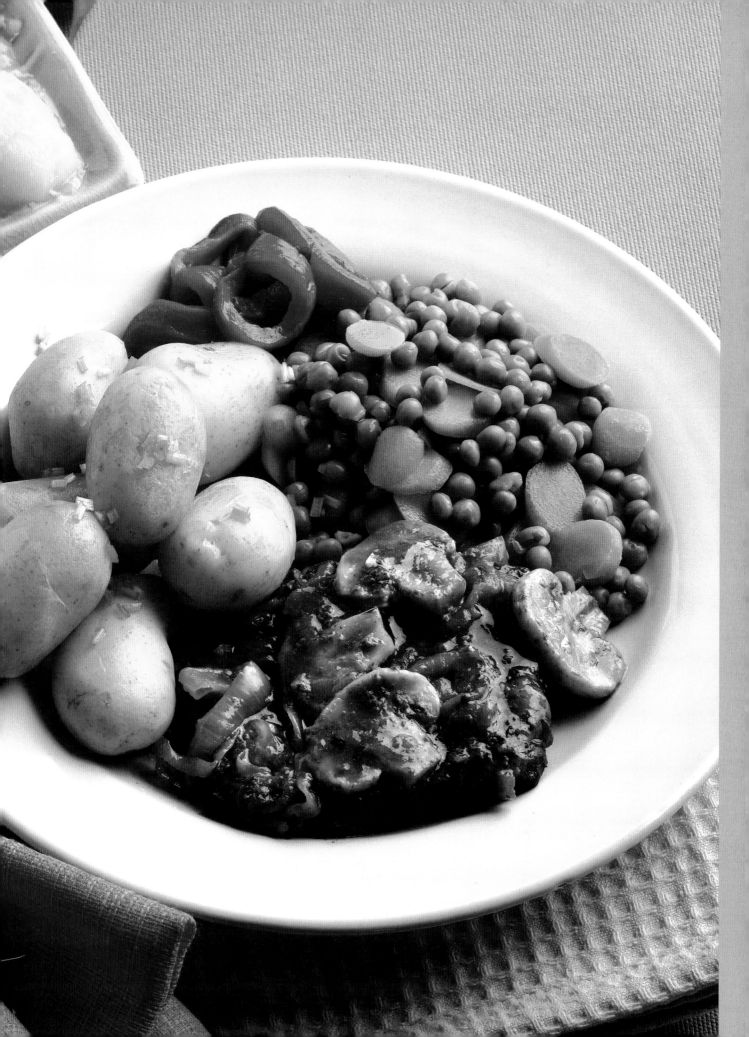

DINNER 33

Thai Chicken

Thai Chicken

Makes 3½ cups (875 mL)
(3½ large or 4½ small servings)

6 chicken thighs (or 4 small breasts), skin and visible fat removed and bones cut out, cut into strips

1 small onion, chopped

2 tbsp (30 mL) water

¾ cup (175 mL) salsa (mild or hot)

2 tbsp (30 mL) chopped fresh cilantro

3 tbsp (45 mL) peanut butter

1 tbsp (15 mL) oyster sauce

1 cup (250 mL) skim (non-fat) evaporated canned milk

1 tsp (5 mL) cornstarch

Cilantro or lime wedges, for garnish

PER 1 CUP (250 ML)	
Calories	311
Carbohydrate	20 g
Fiber	2 g
Net carbs	18 g
Protein	32 g
Fat, total	11 g
Fat, saturated	3 g
Cholesterol	88 mg
Sodium	620 mg

1. In a large, nonstick frying pan, place the chicken strips and chopped onions with the water. Cook on medium-low heat until there is no pink inside the chicken.
2. In a bowl, mix together the salsa, cilantro, peanut butter and oyster sauce.
3. In another bowl, whisk the cornstarch into the evaporated milk until well blended.
4. Add the salsa mixture to the chicken, then pour in the milk. Stir until the sauce boils and thickens.

Poppy Seed Spinach Salad

Makes 2 servings

⅓ of a 10-oz (300 g) bag of fresh washed spinach

1 medium tomato, cut into small wedges

¼ small red onion, sliced into rings

½ cup (125 mL) sliced fresh strawberries

1 tbsp (15 mL) sliced almonds, lightly toasted

Sprinkle of poppy seeds, for topping (optional)

Light creamy poppy seed salad dressing (2 tbsp/25 mL for large meal and 1 tbsp/15 mL for small meal)

PER SERVING	
Calories	51
Carbohydrate	7 g
Fiber	3 g
Net carbs	4 g
Protein	3 g
Fat, total	2 g
Fat, saturated	0 g
Cholesterol	0 mg
Sodium	41 mg

1. Wash spinach and arrange in two salad bowls.
2. Place the other ingredients on top of the spinach.

RECIPE TIP

Thai Chicken can be made the night before and reheated the next day. Serve it with rice noodles (as seen in the photo), angel hair pasta or vermicelli pasta.

FOOD FACT

Thai cooking

Did you know? Thailand is the world's largest exporter of rice, and they grow over 5,000 varieties. Thai food is usually flavored with garlic, chiles, lime, cilantro and fish sauce.

HEALTH TIP

Salad goodness

This colorful salad is an excellent source of iron, folic acid and vitamin C. If strawberries are not available, add slices of orange, kiwi, mango or apple instead.

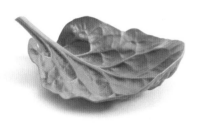

Winter Fruit Cream

Makes 3 servings

14-oz (398 mL) can of fruit, drained
1 tbsp (15 mL) brown sugar
$1/8$ tsp (0.5 mL) cinnamon
$1/3$ cup (75 mL) low-fat sour cream

PER SERVING	
Calories	77
Carbohydrate	19 g
Fiber	1 g
Net carbs	18 g
Protein	1 g
Fat, total	0 g
Fat, saturated	0 g
Cholesterol	0 mg
Sodium	45 mg

1. Place the fruit pieces in a small casserole dish or, if you have three small ovenproof dessert bowls, divide the fruit between the bowls.
2. Mix the brown sugar and cinnamon together in a small bowl. Place about half of the sugar and cinnamon mixture on top of the fruit.
3. Add the sour cream on top of the fruit and sugar. Then top the sour cream with the remainder of the sugar and cinnamon.
4. Place under a hot grill and grill for about 4 to 6 minutes, until it's bubbling around the edges and caramelized on top.

Summer Fruit Cream

Makes 3 servings

$1^1/2$ to 2 cups (375 to 500 mL)
   sliced or chopped fresh fruit
1 tbsp (15 mL) brown sugar
$1/8$ tsp (0.5 mL) cinnamon
$1/3$ cup (75 mL) low-fat sour cream

PER SERVING	
Calories	75
Carbohydrate	18 g
Fiber	2 g
Net carbs	16 g
Protein	1 g
Fat, total	0 g
Fat, saturated	0 g
Cholesterol	0 mg
Sodium	42 mg

1. Divide the fruit between three dessert bowls.
2. Mix brown sugar, cinnamon and sour cream together and place on top of each serving.

HEALTH TIP

Healthy desserts

Dessert is not just a sweet end to a meal, it can contribute to your day's nutrition. Here are two nutritious fruit desserts. Winter Fruit Cream is made with canned fruit (such as apricots, peaches or pears), and is heated under the grill. Summer Fruit Cream is made with fresh fruit (such as sliced strawberries or kiwis, blueberries, orange pieces, melon slices, pomegranate seeds or thin apple slices) and served cold. Both are equally sensational.

Food Choices	Large Meal	Small Meal
Carbohydrate	5	$3^1/2$
Protein	$3^1/2$	3
Fat	1	$1/2$

Your Dinner Menu	Large Meal (730 calories)	Total Carbs	Net Carbs	Small Meal (550 calories)	Total Carbs	Net Carbs
Thai Chicken	1 cup (250 mL)	20	18	$3/4$ cup (175 mL)	15	13
Noodles or rice, cooked	1 cup (250 mL)	44	42	$2/3$ cup (150 mL)	29	28
Poppy Seed Spinach Salad	1 serving	7	4	1 serving	7	4
Light creamy poppy seed salad dressing	2 tbsp (30 mL)	6	6	1 tbsp (15 mL)	3	3
Winter Fruit Cream or Summer Fruit Cream	1 serving	19	18	1 serving	19	18
		96 g	**88 g**		**73 g**	**66 g**

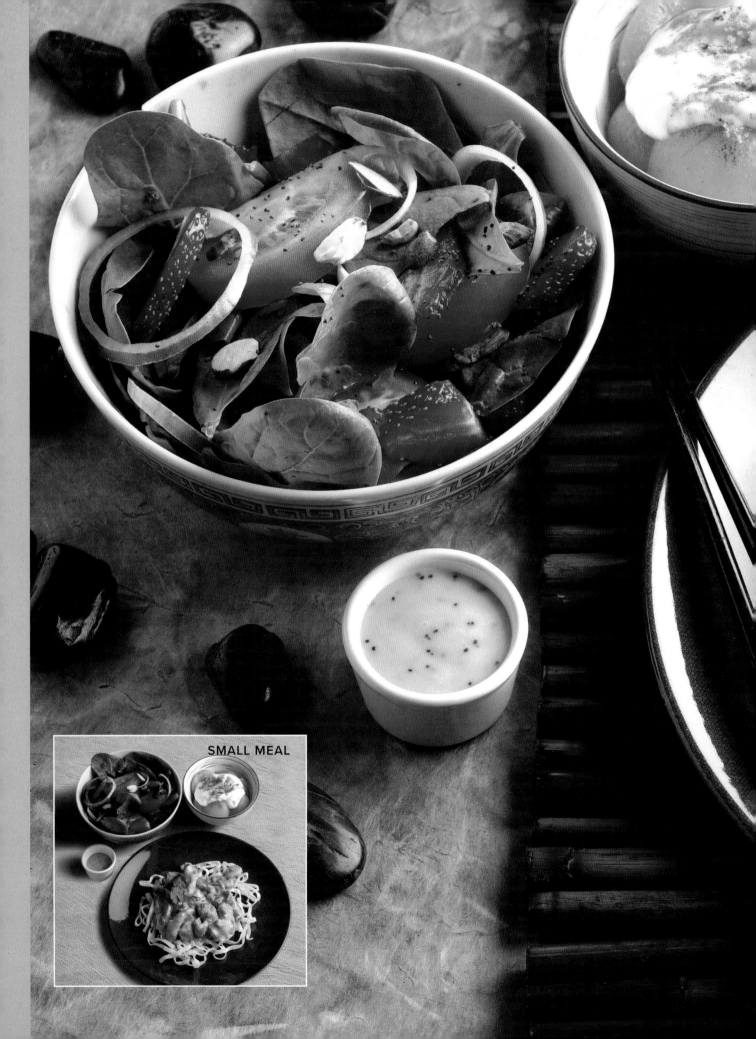

SMALL MEAL

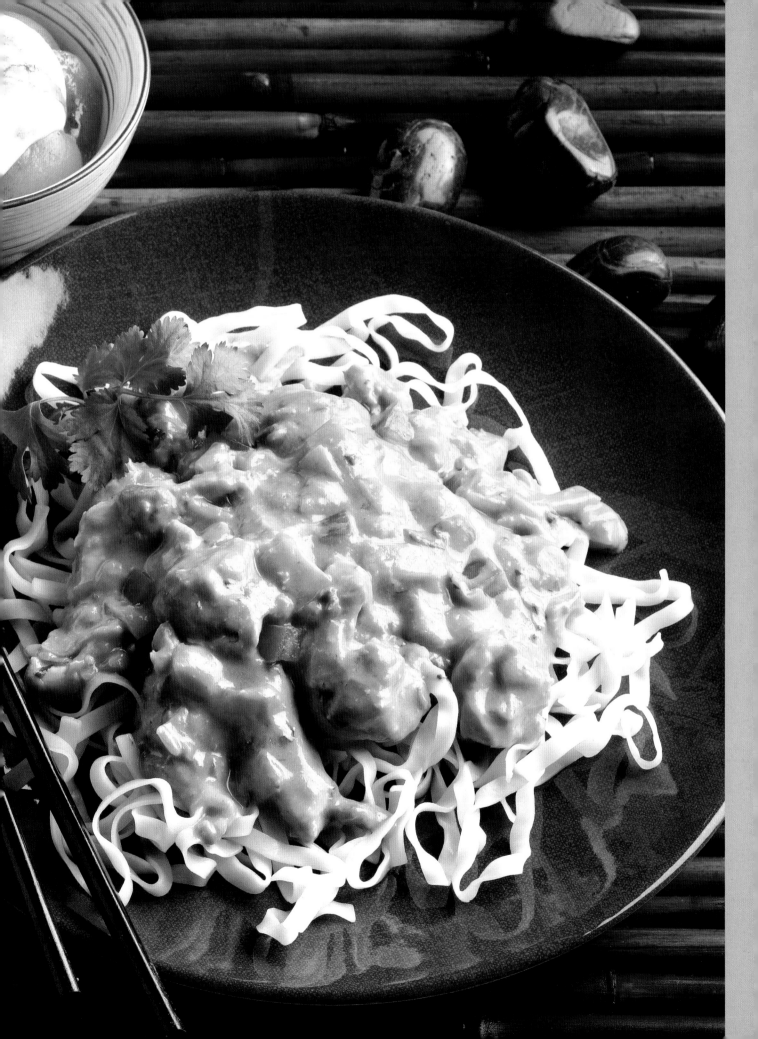

Poached Fish with Dill

OPTIONS

For a list of low-fat and high-fat fish, see page 120.

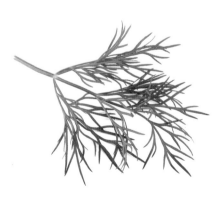

How to Poach Fish

Poaching means cooking in water, and the great thing is, you don't get a fishy smell in your house. You can add peppercorns, bay leaves, whole cloves, garlic, lemon juice or white wine to the poaching water to add flavor to the fish.

1. Place the fish skin side down in a pot or pan. Pour in enough water to cover, and bring to a boil over medium heat. Flavor and salt the water, if desired.
2. Cover with a lid. Fresh fillets take about 5 minutes to cook, while frozen fish fillets take about 10 minutes.
3. Using a slotted spoon, remove the fish from the water and place on your dinner plate. Top fish with Dill Topping. Optional: lemon wedges on the side.

Dill Topping

Makes ¼ cup (60 mL)

¼ cup (60 mL) low-fat mayonnaise
1 tsp (5 mL) dried dill or 1 tbsp (15 mL) finely chopped fresh dill

1. Combine ingredients.

PER 1 TBSP (15 ML)	
Calories	14
Carbohydrate	3 g
Fiber	0 g
Net carbs	3 g
Protein	0 g
Fat, total	0 g
Fat, saturated	0 g
Cholesterol	1 mg
Sodium	127 mg

Alternative Way to Cook Fish

Herb Cheese Fish Topping

Makes about ½ cup (125 mL) packed topping for 1 lb (500 g) of fresh or frozen fish

⅓ cup (75 mL) shredded cheese blend
2 tbsp (30 mL) dry bread crumbs
1 tsp (5 mL) dried basil
1 tsp (5 mL) dried dill or 1 tbsp (15 mL) finely chopped fresh dill
3 tbsp (45 mL) low-fat mayonnaise

PER 1 TBSP (15 ML)	
Calories	32
Carbohydrate	1 g
Fiber	0 g
Net carbs	1 g
Protein	1 g
Fat, total	2 g
Fat, saturated	1 g
Cholesterol	5 mg
Sodium	60 mg

1. Place your fish (thawed first, if frozen) in a flat pan or baking dish.
2. Mix the ingredients in a bowl. Spread the topping on your raw fish fillets.
3. Bake until cooked, about 20 minutes in a 400°F (200°C) oven, or about 10 minutes in a microwave.

This Walnut Barley Medley has a wonderful nutty flavor. It can be cooked a day ahead, cooled, covered and refrigerated, then reheated in the microwave or eaten cold.

Walnut Barley Medley

Makes 2¹/₂ cups (625 mL)

¹/₂ cup (125 mL) pot barley

1 tbsp (15 mL) wild rice

1 packet (4.5 g) reduced-salt beef
   or chicken bouillon powder

1¹/₂ cups (375 mL) water

¹/₄ cup (60 mL) chopped walnuts

¹/₄ cup (60 mL) currants

PER 1 CUP (250 ML)	
Calories	275
Carbohydrate	48 g
Fiber	5 g
Net carbs	43 g
Protein	6 g
Fat, total	8 g
Fat, saturated	1 g
Cholesterol	0 mg
Sodium	218 mg

1. In a small pot over medium-high heat, bring barley, wild rice, bouillon and water to a boil. As soon as it boils, reduce the heat to low, cover with a lid and let simmer for 1 hour, until the liquid has been absorbed. It will still be slightly moist.

2. Once the barley is cooked, stir in the walnuts and currants. Remove from the heat and serve.

Vegetables

Enjoy the meal with green beans or other low-sugar vegetables and pickled beets. Pickled beets have vinegar, spices and some sugar added, but still fit nicely into this meal plan.

Cookies and Milk for Dessert

Enjoy a glass of milk with a couple of cookies. Look for cookies that are labeled as three for less than 100 calories. These cookies will tend to be thinner or smaller than super-sized bakery cookies.

HEALTH TIP

Benefits of barley

Barley is rich in soluble fiber, which helps absorb the bad cholesterol out of your bloodstream. Soluble fiber also helps to manage diabetes by slowing the absorption of carbohydrates into your bloodstream.

  Pot barley is higher in fiber than pearl barley and quick-cooking barley, but will need an hour to cook to tenderness.

Food Choices	Large Meal	Small Meal
Carbohydrate	4¹/₂	3¹/₂
Protein	3¹/₂	2¹/₂
Fat	2	1

Your Dinner Menu	Large Meal (730 calories)	Total Carbs	Net Carbs	Small Meal (550 calories)	Total Carbs	Net Carbs
Poached fish (salmon is shown)	3¹/₂ oz (105 g) high-fat fish or 6 oz (175 g) low-fat fish	0	0	2¹/₂ oz (75 g) high-fat fish or 4 oz (125 g) low-fat fish	0	0
Dill Topping	2 tbsp (30 mL)	5	4	2 tbsp (30 mL)	5	4
Walnut Barley Medley	³/₄ cup (175 mL)	36	33	¹/₂ cup (125 mL)	24	22
Green beans	1 cup (250 mL)	10	7	1 cup (250 mL)	10	7
Pickled beets	¹/₂ cup (125 mL)	13	12	¹/₂ cup (125 mL)	13	12
Margarine	1 tsp (5 mL)	0	0	–	–	–
Skim or 1% milk	1 cup (250 mL)	12	12	1 cup (250 mL)	12	12
Thin cookies	2	8	8	2	8	8
		84 g	**76 g**		**72 g**	**65 g**

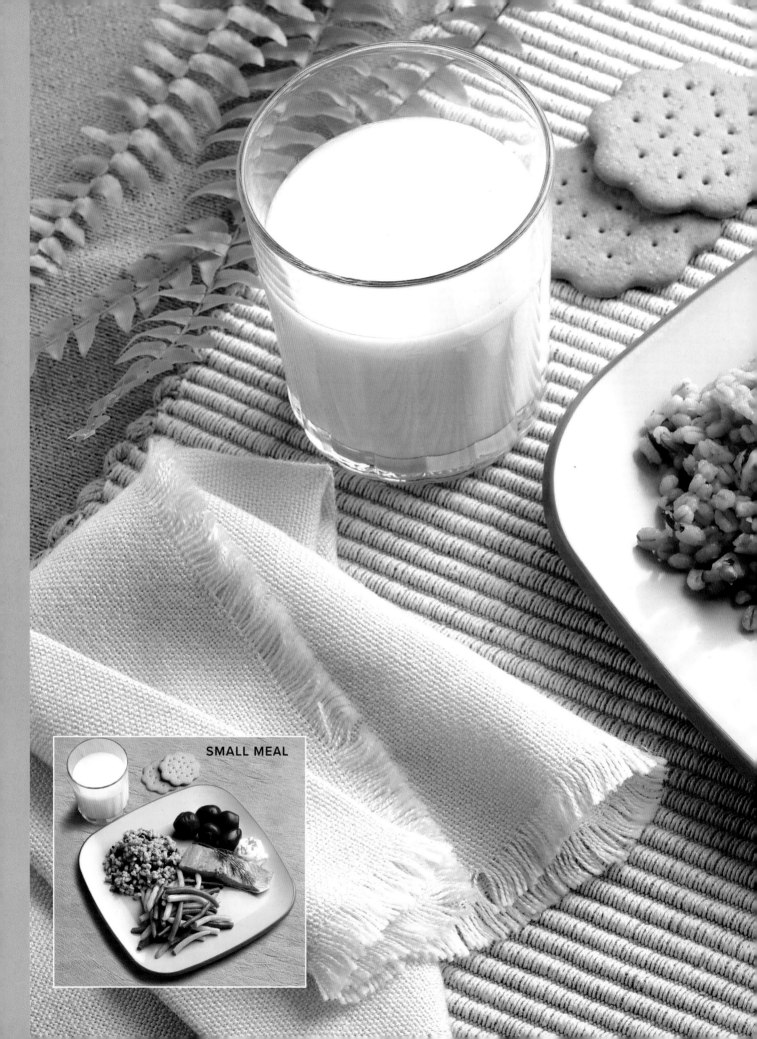

SMALL MEAL

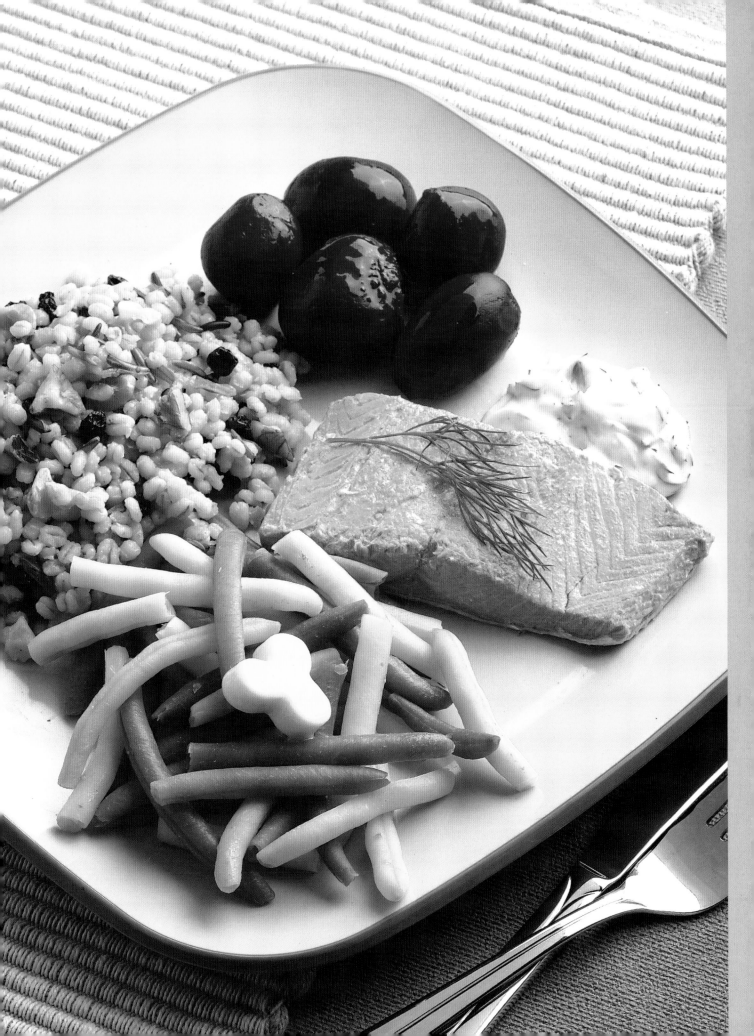

Sub Sandwich

When ordering a sub sandwich at a fast food restaurant, go light on the dressing and beware of supersizing, and of large-size soft drinks, juices and sweetened milk.

Sugar in Beverages

When eating out, your choice of beverage can add many extra calories (from sugar and fat) to your meal. we suggest water or a diet drink with this meal. See page 22 for a table that shows a breakdown of the amount of sugar in beverages.

Nutrient Guides

Visit the website of the fast-food restaurant where you like to eat most often. There you will find the nutrient guides for their meals. Some restaurants have the information on their menu, or you can ask at the counter. Keep in mind that they may not list the extras, such as mayonnaise, that we add to our sub sandwiches. Also, products like potato chips or corn chips come in various package sizes. A $1\frac{1}{2}$-oz (45 g) bag of regular chips will have about 240 calories. Doritos have 260 calories, Sun Chips 210 calories and baked chips 130 calories.

FOOD FACT

The apps with the most accurate nutritional content will be based on the federal government searchable nutrient databases. These are available online: USDA FoodData Central (American) or Nutrient Value of Some Common Foods (Canadian).

Food Apps for Your Phone

If you are phone savvy, you probably already have a variety of apps on your phone. You might want to search the web for some of the latest food and exercise apps. MyFitnessPal is a comprehensive and accurate app, and one of the most popular.

Here are some examples of topics that apps cover:

- Places to eat in a new city
- Nutritional content of restaurant foods
- Calorie and carb counters
- Nutrient content of individual foods
- Exercise apps, to give you exercise suggestions and also to calculate calories burned

Apps on their own won't make you healthy. But they are a tool to give you information. Typically, the more time you spend inputting data into your app, the more benefit you'll get.

Once you've established a healthy lifestyle of eating consistent smaller portions with lots of vegetables, and walking or doing other exercise daily, you may find you don't need the apps. This is good. Then you can spend less time on your phone, and you'll have more time to go for a walk, cook and eat a meal, and just enjoy time for yourself and those around you.

Here is a quick sub sandwich to make at home. It has the same calories as a commercial 6-inch (15 cm) sub, but without all the extras.

Homemade Sub Sandwich

(made with 3 oz/90 g roast chicken)

6-inch (15 cm) whole wheat sub bun
3 oz (90 g) thinly sliced meat
    of your choice
1½ oz (45 g) sliced cheese of your choice
A variety of vegetables of your choice
Black pepper
1 tbsp (15 mL) light mayonnaise or
    2 tbsp (30 mL) fat-free mayonnaise
1 tbsp (15 mL) fat-free honey mustard

PER SANDWICH	
Calories	484
Carbohydrate	40 g
Fiber	6 g
Net carbs	34 g
Protein	44 g
Fat, total	16 g
Fat, saturated	8 g
Cholesterol	105 mg
Sodium	773 mg

RECIPE TIP

Cold cuts contain a lot of salt. For example, 1 oz (30 g) of ham has about 300 mg of sodium. In comparison, 1 oz (30 g) of leftover roast chicken has only 25 mg of sodium, so use leftover roast meat when you can.

1. Cut the sub bun in half crosswise. If desired, toast under the broiler.
2. Evenly spread the meat and cheese on the bottom half of the bun.
3. Add the vegetables, pepper and condiments. Cover with the top half of the bun.

Food Choices	Large Meal	Small Meal
Carbohydrate	4½	3
Protein	4½	4½
Fat	3	1

Your Dinner Menu	Large Meal (730 calories)	Total Carbs	Net Carbs	Small Meal (550 calories)	Total Carbs	Net Carbs
Homemade Sub Sandwich or Purchased sub sandwich	1 sandwich (6 inch/15 cm) or up to 450 calories, plus 1 tbsp (15 mL) each light mayonnaise and honey mustard	48	42	1 sandwich (6 inch/15 cm) or up to 450 calories, plus 1 tbsp (15 mL) each light mayonnaise and honey mustard	48	42
1 bag of chips or nachos or 1 large cookie	1 choice (200–210 calories)	28	25	–	–	–
Diet drink	Medium	1	1	Diet drink Medium	1	1
		77 g	**68 g**		**49 g**	**43 g**

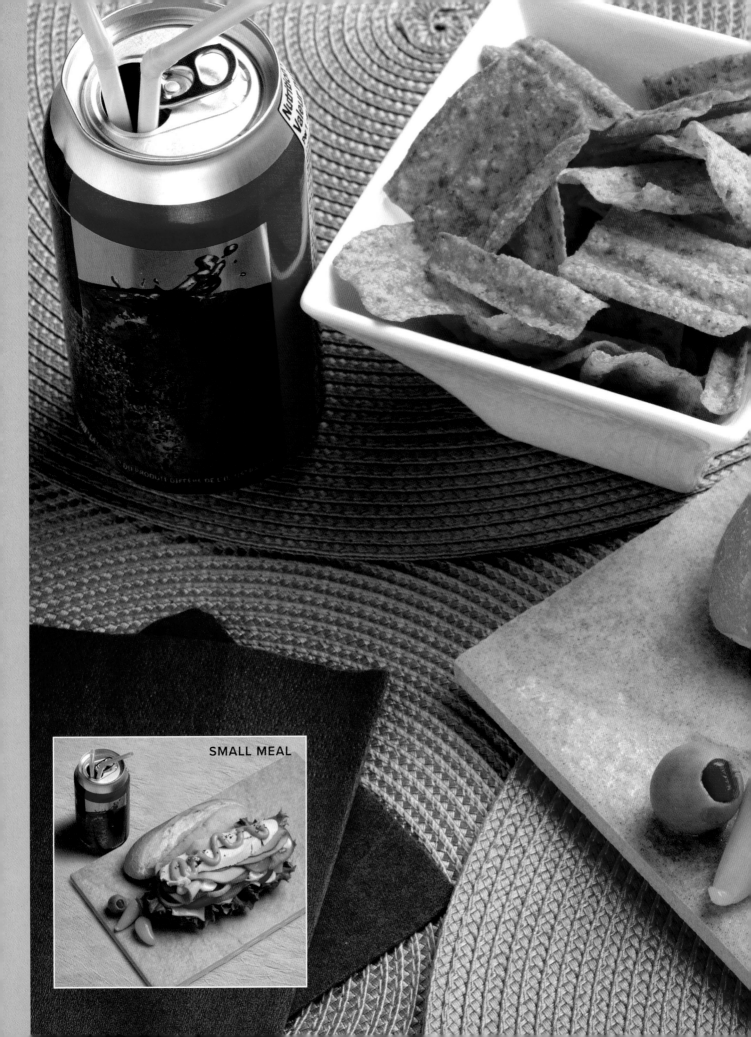

SMALL MEAL

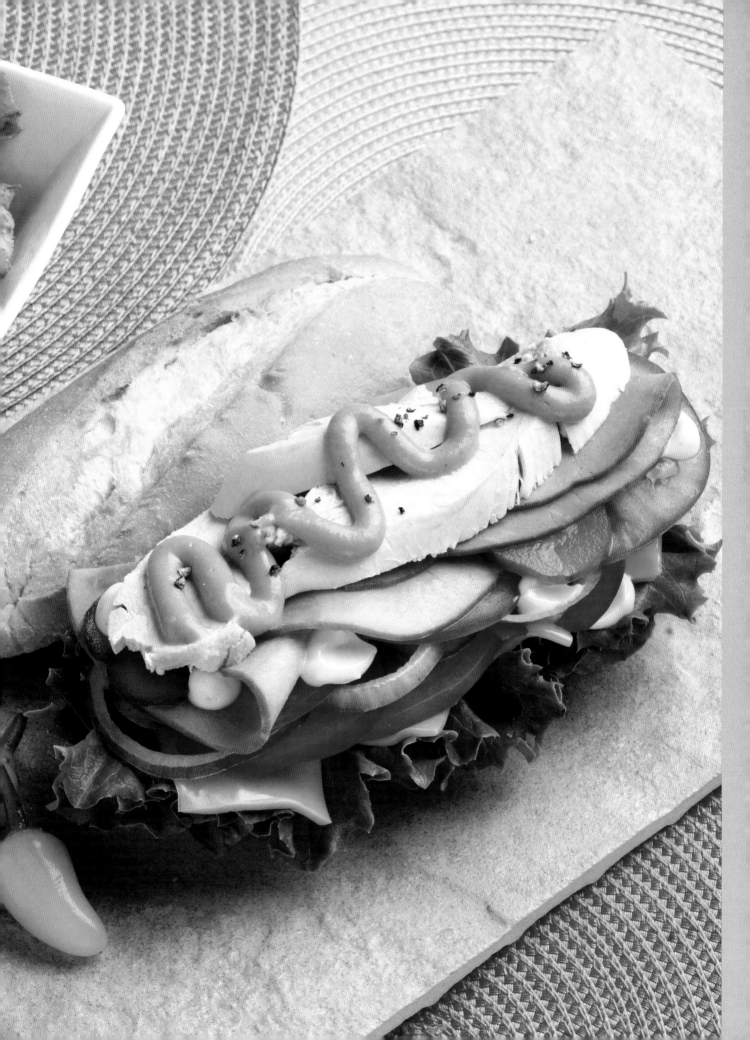

DINNER 36

Beef Parmesan

This meal has lots of variations, because you can use the Classic Beef Patties below, or frozen beef patties, breaded chicken cutlets, veal cutlets, pork cutlets or pounded minute steak. The Beef Parmesan is served with Low-Fat Mashed Potatoes (see Dinner 8), broccoli, a tossed salad and ice cream for dessert.

(see Dinner 8)

FOOD FACT

Pasta sauces vary in calories

Some pasta sauces have more oil or sugar added. Check the Nutrition Facts on the pasta sauce label and look for a mid-range to lower-calorie choice, such as 30 to 60 calories per ½-cup (125 mL) serving.

Beef Parmesan

For each patty:

Meat patty or cutlet of your choice

3 tbsp (45 mL) pasta sauce

Dash of hot pepper sauce or
   hot pepper flakes (optional)

1½ tbsp (22 mL) grated Parmesan,
   Cheddar or mozzarella cheese

PER PATTY WITH TOPPINGS	
Calories	278
Carbohydrate	10 g
Fiber	0 g
Net carbs	10 g
Protein	24 g
Fat, total	15 g
Fat, saturated	6 g
Cholesterol	95 mg
Sodium	507 mg

1. If using a store-bought frozen patty or cutlet, cook in a frying pan, oven or barbecue according to the package directions. If making homemade beef patties, cook according to directions below.
2. Heat pasta sauce in the microwave or on the stovetop over medium heat until hot and bubbling. Add hot pepper sauce or flakes, if using.
3. Place meat patty or cutlet on your plate and top with the pasta sauce, then the shredded cheese.

RECIPE TIP

Seasoning salt

If you add ½ tsp (2 mL) Hy's Seasoning Salt to the recipe, you will add 85 mg more sodium per patty.

Classic Beef Patties

Makes 10 large patties

12 unsalted soda crackers, crumbled

2 lbs (1 kg) lean ground beef

2 eggs

1 small onion, finely chopped

2 tsp (10 mL) Worcestershire sauce

Hy's Seasoning Salt (optional)

¼ tsp (1 mL) black pepper

PER PATTY	
Calories	182
Carbohydrate	4 g
Fiber	0 g
Net carbs	4 g
Protein	18 g
Fat, total	10 g
Fat, saturated	4 g
Cholesterol	85 mg
Sodium	94 mg

1. In a large mixing bowl, combine all ingredients together with your hands.
2. Form into 10 patties and place on a plate or tray.
3. Fry patties in a pan over medium heat, or cook under a grill or on the barbecue, until no longer pink inside.

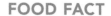

Different Kinds of Ice Cream

Regular ice cream is an easy light dessert; a $\frac{1}{2}$-cup (125 mL) serving will have 125 to 150 calories. Served in a regular ice cream cone will only add another 20 calories.

Limit or Avoid Rich Ice Cream

Decadent ice creams get their reputation for a reason. Up to $\frac{1}{3}$ of their calories comes from unhealthy saturated fat, and a $\frac{1}{2}$-cup (125 mL) serving can have up to 4 tsp (20 mL) of sugar. At 200 to 300 (or more) calories per $\frac{1}{2}$ cup (125 mL), they contain up to double the calories of regular ice cream.

Bowl Sizes Affect How Much You Eat

When you eat from a smaller bowl, you will eat less. Take a look at these three bowls, which each hold a $\frac{1}{2}$-cup (125 mL) scoop of regular ice cream. By putting the ice cream in the small bowl, it looks more filling. If you use the large bowl, you just might fill it up with three or four scoops of ice cream, and you would overeat.

FOOD FACT

Low-fat or sugar-free ice creams

These ice creams have 100 to 120 calories per $\frac{1}{2}$ cup/125 mL), so, are only a little lower than regular ice cream at 125 to 150. Frozen yogurt, with no more than 3 grams of fat per $\frac{1}{2}$ cup (125 mL), contains around 100 to 110 calories in that amount. Check the carb values, as these can vary.

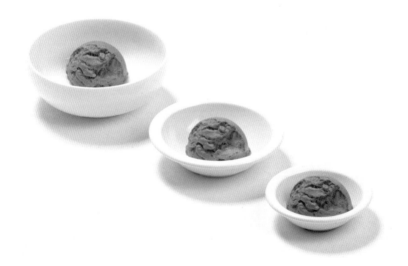

Food Choices	Large Meal	Small Meal
Carbohydrate	3	2
Protein	5	$3\frac{1}{2}$

Your Dinner Menu	Large Meal (730 calories)	Total Carbs	Net Carbs	Small Meal (550 calories)	Total Carbs	Net Carbs
Beef Parmesan	$1\frac{1}{2}$ patties with sauce and cheese	14	14	1 patty with sauce and cheese	9	9
Low-Fat Mashed Potatoes	1 cup (250 mL)	38	35	$\frac{1}{2}$ cup (125 mL)	19	18
Broccoli	1 to 2 cups (250 to 500 mL)	6	4	1 to 2 cups (250 to 500 mL)	6	4
Tossed salad	Medium	5	4	Medium	5	4
Fat-free Italian salad dressing	1 tbsp (15 mL)	2	2	1 tbsp (15 mL)	2	2
Frozen yogurt or ice cream (light or regular)	$\frac{1}{2}$ cup (125 mL)	19	19	$\frac{1}{2}$ cup (125 mL)	19	19
		84 g	**78 g**		**60 g**	**56 g**

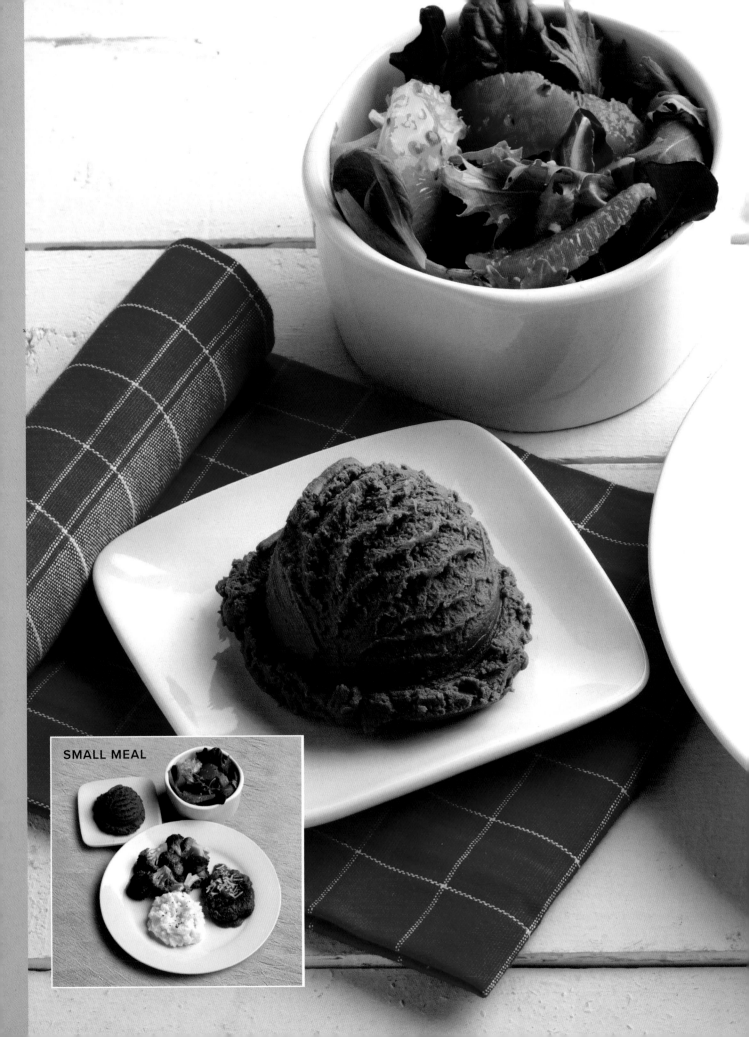

SMALL MEAL

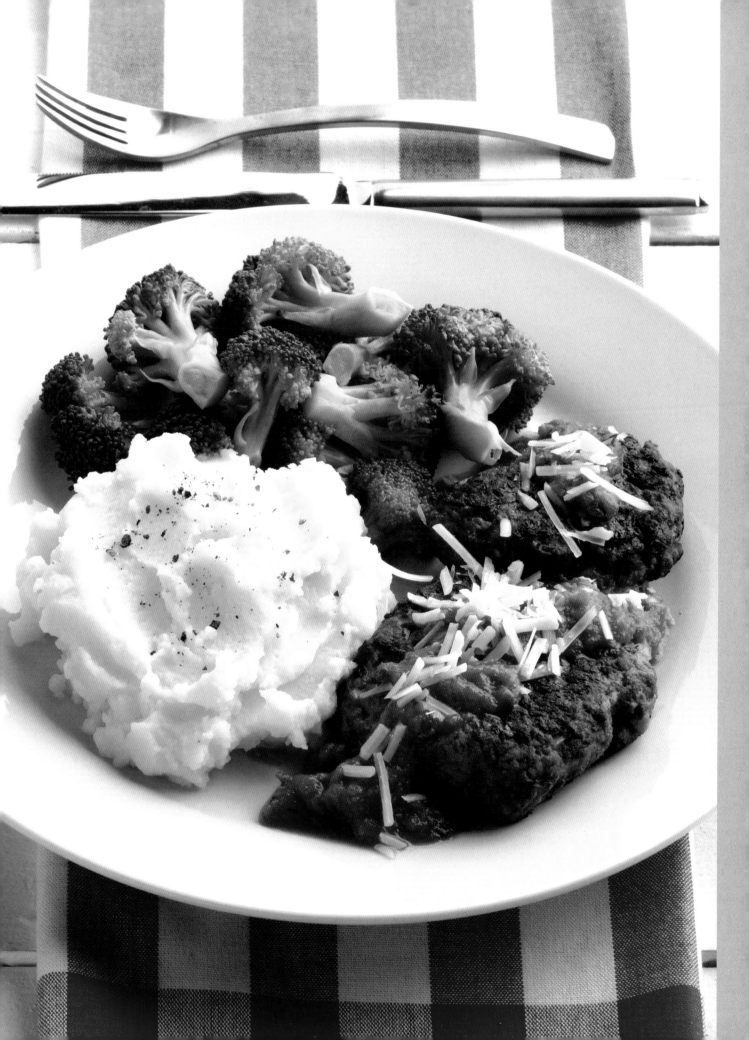

DINNER 37

Santa Fe Salad

This flavorful and colorful salad includes corn, beans and chicken, and is inspired by Mexican-American cuisine. It is served with tortilla chips and Banana Bread.

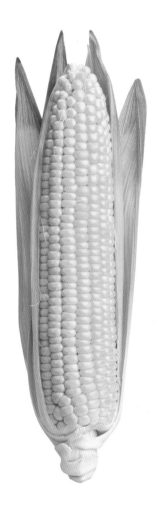

Santa Fe Salad

Makes 4 servings

12-oz (341 mL) can of corn, drained

19-oz (540 mL) can of black beans, rinsed in cold water and drained

1 tbsp (15 mL) fresh cilantro or parsley, finely chopped

2 to 3 green onions, chopped

1 red pepper, cut into thin 1-inch (2.5 cm) slices

½ head of lettuce, torn into bite-size pieces

½ cup (125 mL) shredded or grated cheese

3 tbsp (45 mL) light coleslaw dressing

10 oz (300 g) chicken breasts or thighs, boneless and skin removed, sliced into thin pieces

2 tbsp (30 mL) hickory smoke barbecue sauce

PER SERVING	
Calories	348
Carbohydrate	43 g
Fiber	9 g
Net carbs	34 g
Protein	29 g
Fat, total	8 g
Fat, saturated	4 g
Cholesterol	60 mg
Sodium	860 mg

1. In a large bowl, gently toss corn, black beans, cilantro, green onions, red pepper, lettuce and cheese. Mix in the coleslaw dressing. Divide salad onto four dinner plates (or large salad bowls).
2. In a nonstick pan over medium heat, cook chicken pieces with about 2 tbsp (30 mL) of water. When the chicken is no longer pink inside, add the barbecue sauce. Reduce heat and simmer for a couple of minutes.
3. Divide chicken between the four plates, placing on top of the salad.

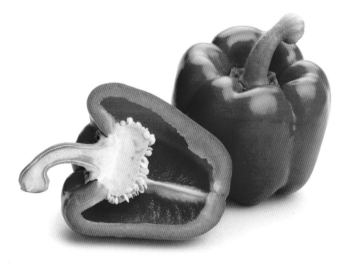

Banana Bread is a heart-warming accompaniment to the Santa Fe Salad. It serves as a starch and a sweet dessert. One slice of Banana Bread can be eaten as a large snack (200 calories); see the snack section, pages 276–285. Banana Bread can also nicely substitute for 1 cup (250 mL) of Rice Pudding (Dinner 5).

Banana Bread

Makes 12 slices

2¼ cups (550 mL) flour

1 tbsp (15 mL) baking powder

½ tsp (2 mL) salt

½ tsp (2 mL) nutmeg

¼ cup (60 mL) margarine or butter

⅓ cup (75 mL) sugar

1 large egg

¼ cup (60 mL) skim milk

3 small bananas

½ cup (125 mL) raisins

¼ cup (60 mL) chopped walnuts or pecans

PER SLICE	
Calories	211
Carbohydrate	36 g
Fiber	2 g
Net carbs	34 g
Protein	4 g
Fat, total	6 g
Fat, saturated	1 g
Cholesterol	16 mg
Sodium	239 mg

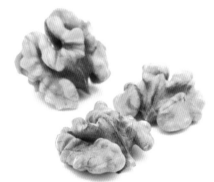

1. Mix flour with baking powder, salt and nutmeg in a medium bowl.
2. In a large bowl, cream margarine and sugar with a wooden spoon. Beat in the egg and milk until smooth.
3. In a small bowl, mash the bananas with a fork.
4. Add mashed bananas and the flour mixture to the large bowl, and stir together. Then add the nuts and raisins.
5. Scrape into a lightly greased 9- by 5-inch (2 L) loaf pan and bake for 50 minutes to 1 hour at 350°F (180°C), until a knife inserted in the center comes out clean. Let cool in the pan, then remove and cut into 12 slices.

Food Choices	Large Meal	Small Meal
Carbohydrate	4½	4
Protein	3½	3½
Fat	1½	–

Your Dinner Menu	Large Meal (730 calories)	Total Carbs	Net Carbs	Small Meal (550 calories)	Total Carbs	Net Carbs
Santa Fe Salad	1 serving	43	34	1 serving	43	34
Tortilla chips	8 chips	11	9	5 chips	7	6
Banana Bread	1 slice	36	34	1 slice	36	34
Margarine or butter	1½ tsp (7 mL)	0	0	–	–	–
		90 g	**77 g**		**86 g**	**74 g**

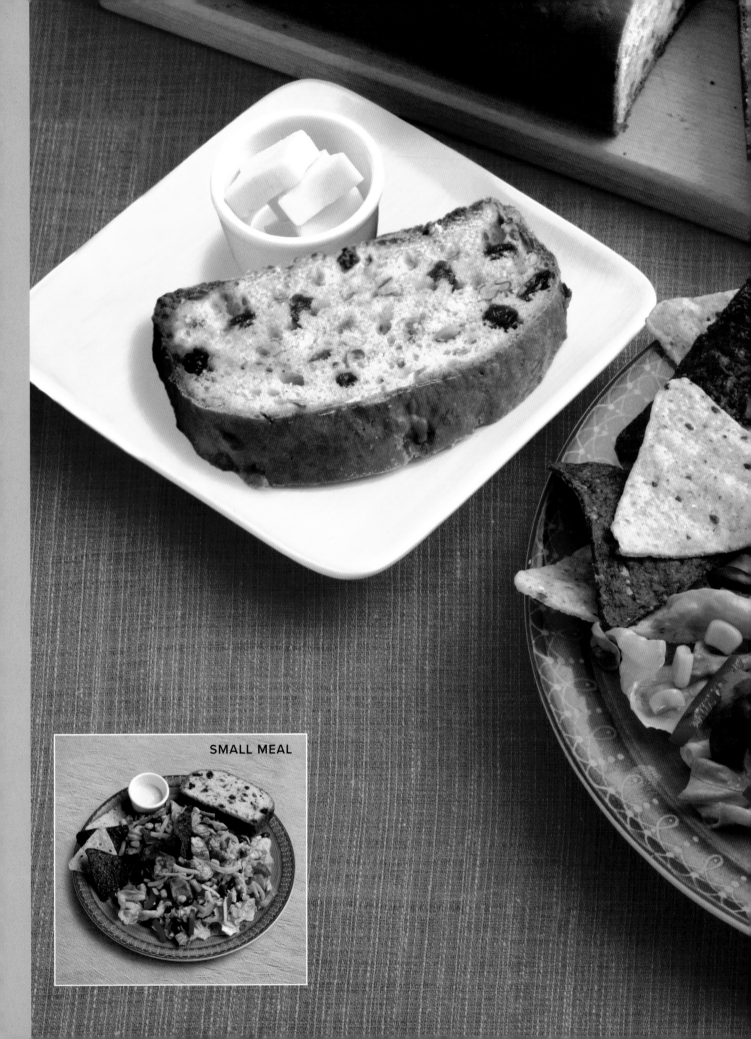

SMALL MEAL

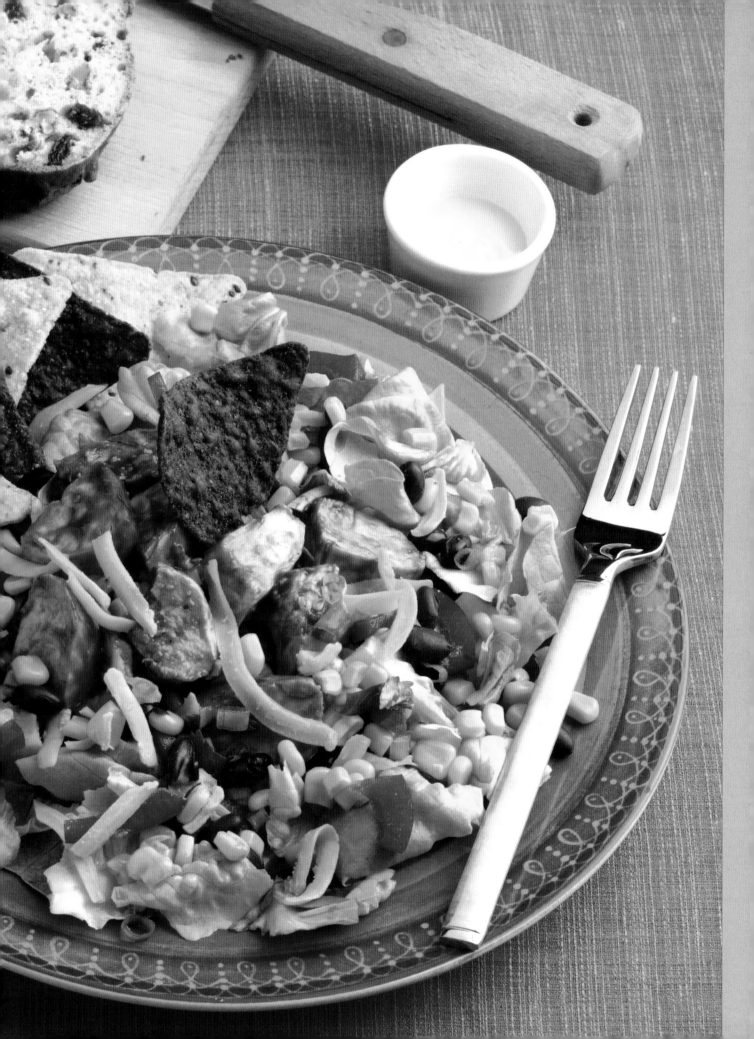

DINNER 38

Pork Chop Casserole

This scrumptious and uncomplicated, no-fail casserole will take an hour to cook. After it has cooked for 40 minutes, put the rice on to cook. At this time, prepare the Grilled Tomato halves. They can go into the oven alongside the casserole dish and cook for the last 15 minutes. The plan is to have the rice, pork chops and tomatoes ready at the same time.

Pork Chop Casserole

Makes 3 large or 5 small meals

5 pork chops (thin loin cut), total raw weight with bone about 1¾ lbs (875 g)

1 small onion, thinly sliced

3 stalks celery, sliced

10-ounce (284 mL) can cream soup

PER PORK CHOP WITH SAUCE	
Calories	192
Carbohydrate	6 g
Fiber	1 g
Net carbs	5 g
Protein	21 g
Fat, total	8 g
Fat, saturated	3 g
Cholesterol	62 mg
Sodium	439 mg

1. Trim visible fat from the pork chops. Place in a casserole dish. Evenly add onion and celery on top of the pork chops. Spread the cream soup on top.
2. Bake in a covered casserole dish at 350°F (180°C) for 1 hour, or more if needed, until the pork chops are fork-tender.

Grilled Tomato

Makes 2 servings

1 medium tomato, washed

1 tsp (5 mL) dry bread crumbs

1 tsp (5 mL) ground flax seeds (flaxseed meal)

2 tsp (10 mL) store-bought pre-grated Parmesan cheese

½ tsp (2 mL) dried oregano

1 tsp (5 mL) butter or margarine

PER SERVING	
Calories	51
Carbohydrate	4 g
Fiber	1 g
Net carbs	3 g
Protein	2 g
Fat, total	3 g
Fat, saturated	2 g
Cholesterol	7 mg
Sodium	72 mg

1. Cut the tomato in half crosswise. Place cut side up in a casserole or small baking pan.
2. In a small bowl, combine bread crumbs, flax seeds, Parmesan cheese, oregano and butter. Spoon over the open tomato halves and, with the back of the spoon, press down gently.
3. Bake at 350°F (180°C) for 15 minutes. Then put under the broiler until the topping is golden brown. The broiling will take only a minute or less — watch it carefully so it doesn't burn.

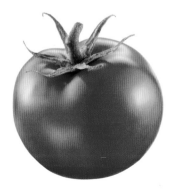

Sugar Snap Peas

This meal is served with raw sugar snap peas on the side. These crunchy peas are great raw or lightly steamed. They are low-calorie, with just 14 calories in 10 snap peas. Sugar snap peas can be added anytime to a stir-fry, or sliced and added to a salad or casserole. They are also great as a snack in the middle of the day or in the evening. If you can't find sugar snap peas, you can substitute any other low-calorie vegetable (see page 149).

Mandarins & Cottage Cheese is a simple, delicious dessert.

Mandarins & Cottage Cheese

Makes 4 servings

1 cup (250 mL) canned mandarin orange segments in light syrup, drained
¾ cup (175 mL) 1 or 2% cottage cheese
Pinch of ground nutmeg (optional)

PER SERVING	
Calories	59
Carbohydrate	9 g
Fiber	0 g
Net carbs	9 g
Protein	6 g
Fat, total	0 g
Fat, saturated	0 g
Cholesterol	2 mg
Sodium	180 mg

1. Gently combine the orange pieces and cottage cheese, reserving a few mandarin segments to decorate the top of each serving.
2. Divide among three dessert-size dishes and decorate with the reserved orange segments. Add nutmeg, if desired.

This meal is served with a cup of antioxidant-rich green tea.

HEALTH TIP
Benefits of tea

Black tea and green tea contain heart-healthy antioxidants. Green teas appear to have the greatest health benefit, which will come from drinking tea every day. There are significantly fewer antioxidants in tea when it is decaffeinated, since the process of removing the caffeine also removes many of the antioxidants. However, if you wish to limit or avoid caffeine, feel free to choose a cup of decaffeinated black tea or coffee, or one of the many delicious flavors of herbal tea.

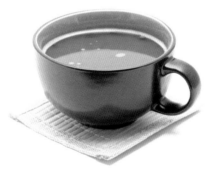

Food Choices	Large Meal	Small Meal
Carbohydrate	5	3½
Protein	5	3½

Your Dinner Menu	Large Meal (730 calories)	Total Carbs	Net Carbs	Small Meal (550 calories)	Total Carbs	Net Carbs
Pork chops with sauce	1½ chops	10	9	1 chop	6	5
Rice	1⅓ cups (325 mL)	59	58	1 cup (250 mL)	45	44
Grilled Tomato	1 half	4	3	1 half	4	3
Sugar snap peas	15	4	3	15	4	3
Mandarins & Cottage Cheese	1 serving	9	9	1 serving	9	9
Green tea	1 cup (250 mL)	0	0	1 cup (250 mL)	0	0
		86 g	82 g		68 g	64 g

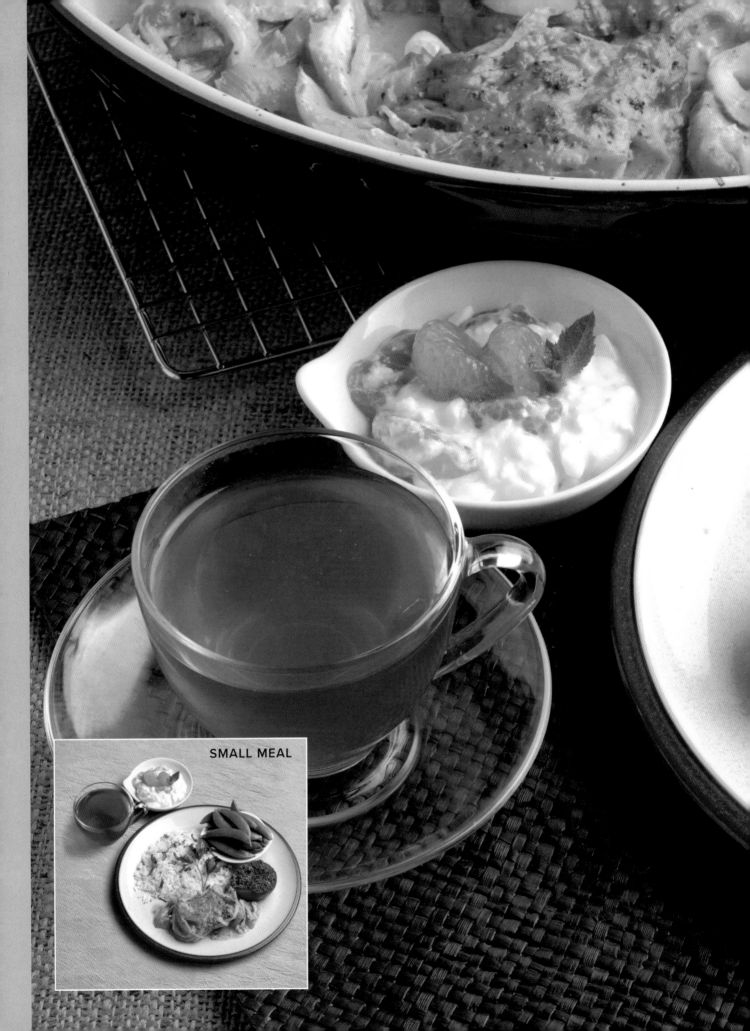

SMALL MEAL

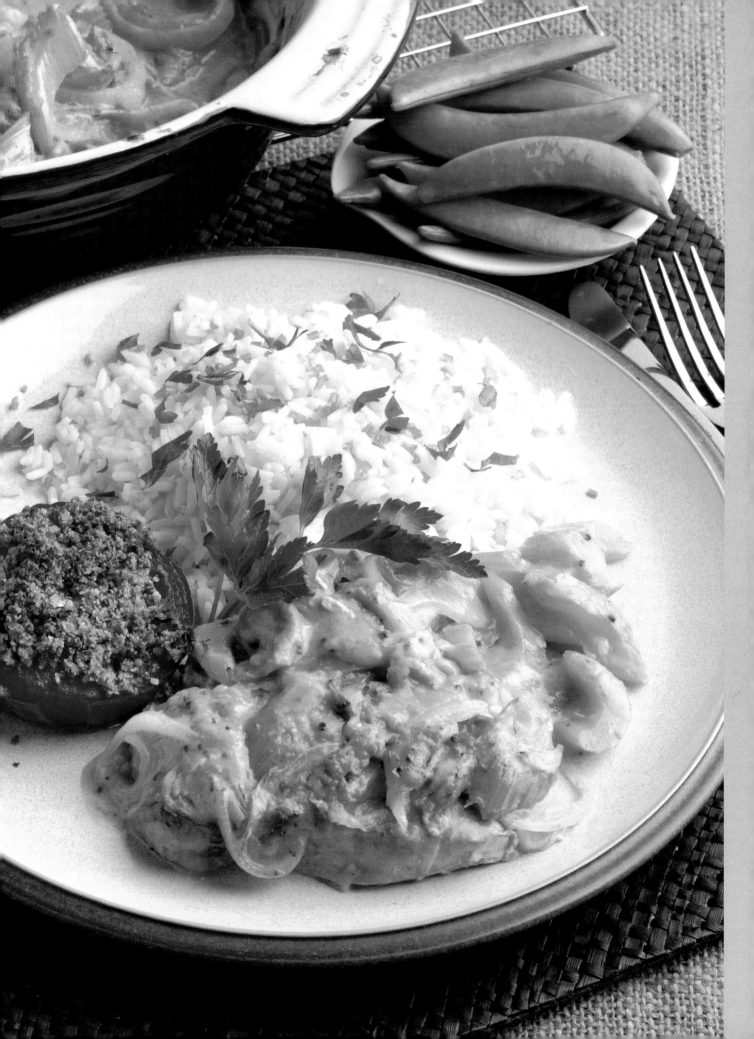

DINNER 39

Shrimp Linguini

Linguini is a flat pasta noodle that, in southern Italy, is traditionally served with a clam or seafood sauce. I have chosen shrimp for the sauce, as it is a delight to eat and is readily available, precooked and frozen. The Shrimp Linguini Sauce will take about 30 minutes to prepare and cook. The Shrimp Linguini is served with Caesar Salad, and the beverage is a refreshing Italian Iced Soda Float.

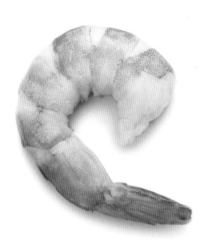

RECIPE TIP

Cooking the pasta

Time the cooking of your pasta so that it will be ready at the same time as the sauce. Cook pasta according to the directions on the package; adding salt to the water is optional.

Shrimp Linguini Sauce

Makes 4 cups (1 L)

1 tbsp (15 mL) olive or vegetable oil

⅓ cup (75 mL) water

1 small onion, chopped

3 large cloves garlic, minced

1 cup (250 mL) sliced fresh mushrooms
   (or one 10-oz/284 mL can, drained)

2 tbsp (30 mL) flour

1 packet (4.5 g) reduced-sodium chicken bouillon powder

⅛ tsp (0.5 mL) black pepper

1 tsp (5 mL) dried dill

1¾ cups (425 mL) skim milk

½ red or green pepper, cut into 1-inch (2.5 cm) thick strips,
   or ½ cup (125 mL) other vegetables of your choice

10 oz (300 g) cooked frozen shrimp, thawed, shells and
   tails removed

¾ cup (175 mL) shredded Italian 4-cheese blend,
   or cheese of your choice

PER 1 CUP (250 ML)	
Calories	251
Carbohydrate	14 g
Fiber	1 g
Net carbs	13 g
Protein	27 g
Fat, total	10 g
Fat, saturated	4 g
Cholesterol	133 mg
Sodium	483 mg

1. In a large pan over medium heat, add olive oil, water, onion and garlic and cook until soft.
2. Meanwhile, in a small pan, sauté the mushrooms in a bit of water over medium heat until soft. Drain off the water and set the mushrooms aside.
3. In a small bowl, mix flour, bouillon powder, pepper and dill. Add this mixture to onion mixture and stir until the flour is absorbed.
4. Gradually whisk in milk and cook, stirring constantly, until the mixture thickens slightly, about 5 minutes. Do not let boil. Mix in vegetables and shrimp, and cook, stirring often, until vegetables are tender, about 5 minutes.
5. Stir in mushrooms and shredded cheese until melted. The sauce will thicken up now.
6. Serve over cooked linguini.

Caesar salad is usually made with dark green romaine lettuce. Dark salad greens are rich in folic acid, a nutrient that is essential for pregnant mothers, but also important for everybody's heart health.

Caesar Salad

For 1 serving:

2 cups (500 mL) dark salad greens, torn into bite-size pieces

2 tbsp (30 mL) shredded fresh Parmesan cheese or 1 tbsp (15 mL) grated dried Parmesan

¼ cup (60 mL) croutons

Squirt of fresh lemon juice (optional)

PER SERVING	
Calories	88
Carbohydrate	9 g
Fiber	2 g
Net carbs	7 g
Protein	6 g
Fat, total	3 g
Fat, saturated	2 g
Cholesterol	7 mg
Sodium	231 mg

1. Combine greens, cheese, croutons and lemon juice, if using.
2. Top with Caesar salad dressing, as shown in menu box.

This cool and delightful beverage is best with crushed ice; however, it can be served over ice cubes.

Italian Iced Soda Float

Makes one 12-oz (375 mL) serving

½ cup (125 mL) crushed ice

¾ cup (175 mL) soda water

½ tsp (2 mL) cherry- or berry-flavored Crystal Light or Diet Kool-Aid

¼ cup (60 mL) 2% milk

PER SERVING	
Calories	37
Carbohydrate	4 g
Fiber	0 g
Net carbs	4 g
Protein	2 g
Fat, total	1 g
Fat, saturated	1 g
Cholesterol	5 mg
Sodium	74 mg

1. Pour ice into a tall glass.
2. Slowly pour the soda water over the ice,
then add the Crystal Light and the milk.
Stir and enjoy.

FOOD FACT

All-in-one Caesar salad packages

The dressing is usually high in calories in these packages, so don't use the full package.

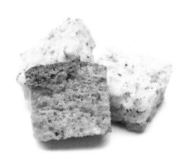

Food Choices	Large Meal	Small Meal
Carbohydrate	4½	3½
Protein	3	2½

Your Dinner Menu	Large Meal (730 calories)	Total Carbs	Net Carbs	Small Meal (550 calories)	Total Carbs	Net Carbs
Shrimp Linguini Sauce	1 cup (250 mL)	14	13	¾ cup (175 mL)	10	9
Cooked pasta (linguini)	1½ cups (375 mL)	59	55	1 cup (250 mL)	40	38
Caesar Salad	1 serving	9	7	1 serving	9	7
Caesar salad dressing, light	1 tbsp (15 mL)	3	3	1 tbsp (15 mL)	3	3
Italian Iced Soda Float	12 oz (375 mL)	4	4	12 oz (375 mL)	4	4
		89 g	**82 g**		**66 g**	**61 g**

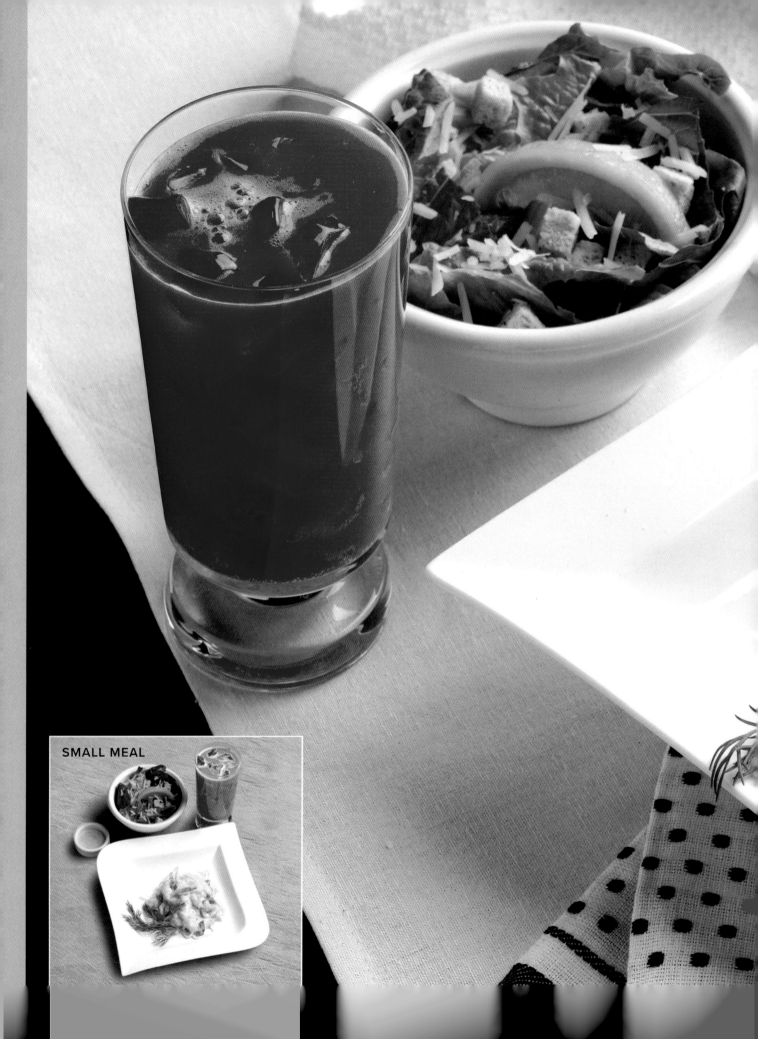

SMALL MEAL

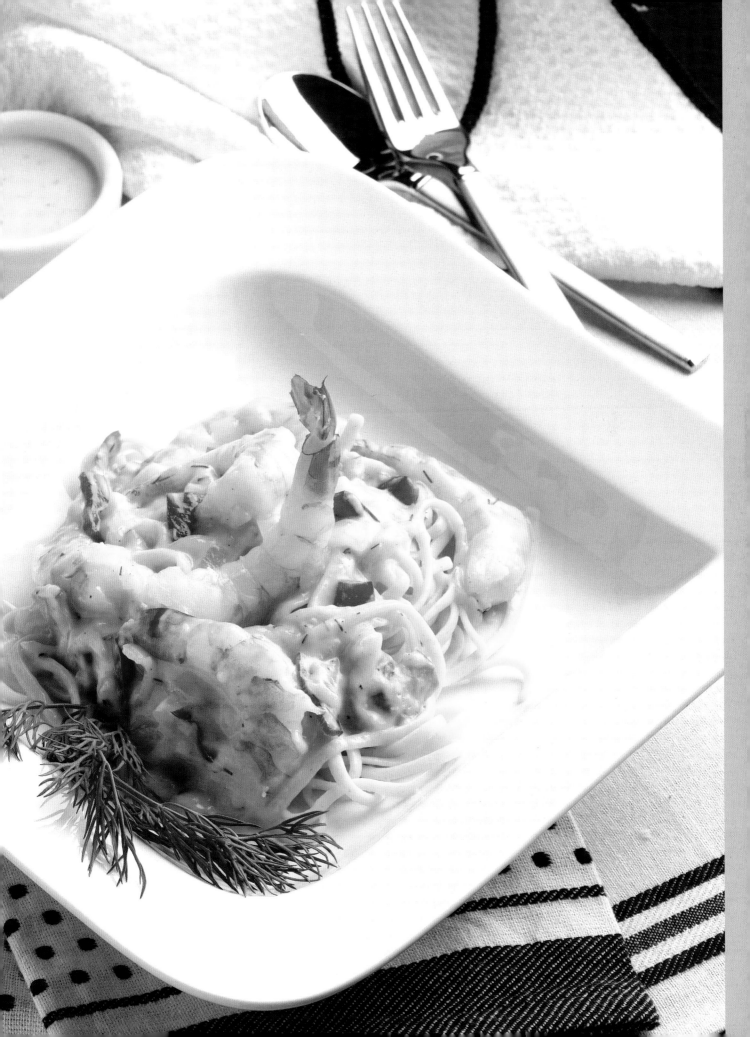

DINNER 40

Chicken Cordon Bleu

Cordon Bleu is French for "Blue Ribbon," which is a famous cooking school in France. Chicken Cordon Bleu has been adapted from the classic French Veal Cordon Bleu.

This dinner includes sweet potatoes, Sesame Vegetables and a small salad. For dessert, treat yourself to the exquisite Cream Cheese Pomegranate Burst (recipe on pages 270–271).

Chicken Cordon Bleu

Makes 3 large or 4 medium pieces

¼ cup (60 mL) fine dry bread crumbs or flour

Shake of salt and black pepper

1 egg

2 slices of ham (½ oz/15 g for each chicken breast)

3 slices of part-skim mozzarella cheese (¾ oz/23 g for each chicken breast)

3 large or 4 medium boneless skinless chicken breasts (14 oz/420 g total)

1 to 2 tbsp (15 to 30 mL) butter or margarine

PER MEDIUM PIECE	
Calories	278
Carbohydrate	6 g
Fiber	0 g
Net carbs	6 g
Protein	39 g
Fat, total	10 g
Fat, saturated	5 g
Cholesterol	150 mg
Sodium	398 mg

1. In a bowl, mix bread crumbs with the salt and pepper.
2. In another bowl, beat the egg with a fork.
3. Slice the ham and cheese into four portions and lay on a plate.
4. Cut each chicken breast in half crosswise, but not all the way through. Gently flatten with a meat pounder or edge of a plate.
5. Inside each piece of chicken, tuck a slice of ham and cheese. Pull the top flap of chicken over to cover the ham and cheese. Dip each piece of chicken in the egg, turning to fully coat in egg both sides and the edges. Next, coat the chicken breasts in the bread crumbs. Put the chicken on a dinner plate.
6. Heat the butter in a nonstick pan. Add the chicken pieces to the pan and cover the pan. Cook over medium heat for 5 to 8 minutes, until nicely browned on one side. Then reduce the heat and cook the other side for 4 to 6 minutes, or until cooked all the way through and there is no pink inside the chicken.

Sweet Potatoes

See Dinner 10 for information about sweet potatoes. For mashed sweet potatoes, poke the potato with a fork and microwave for about 5 minutes, or peel the potato, cut into 2-inch (5 cm) pieces and boil until tender, about 15 minutes. Cooking time will vary depending on the size of the potato. Mash with a small amount of milk or butter, if desired.

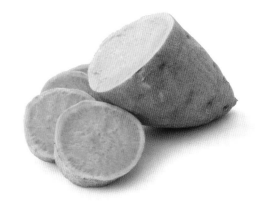

This recipe for Sesame Vegetables provides an easy way to add flavor and texture to steamed vegetables. Make this recipe with your favorite vegetables; we've used parsnips and yellow and green zucchini. For convenience, you can use frozen mixed vegetables.

Sesame Vegetables

Makes 4 servings

1 tbsp (15 mL) sesame seeds

2 to 3 cups (500 to 750 mL) sliced or diced vegetables

1 tsp (5 mL) olive oil, margarine or butter

1 tsp (5 mL) brown sugar

PER SERVING	
Calories	56
Carbohydrate	8 g
Fiber	2 g
Net carbs	6 g
Protein	2 g
Fat, total	2 g
Fat, saturated	0 g
Cholesterol	0 mg
Sodium	4 mg

RECIPE TIP

Instead of sesame seeds, an equal amount of sunflower seeds and a squirt of lemon juice is delicious on vegetables.

1. Toast sesame seeds in the microwave for 2 to 3 minutes, stirring several times. Or put the sesame seeds in a dry frying pan and toast for a few minutes over medium heat, stirring constantly, until lightly browned.
2. Steam or boil the vegetables until tender-crisp. Drain water.
3. Add the olive oil and brown sugar to the vegetables and mix gently. Then add the toasted sesame seeds to coat the vegetables.

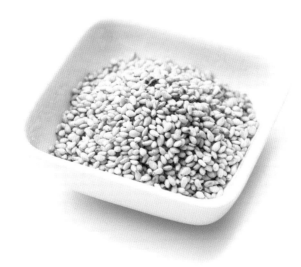

Meal continued on next page...

DINNER 40

It is the flavor and crunch of the pomegranate seeds that make this delicate dessert special. Your family or guests will never guess that this dessert has only 100 calories per serving! If pomegranates are out of season, you can make this dessert with finely chopped apple or other chopped fruit.

Cream Cheese Pomegranate Burst

Makes 4 servings

1 package (4-serving size) raspberry-flavored diet gelatin (or any red flavor will do)

¾ cup (175 mL) boiling water

¾ cup (175 mL) cold water

Seeds of 1 large pomegranate (see sidebar) or 1 cup frozen pomegranate arils (seeds)

¼ tsp (1 mL) cinnamon

½ package (4 oz/125 g) light cream cheese, softened at room temperature

PER SERVING	
Calories	100
Carbohydrate	9 g
Fiber	0 g
Net carbs	9 g
Protein	4 g
Fat, total	6 g
Fat, saturated	4 g
Cholesterol	20 mg
Sodium	237 mg

1. In a glass or metal bowl, add gelatin and pour the boiling water on top. Stir for about 1 minute, until the gelatin is completely dissolved. Add the cold water to the gelatin mixture.

2. Put ¼ cup (60 mL) of the gelatin mixture into each of four small dessert dishes. Place the dessert dishes in the fridge for about 15 minutes, until they are just slightly set. Leave the remaining gelatin mixture (about ½ cup/125 mL) in the bowl on the counter.

3. Take the dessert dishes out of the fridge. Divide the pomegranate seeds among the dishes, letting them sink into the partially set gelatin. Set 1 tbsp (15 mL) of seeds aside for decorating the finished dessert. Return the dessert dishes to the fridge.

4. Add cinnamon to the softened cream cheese and beat with a wooden spoon until smooth. Add gelatin mixture that was in the bowl on the counter. Beat with an electric beater for several minutes, until well blended and only small flecks of cream cheese are seen. It will be semi-liquid.

5. Once gelatin is set, take dessert dishes out of the fridge and evenly divide the cream cheese mixture among them, pouring it on top of the gelatin and pomegranate mixture. Return to the fridge. After about 15 minutes, it should be completely set. Add the extra seeds on top for decoration.

6. It can be served now, or returned to the fridge for serving later, in which case, cover each dessert dish with plastic wrap to keep it fresh. It is best if eaten within 3 or 4 hours of making it.

FOOD TIP

Pomegranate seeds are bursting with extraordinary flavor, and are full of vitamin C and antioxidants that help fight cancer and keep your skin healthy. They are wonderful in desserts and added to fruit salads and green salads.

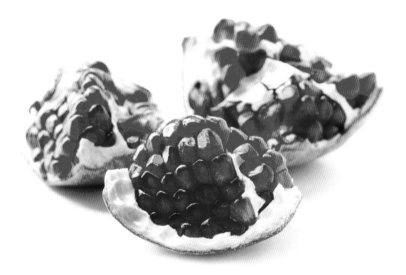

Food Choices	Large Meal	Small Meal
Carbohydrate	3	2
Protein	7	5½
Fat	2	2

Your Dinner Menu	Large Meal (730 calories)	Total Carbs	Net Carbs	Small Meal (550 calories)	Total Carbs	Net Carbs
Chicken Cordon Bleu	1 large piece	8	8	1 medium piece	6	6
Mashed sweet potato	⅔ cup (150 mL)	39	34	⅓ cup (75 mL)	19	16
Sesame Vegetables	1 serving	8	6	1 serving	8	6
Tossed salad	Small	3	3	Small	3	3
Fat-free Italian salad dressing	1 tbsp (15 mL)	2	2	1 tbsp (15 mL)	2	2
Cream Cheese Pomegranate Burst	1 serving	9	9	1 serving	9	9
		69 g	**62 g**		**47 g**	**42 g**

271

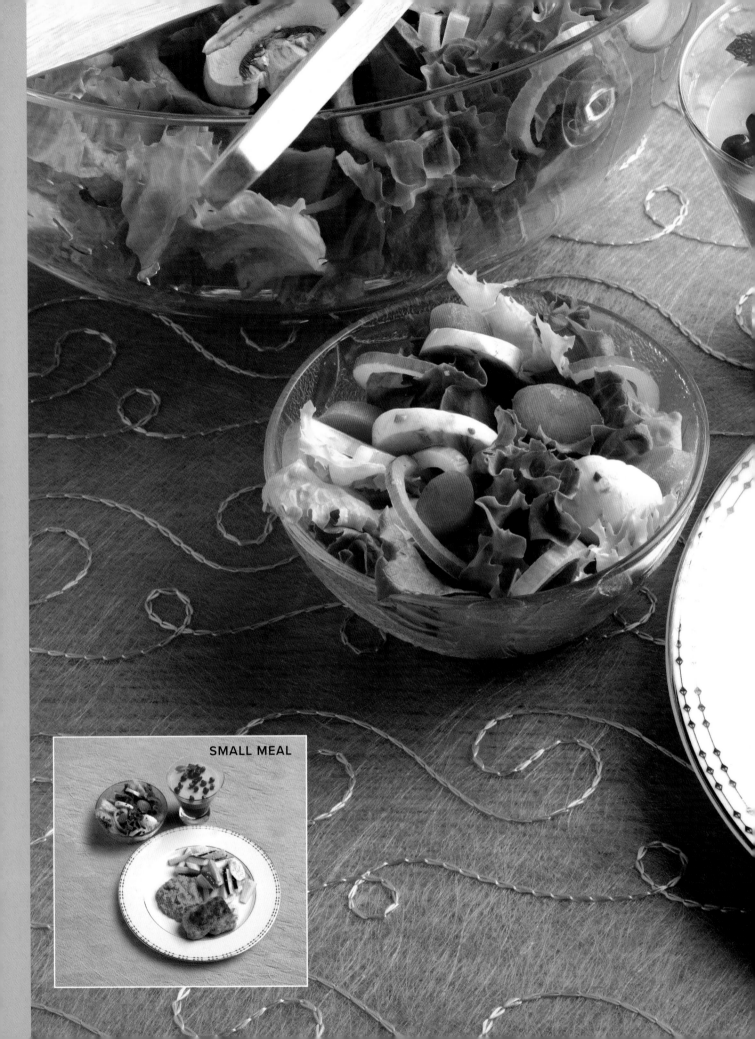

SMALL MEAL

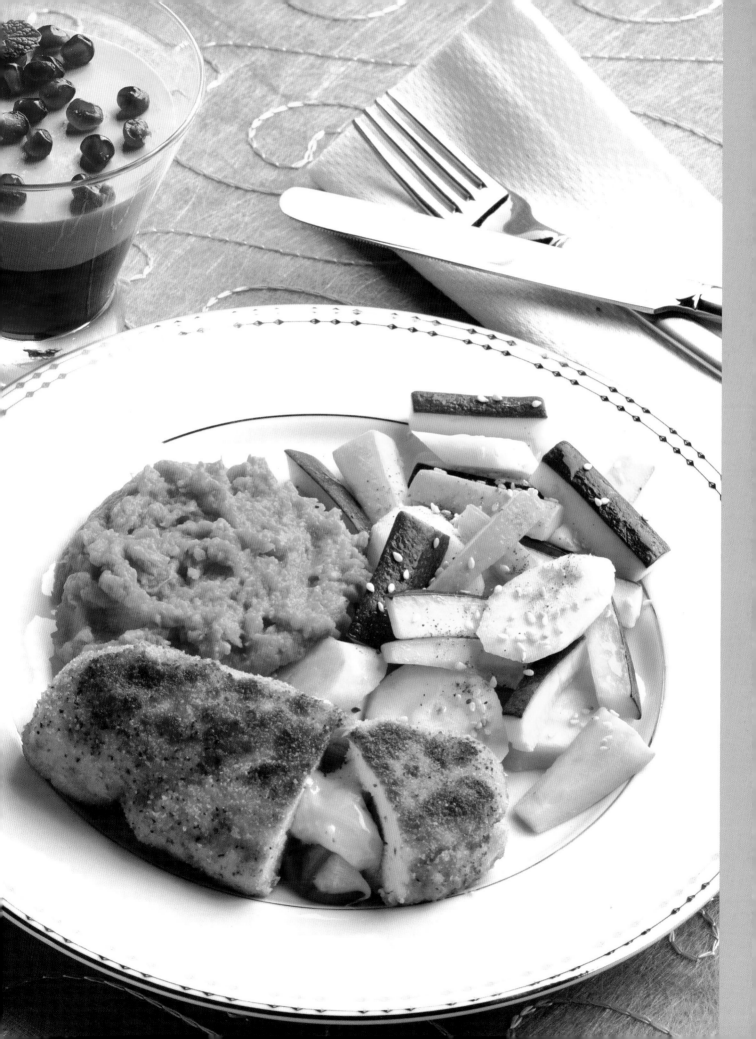

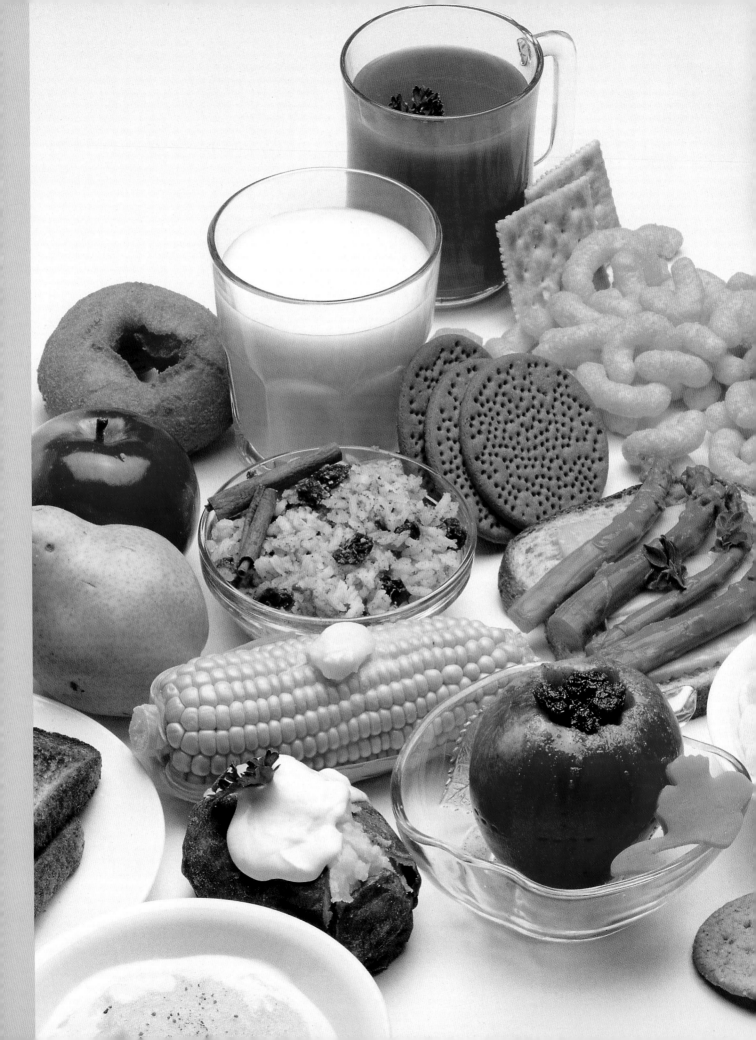

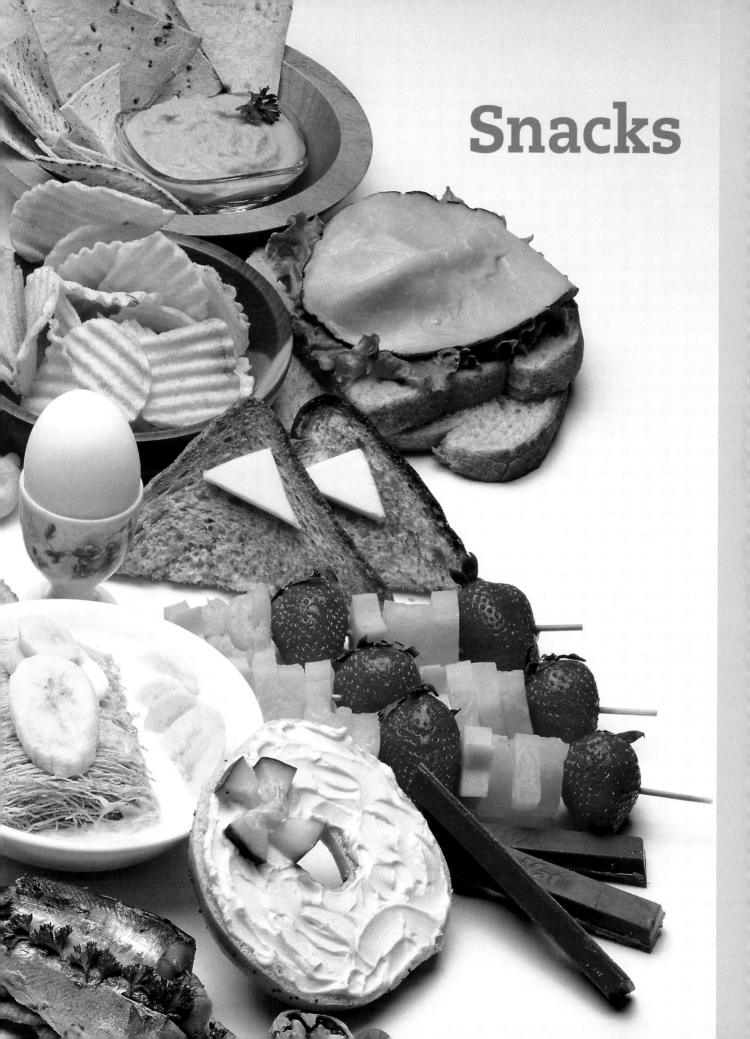

Snacks

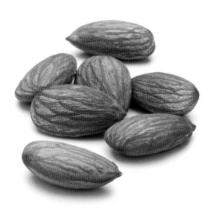

Four Snack Groups

In this section you will find photographs of four groups of snacks. The groups are low-calorie snacks, small snacks, medium snacks and large snacks. The calories for each snack within each group are about the same. The number of snacks you choose will depend on how many calories a day you want. Look at the chart on page 37 that shows the calories of the small and large meals and of different snacks.

For most of us, it's good to choose no more than three of the small, medium or large snacks a day.

Three small snacks add up to 150 calories, three medium snacks add up to 300 calories and three large snacks add up to 600 calories.

Low-calorie snacks

- These snacks have just 20 calories or less.
- These foods are not fattening. A few of these a day will have little effect on your weight or blood sugar. You may add them to your meals or snacks.

Small snacks

- These snacks have 50 calories.

Medium snacks

- These snacks have 100 calories.
- Two small snacks would equal one medium snack.

Large snacks

- These snacks have 200 calories.
- Two medium snacks, or four small snacks, would equal one large snack.

Carbs in snacks

In the photograph of each snack group are snacks with about the same number of calories. However, the snacks have different amounts of sugar or starch, protein or fat. The grams of total Net (Available) Carbohydrates in each snack are listed in red.

Note: In the Low-Calorie snacks on pages 278 to 279, only total carbs are shown, as the total carbs and net carbs are the same due to the small portions and the insignificant amount of fiber.

Remember:
- 1 medium snack =
  2 small snacks

- 1 large snack =
  2 medium snacks, or
  4 small snacks

Choose a variety of snacks and you won't get bored. When you eat a snack between meals you will not feel so hungry at meal times. Most of the snacks shown here are low in fat and sugar, just like the meals. A snack made from a milk food will give you important calcium, a vegetable will give you fiber, and a fruit is full of vitamins.

In the small, medium and large photographs, you will find:

- starchy snacks, which have mostly starch
- fruit and vegetable snacks, which have natural sugar
- milk snacks, which have natural milk sugar and protein, and some may have some fat
- mixed snacks, which are a mix of foods from different food groups, such as a starch and a protein
- occasional snacks: these are high in fat, sugar or salt, or that have alcohol.

Candy, chocolates and chips

What about eating candy, chocolates and chips and other foods that are made with lots of fat or sugar? It is okay to have a small amount of these once in a while. But these shouldn't be eaten often, as they give you calories but little nutrition. On the photographs on pages 280–285 you will find these kinds of foods marked as occasional snacks.

Alcoholic drinks

Alcoholic drinks are also marked as an occasional snack choice. Remember the cautions about alcohol (see pages 25–26).

Salty snacks

Salty snacks with 300 to 499 mg of salt are shown with one salt shaker. These should be limited to no more than once a day or even a couple of times a week.

Snacks with 500 mg or more are shown with two salt shakers and should be limited to no more than once a week.

DOCTOR'S TIP

If you have diabetes and you take insulin or a diabetes pill in the evening, read this: An evening snack that has some protein or fat may help prevent low blood sugar in the middle of the night. Ask your doctor or dietitian for more advice.

Have a glass of water when you have a snack. And try to avoid late-night snacking.

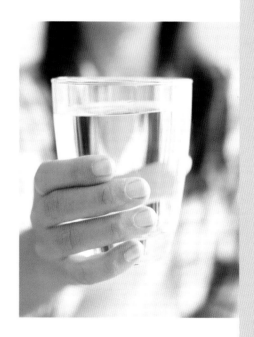

Low-Calorie Snacks
20 calories or less in each snack

Because the portions are small, the total carbs and net carbs are the same in the low-calorie snacks. These are shown in grams and are marked in red.

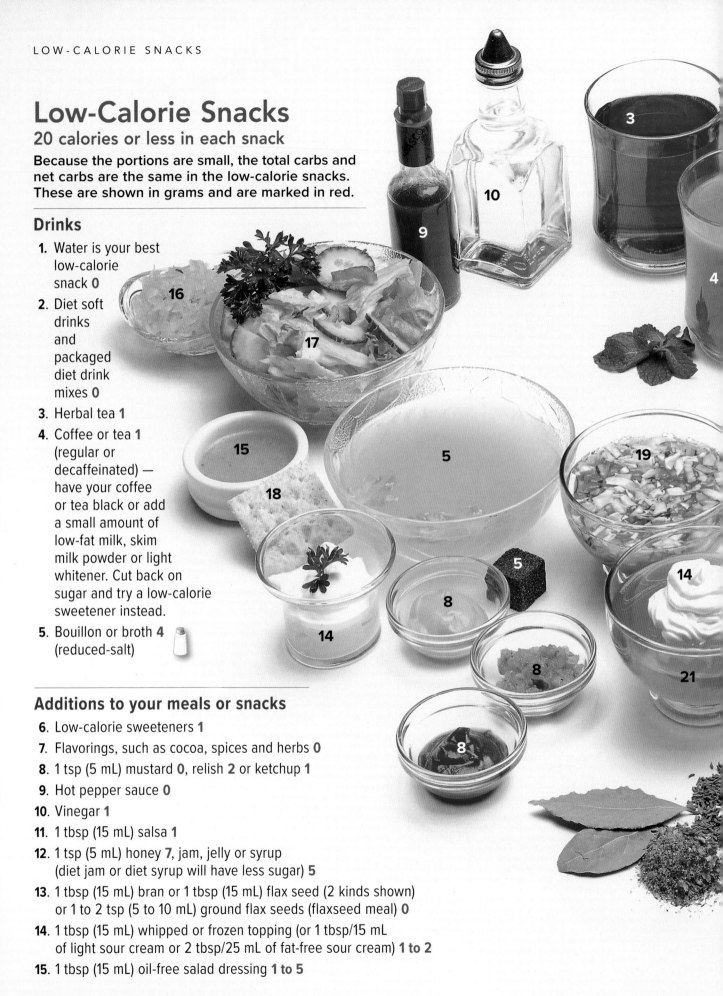

Drinks

1. Water is your best low-calorie snack **0**

2. Diet soft drinks and packaged diet drink mixes **0**

3. Herbal tea **1**

4. Coffee or tea **1** (regular or decaffeinated) — have your coffee or tea black or add a small amount of low-fat milk, skim milk powder or light whitener. Cut back on sugar and try a low-calorie sweetener instead.

5. Bouillon or broth **4** (reduced-salt)

Additions to your meals or snacks

6. Low-calorie sweeteners **1**

7. Flavorings, such as cocoa, spices and herbs **0**

8. 1 tsp (5 mL) mustard **0**, relish **2** or ketchup **1**

9. Hot pepper sauce **0**

10. Vinegar **1**

11. 1 tbsp (15 mL) salsa **1**

12. 1 tsp (5 mL) honey **7**, jam, jelly or syrup (diet jam or diet syrup will have less sugar) **5**

13. 1 tbsp (15 mL) bran or 1 tbsp (15 mL) flax seed (2 kinds shown) or 1 to 2 tsp (5 to 10 mL) ground flax seeds (flaxseed meal) **0**

14. 1 tbsp (15 mL) whipped or frozen topping (or 1 tbsp/15 mL of light sour cream or 2 tbsp/25 mL of fat-free sour cream) **1 to 2**

15. 1 tbsp (15 mL) oil-free salad dressing **1 to 5**

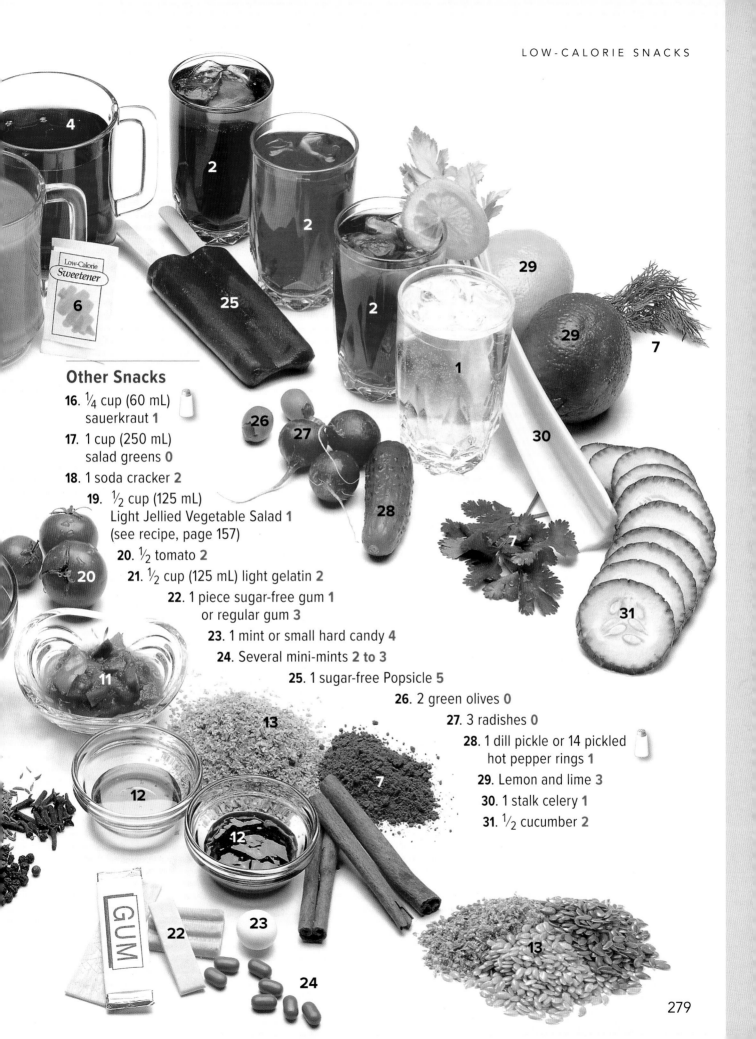

Other Snacks

16. ¼ cup (60 mL) sauerkraut **1**

17. 1 cup (250 mL) salad greens **0**

18. 1 soda cracker **2**

19. ½ cup (125 mL) Light Jellied Vegetable Salad **1** (see recipe, page 157)

20. ½ tomato **2**

21. ½ cup (125 mL) light gelatin **2**

22. 1 piece sugar-free gum **1** or regular gum **3**

23. 1 mint or small hard candy **4**

24. Several mini-mints **2 to 3**

25. 1 sugar-free Popsicle **5**

26. 2 green olives **0**

27. 3 radishes **0**

28. 1 dill pickle or 14 pickled hot pepper rings **1**

29. Lemon and lime **3**

30. 1 stalk celery **1**

31. ½ cucumber **2**

Small Snacks
50 calories or less in each snack

Total carbs are shown in dark blue and net carbs follow in red. Both are in grams.

Vegetables

Always have raw, washed vegetables in the fridge. The vegetables should be ready to eat and easy to grab.

1. ¾ cup (175 mL) Coleslaw (page 84) **8/6**
2. 1 stalk celery with 1 tbsp (15 mL) cheese spread **2/2**
3. Large salad with 1 tbsp (15 mL) fat-free salad dressing **4/3**
4. 1 medium carrot **8/6**
5. 1 cup (250 mL) canned tomatoes **10/7**

Fruit

6. 1 cup (250 mL) strawberries **12/8**
7. 1 small orange **14/12**
8. ½ large grapefruit **12/10**
9. ½ medium apple **11/10**
10. 1 medium plum **10/9**
11. 1 medium kiwi **12/9**
12. 2 prunes (or figs) **11/10**
13. 2 tbsp (30 mL) raisins **16/15**
14. 2-inch (5 cm) piece of banana **13/12**
15. ¾ cup (175 mL) Light Gelatin with Fruit (page 205) **13/12**
16. ¾ cup (175 mL) Stewed Rhubarb (page 125) **10/6**

Juice

17. 1 cup (250 mL) tomato or vegetable juice **10/8**
18. ½ cup (125 mL) unsweetened fruit juice **13/13** (try mixing the juice with some sparkling water or diet ginger ale)

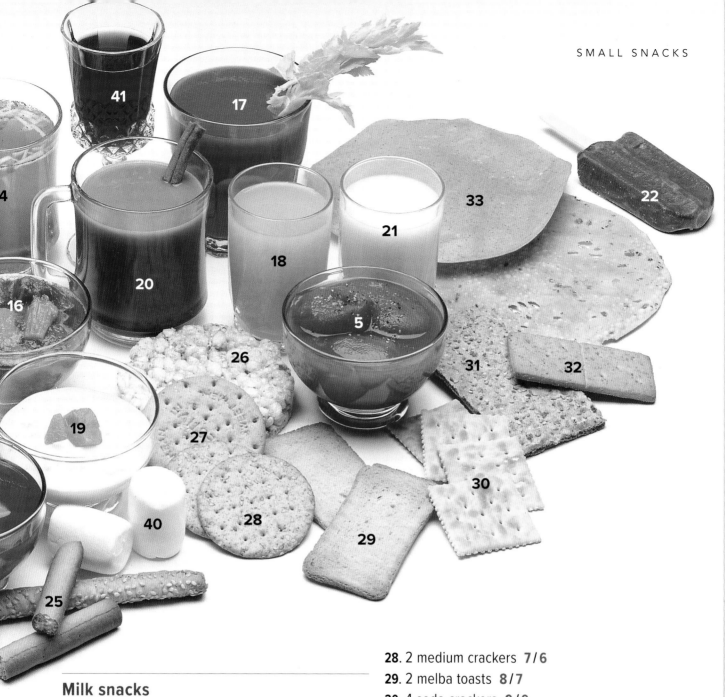

Milk snacks

19. ½ cup (125 mL) low-fat fruit yogurt, sweetened with a low-calorie sweetener **8/8**

20. 1 cup (250 mL) light hot cocoa **8/8**

21. ½ cup (125 mL) low-fat milk (skim or 1%) **6/6**

22. 1 light fudge ice cream bar, Revello (with low-calorie sweetener) **12/12**

Starchy snacks

23. 1 cup (250 mL) puffed wheat cereal **10/9**

24. 1 cup (250 mL) Reduced-Salt Instant Cup-of-Soup (page 86) **6/6**

25. 2 bread sticks **8/7**

26. 1 rice cake **12/11**

27. 1 digestive or other plain cookie **7/7**

28. 2 medium crackers **7/6**

29. 2 melba toasts **8/7**

30. 4 soda crackers **9/9**

31. 1 fiber crispbread **7/4**

32. 2 Graham wafer halves **11/11**

33. 2 poppadoms **9/7**

Occasional snacks

34. 1 chocolate chip cookie **7/7**

35. 1 fig bar **11/10**

36. ¼ cup (60 mL) (21) fish crackers **6/6**

37. 3 hard candy mints **12/12**

38. 5 LifeSavers **15/15**

39. 1 small chocolate **6/6**

40. 2 marshmallows **12/12**

41. 3 oz (90 g) dry table wine **9/3 + 6 g alcohol**

Medium Snacks

100 calories in each snack
(two small snacks = one medium snack)

Total carbs are shown in dark blue and
net carbs follow in red. Both are in grams.

Vegetables

1. 2 to 3 cups (500 to 750 mL) raw
   vegetables with 2 tbsp (30 mL)
   Vegetable Dip (page 189) **20/14**

Fruit

2. ½ medium cantaloupe **22/20**
3. 1 cup (250 mL) applesauce **28/24**
4. 4 pineapple rings plus
   2 tbsp (30 mL) juice **24/22**
5. 1 small banana **16/15**
6. 3 figs **29/24**
7. 5 dried apricots **22/19**
8. 1 pear **26/21**
9. 1 cup (250 mL) fresh
   fruit salad **27/23**
10. 4 thin slices watermelon **22/21**
11. 1½ cups (375 mL) grapes **24/23**

Starchy snacks

12. 1 slice raisin bread
    with 1 tsp (5 mL) of
    margarine **14/13**
13. 3 arrowroots or other
    plain cookies **17/16**
14. 6 pretzels **24/23**
15. 1 waffle or crumpet
    with 1 tsp (5 mL) jam
    21/20
16. 3 cups (750 mL)
    air-popped popcorn **19/15**
17. 1 whole wheat roll with
    cucumber, tomato, lettuce **19/16**
18. ⅓ of a 3-oz/80 g package of oriental noodles
    (made with salt-free spice blend) **20/19**
19. 1 slice matzo bread **27/26**
20. 8 baked tortilla chips or other baked chips
    with 1 tbsp (15 mL) salsa sauce **12/10**

Mixed snacks

21. ½ pizza bun **13/12**
22. 1 piece toast with
    1 tsp (5 mL) peanut
    butter **15/12**
23. ½ cup (125 mL) 1%
    or 2% cottage cheese and ½ tomato **6/5**
24. 1 cup (250 mL) canned tomatoes and 2 tbsp
    (30 mL) shredded cheese **10/7**
25. ⅔ cup (150 mL) round oat cereal and ½ cup
    (125 mL) low-fat milk **17/16**
26. ½ cup (125 mL) low-fat milk and 2 gingersnaps **18/18**
27. 8 jumbo shrimp and 2 tbsp (30 mL) shrimp cocktail
    sauce **3/2**

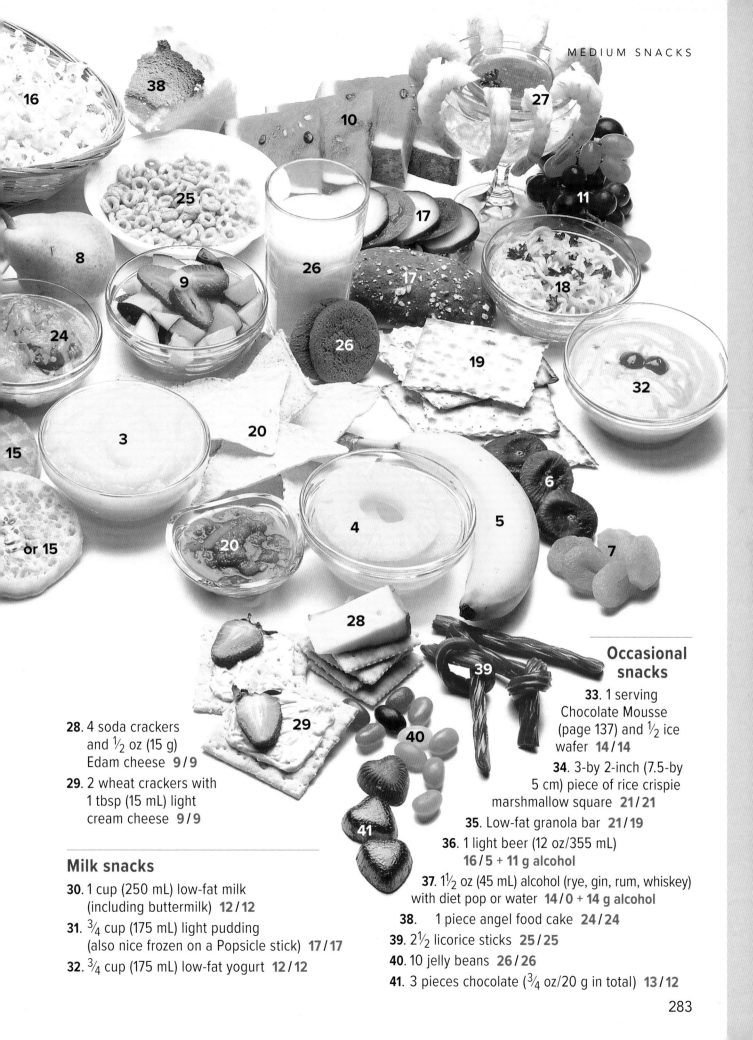

28. 4 soda crackers
and ½ oz (15 g)
Edam cheese **9/9**

29. 2 wheat crackers with
1 tbsp (15 mL) light
cream cheese **9/9**

Milk snacks

30. 1 cup (250 mL) low-fat milk
(including buttermilk) **12/12**

31. ¾ cup (175 mL) light pudding
(also nice frozen on a Popsicle stick) **17/17**

32. ¾ cup (175 mL) low-fat yogurt **12/12**

Occasional snacks

33. 1 serving
Chocolate Mousse
(page 137) and ½ ice
wafer **14/14**

34. 3-by 2-inch (7.5-by
5 cm) piece of rice crispie
marshmallow square **21/21**

35. Low-fat granola bar **21/19**

36. 1 light beer (12 oz/355 mL)
16/5 + 11 g alcohol

37. 1½ oz (45 mL) alcohol (rye, gin, rum, whiskey)
with diet pop or water **14/0 + 14 g alcohol**

38. 1 piece angel food cake **24/24**

39. 2½ licorice sticks **25/25**

40. 10 jelly beans **26/26**

41. 3 pieces chocolate (¾ oz/20 g in total) **13/12**

283

Large Snacks
200 calories in each snack
(two medium snacks = one large snack)

Total carbs are shown in dark blue and net carbs follow in red. Both are in grams.

Mixed snacks

1. Vegetable and cracker bowl: 2 cups (500 mL) any kind of raw vegetables with 3 snackbreads, 2 bread sticks and 3 tbsp (45 mL) Garlic Vegetable Dip (page 189). **42/35**

2. 2 slices toast with 1 tsp (5 mL) butter or margarine and 2 tsp (10 mL) jam **38/32**

3. 1 cup (250 mL) cream of wheat hot cereal and ¾ cup (175 mL) low-fat milk **36/33**

4. 1 piece Crustless Pumpkin Pie (page 177) with 2 tbsp (30 mL) whipped topping **25/23**

5. 1 small cone with ¾ cup (175 mL) light ice cream **26/26**

6. 1 Bran Muffin (page 56) and ½ oz (15 g) cheese **27/24**

7. 1 piece Bannock (page 133) and 1 tsp (5 mL) jam **36/35**

8. 16 fresh peanuts **6/4**

9. 1 slice pumpernickel bread with 1 tsp (5 mL) margarine and 1½ oz (45 g) pickled herring **16/14**

10. 1 cup (250 mL) low-fat milk or buttermilk plus 3 plain cookies **30/30**

11. 1 cup (250 mL) Rice Pudding (page 129) **42/40**

12. 1 large cob of corn with 1 tsp (5 mL) butter or margarine **40/37**

13. 1 small baked potato with 1 tbsp (15 mL) light sour cream **47/43**

14. 1 Baked Apple (page 165) plus ½ oz (15 g) cheese **29/26**

15. 4 crackers with 2 large sardines **10/9**

16. ½ can cream of tomato soup made with low-fat milk, and 2 soda crackers **33/31**

17. 1 oz (30 g) cheese and fresh-steamed asparagus on bread **16/12**

18. 1 shredded wheat biscuit with ½ small banana and ½ cup almond beverage **33/28**

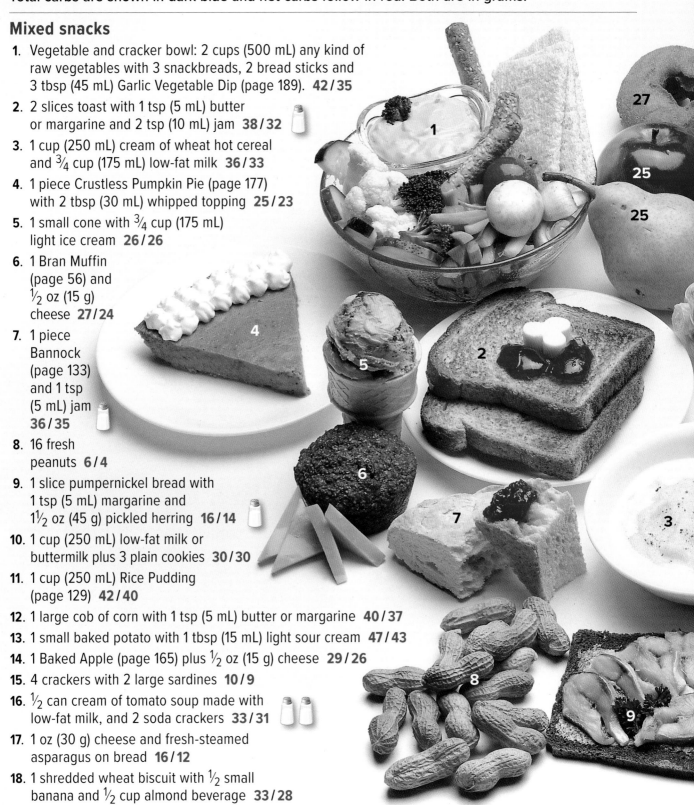

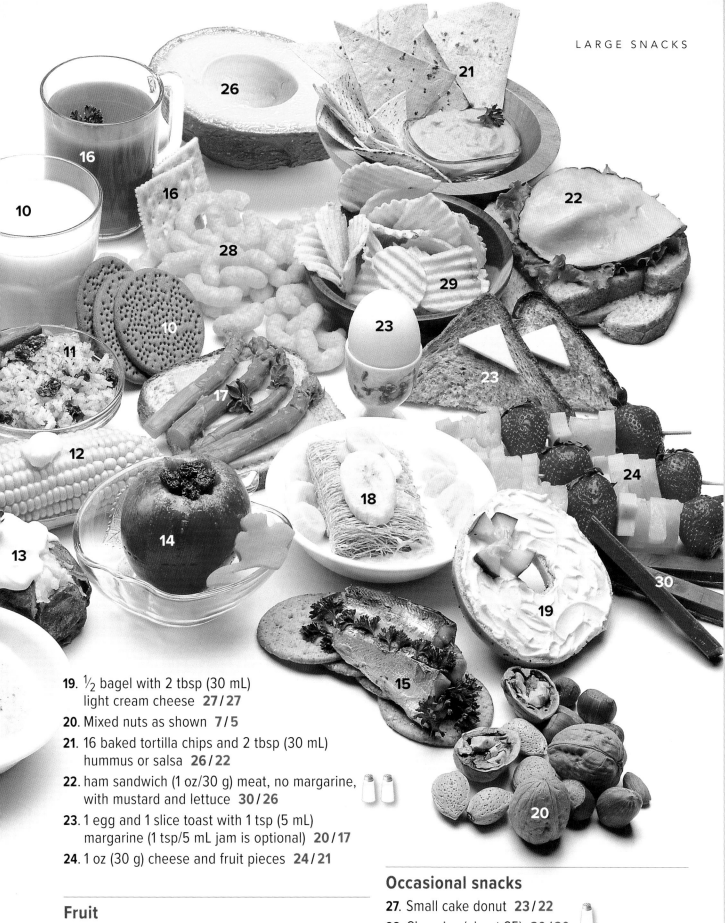

19. ½ bagel with 2 tbsp (30 mL) light cream cheese **27 / 27**

20. Mixed nuts as shown **7 / 5**

21. 16 baked tortilla chips and 2 tbsp (30 mL) hummus or salsa **26 / 22**

22. ham sandwich (1 oz/30 g) meat, no margarine, with mustard and lettuce **30 / 26**

23. 1 egg and 1 slice toast with 1 tsp (5 mL) margarine (1 tsp/5 mL jam is optional) **20 / 17**

24. 1 oz (30 g) cheese and fruit pieces **24 / 21**

Fruit

25. 2 fruits, such as a small apple and a pear **51 / 43**

26. ½ large avocado (try with a sprinkle of Worcestershire sauce or lemon) **9 / 2**

Occasional snacks

27. Small cake donut **23 / 22**

28. Cheesies (about 25) **20 / 20**

29. Potato chips (about 18) **18 / 16**

30. 1⅓-oz (40 g) chocolate bar **24 / 23**

285

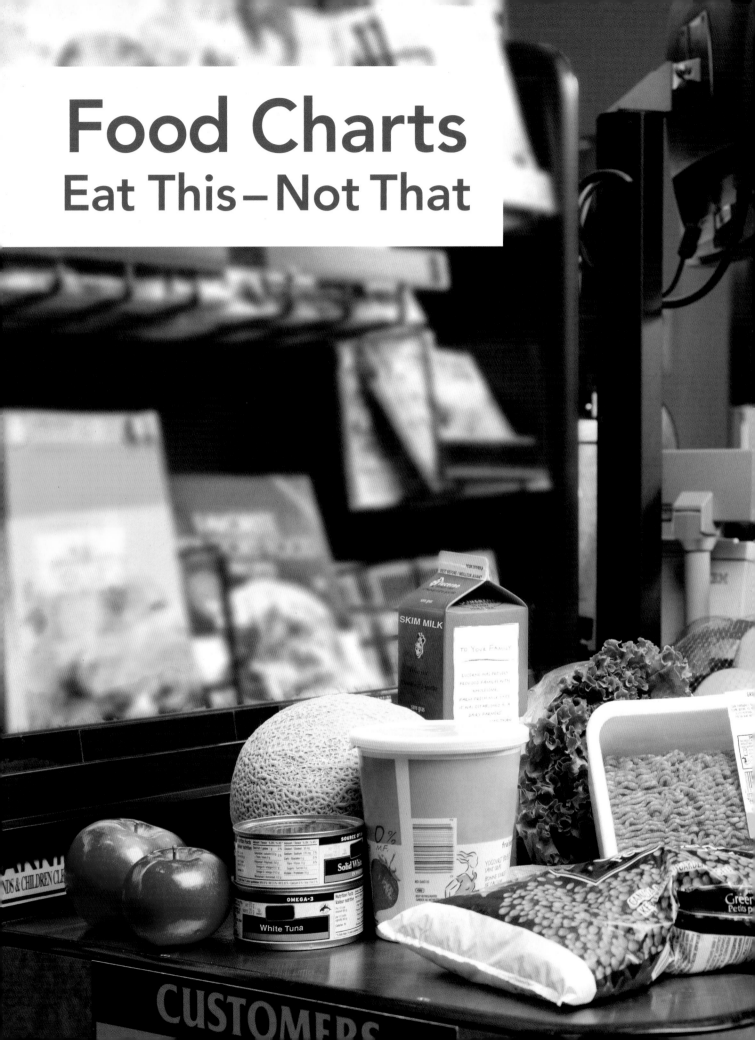

Food Charts
Eat This – Not That

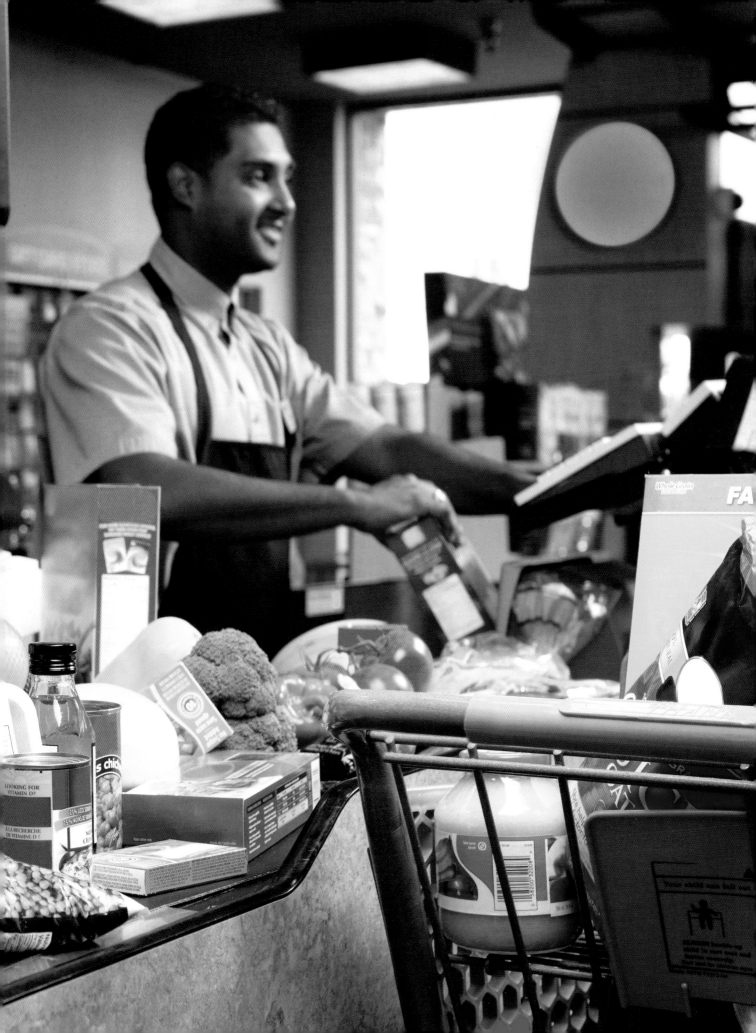

Does your shopping cart look like this?

This cart holds groceries for a week for two people, with many unhealthy food choices.

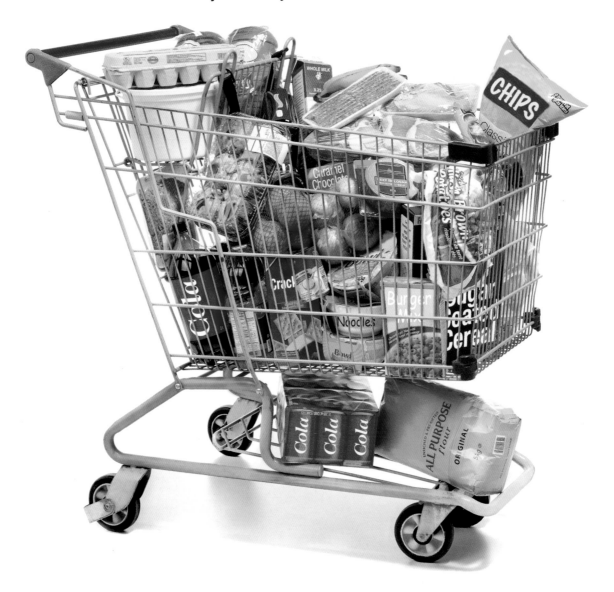

Compare this grocery cart to the healthier cart on page 289. You may be amazed by the difference.

Compared to the healthy cart on the next page, this cart has about:

- Eleven cups (2.75 L) of extra added table sugar — that's 513 teaspoons! This includes sugar added by the manufacturer to foods such as soft drinks, cookies, muffins, ice cream and chocolates. It also includes the sugar that comes from fruit juice.
- Half a pound (250 g), or 200 teaspoons (1 L), of extra fat. That would be like half a pound of butter.
- About 27,000 mg of extra sodium — as much as you would find in almost 12 teaspoons (60 mL) of salt.

Out with the old, in with the new

Here are healthier food choices:

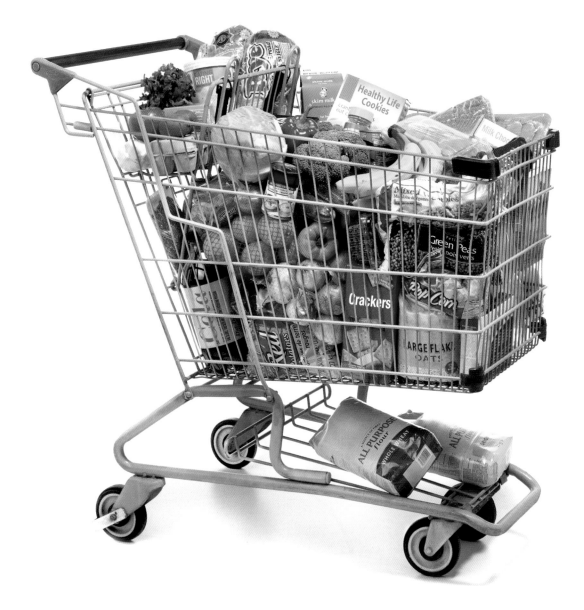

This cart holds groceries for a week for two people, with many healthy food choices. Compare this grocery cart to the unhealthier cart on page 288.

Compared to the unhealthy cart, this cart has:

- 486 g *more* fiber
- 450% *more* vitamin A
- 1400% *more* vitamin C
- 410% *more* calcium

Eat This — Not That

Move from unhealthy to healthy choices using the Food Charts on pages 291–317.

Each page shows four different versions of a food or drink.

- The option at the top of the page is the least healthy.
- Generally, the bottom two choices are healthier than the top two choices.
- The bottom option, Healthy Choice, is generally the healthiest of the four possibilities.
- Keep in mind that nutrients differ among brands and sometimes between American and Canadian producers.

These charts are meant as a guideline only. When you're shopping, look carefully at food labels before deciding what to buy.

The following nutrients are listed for each food or drink:

- **Calories.** When you look at the calories in these charts, it's important to also consider the total amount of food you need each day. The small meals in this book provide about 1,200 calories per day and the large meals about 1,620 calories. Depending on your calorie requirements, you may be able to add 100 to 350 calories of snacks to the small meals and 100 to 600 calories of snacks to the large meals (see page 37).
- **Carbohydrates.** Carbs include starch from foods such as rice, wheat or pasta, the natural sugars found in fruits, vegetables and milk, and added sugar. One teaspoon (5 mL) of added sugar equals 4 g of sugar. Labels list the amount of sugar separately under carbohydrate, but this still gives no indication of how much is added sugar and how much is natural sugar. If the product is a soft drink, you'll know that all of the sugar is added sugar.
- **Net (Available) Carbohydrates.** Net carbs are total carbs minus fiber. This is the amount that mostly affects your blood sugar.
- **Fiber.** Fiber is very good for you, especially when you have diabetes. Adults with diabetes should eat 25 to 50 g of fiber a day.
- **Fat.** One teaspoon (5 mL) of butter, margarine, lard or oil has 5 g of fat. Fat should make up no more than one-third of your daily calories.
  - A daily meal plan of 1,200 calories a day should include no more than about 9 tsp (45 g) of fat, including hidden fat.
  - A daily meal plan of 1,620 calories a day should include no more than about 13 tsp (65 g) of fat, including hidden fat.
  - Limit saturated fats. See page 18 for information about healthy fats.
- **Sodium.** It is best to limit your total sodium intake to 2,300 mg a day (about 1 tsp/5 mL of salt). This is often a challenge: most food products have salt added, sometimes large amounts.

Choosing the healthiest option was in some cases challenging.

This is because one food product might be lower in sugar or fat (which is good) but higher in sodium or lower in fiber (not so good).

Caffeine

Caffeine content is listed only for food products that have more than 45 mg of caffeine. Because caffeine is an addictive drug, consider limiting it to 400 mg a day (300 mg if pregnant or breastfeeding). Children and teenagers should limit caffeine even more — or avoid it altogether.

Oatmeal

½ cup (125 mL) instant sweetened oatmeal (made from a 38-g package) with ½ cup (125 mL) 2% milk

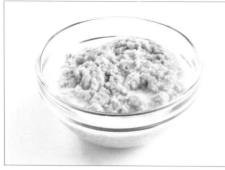

Calories	Carbs	Fiber	Fat	Sodium
213	35 g	2 g	5 g	294 mg

These are super-sweetened packages of oatmeal. Cut back on the sugar by mixing half a package with plain oatmeal. **Note:** 1 package only makes ½ cup (125 mL) of oatmeal, so it will not be as filling as the healthy choice where you get a full cup of porridge with fewer calories. **Net Carbs 33 g**

½ cup (125 mL) instant unsweetened (plain) oatmeal (made from a 28-g package) with ½ tsp (2 mL) brown sugar and ½ cup (125 mL) 2% milk

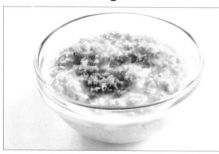

Calories	Carbs	Fiber	Fat	Sodium
171	26 g	3 g	4 g	274 mg

With 1 tsp (5 mL) brown sugar added, this still has less sugar than the presweetened package of oatmeal above. **Net Carbs 23 g**

¾ cup (175 mL) cooked minute oats with ½ tsp (2 mL) brown sugar and ½ cup (125 mL) 1% milk

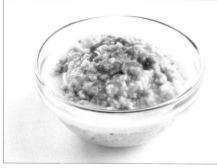

Calories	Carbs	Fiber	Fat	Sodium
173	28 g	3 g	3 g	55 mg

Minute oats are healthier than individual packages, as they are less processed (fiber is less chopped) and they have less sodium. They only take a few minutes longer to cook than the instant oats and can still be cooked in the microwave in your bowl. **Net Carbs 25 g**

1 cup (250 mL) old-fashioned oats with ½ tsp (2 mL) brown sugar and ½ cup (125 mL) skim milk

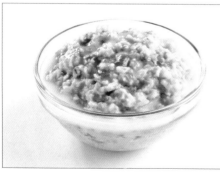

Calories	Carbs	Fiber	Fat	Sodium
180	31 g	4 g	2 g	53 mg

Cook these oats on the stove or in the microwave. They are an excellent choice, as they raise your blood sugar a bit more slowly than minute oats and instant oats. When you choose skim milk, you have all the nutrients with no fat. **Net Carbs 27 g**

HEALTHY CHOICE

FOOD FACT Oats can help reduce your cholesterol. A low-calorie brown sugar substitute can be added to your oatmeal instead of sugar.

Cold Cereal

1½ cups (375 mL) store-bought granola with ¾ cup (175 mL) 2% milk

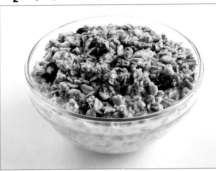

Calories	Carbs	Fiber	Fat	Sodium
710	97 g	9 g	30 g	203 mg

Granola is an excellent source of fiber and is lower in sodium than other cereal choices, but it is very high in calories, sugar and saturated fat. Limit your serving to ¼ to ½ cup (60 to 125 mL), or use it as a topping on plain cereal. **Net Carbs 88 g**

1½ cups (375 mL) frosted flakes with ¾ cup (175 mL) 1% milk

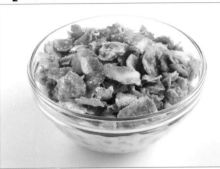

Calories	Carbs	Fiber	Fat	Sodium
279	57 g	1 g	2 g	359 mg

Frosted flakes are high in sugar — 6 tsp (30 mL) of sugar have been added to this serving. Sugar-coated cereals are best sprinkled on top of your corn flakes or bran flakes. **Net Carbs 56 g**

1½ cups (375 mL) corn flakes with ¾ cup (175 mL) skim milk

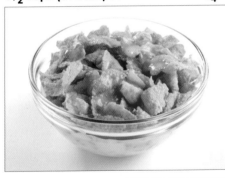

Calories	Carbs	Fiber	Fat	Sodium
208	41 g	1 g	0 g	347 mg

Corn flakes have lower carbs and sodium than the other cereal choices in this chart. This makes them a good choice. However, they have little fiber. You could boost the fiber with a sprinkle of natural bran or bran buds on top. **Net Carbs 40 g**

1½ cups (375 mL) bran flakes with ¾ cup (175 mL) skim milk

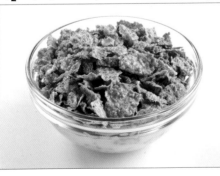

Calories	Carbs	Fiber	Fat	Sodium
209	44 g	6 g	1 g	467 mg

All-Bran Flakes are a good choice; they are an excellent source of fiber. Yet compared to frosted flakes and corn flakes, they are higher in sodium. If reducing sodium is your priority, choose the corn flakes. **Net Carbs 38 g**

HEALTHY CHOICE

FOOD FACT

Having a piece of fruit with your cereal adds healthy antioxidants and 2 to 5 g of fiber.

Milk

1 cup (250 mL) 2% chocolate milk

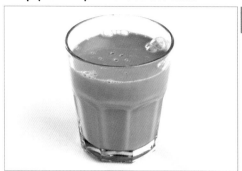

Calories	Carbs	Fiber	Fat	Sodium
180	26 g	1 g	5 g	150 mg

Chocolate milk has good nutrients, including calcium and vitamin D. But it has 3½ tsp (14 g) of added sugar. To cut back on the added sugar, mix ½ cup (125 mL) chocolate milk with ½ cup (125 mL) skim milk. **Net Carbs 25 g**

1 cup (250 mL) 3.3% (homogenized) milk

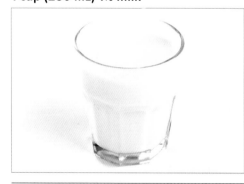

Calories	Carbs	Fiber	Fat	Sodium
146	11 g	0 g	8 g	98 mg

If you are used to drinking whole milk, try mixing it half and half with 2% milk. Eventually you may drink 2% milk and lower your fat intake. **Net Carbs 11 g**

1 cup (250 mL) 1% milk

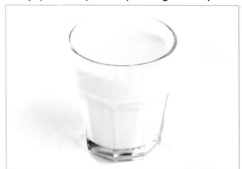

Calories	Carbs	Fiber	Fat	Sodium
102	12 g	0 g	2 g	107 mg

This is a great lower-fat milk choice. **Net Carbs 12 g**

1 cup (250 mL) skim milk

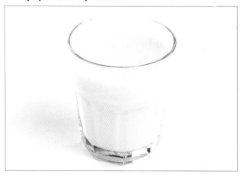

Calories	Carbs	Fiber	Fat	Sodium
83	12 g	0 g	0	103 mg

Skim milk has zero fat. Plus, it has all the protein, calcium, vitamin D and other nutrients found in whole milk that are so important for your health. Try the delicious Fruit Milkshake on page 121. **Net Carbs 12 g**

HEALTHY CHOICE

FOOD FACT A small glass of milk at the end of your meal can decrease the amount of acid in your mouth. This helps reduce the build-up of plaque on your teeth.

Restaurant Egg Breakfast

2 fried eggs, 2 slices of buttered white toast, 2 jams, 2 sausages, 1 cup (250 mL) hash browns, 1 tbsp (15 mL) ketchup, 20-oz (600 mL) coffee with 4 creamers (4 tbsp/60 mL) and 4 tsp (20 mL) sugar

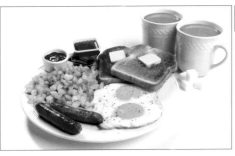

Calories	Carbs	Fiber	Fat	Sodium
1,147	123 g	6 g	62 g	1,194 mg

This "breakfast special" gives you a whole day's fat intake. Save this meal for special occasions. (Note: 1 package of jam equals 2 tsp/10 mL and 1 creamer equals 1 tbsp/15 mL) **Caffeine: 343 mg** (based on filter drip). **Net Carbs 117 g**

2 poached eggs, 2 slices of buttered brown toast, 1 jam, 2 sausages, ½ cup (125 mL) hash browns, 10-oz (300 mL) coffee with 2 tbsp (30 mL) whole milk and 1 tsp (5 mL) sugar

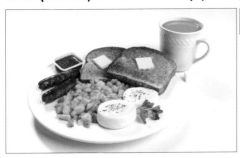

Calories	Carbs	Fiber	Fat	Sodium
705	66 g	6 g	39 g	886 mg

Poached eggs, less jam on your toast, no ketchup and just one mug of coffee are good changes. You will eat less fat and sugar at one meal. **Caffeine: 171 mg.** **Net Carbs 60 g**

2 poached eggs, 2 slices of buttered brown toast, 1 jam, 2 sausages, tomato slices, 10-oz (300 mL) coffee with 2 tbsp (30 mL) whole milk

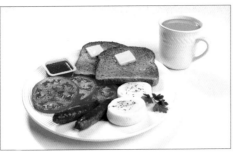

Calories	Carbs	Fiber	Fat	Sodium
530	43 g	5 g	30 g	862 mg

This breakfast replaces hash browns with tomato slices and cuts out almost 2 tsp (10 mL) of fat and more than 150 calories. **Caffeine: 171 mg.** (Switching to instant coffee reduces caffeine to about 114 mg.) **Net Carbs 38 g**

1 poached egg, 2 slices of unbuttered brown toast, 1 jam, tomato slices, 10-oz (300 mL) tea with 2 tbsp (30 mL) 2% milk

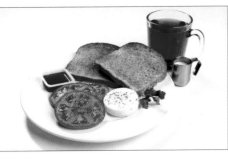

Calories	Carbs	Fiber	Fat	Sodium
286	42 g	5 g	8 g	480 mg

This is a trimmed-down, healthier breakfast. Choose a low-calorie sweetener for your tea (or coffee) if desired. **Caffeine: 59 mg.** (Decaf tea and most herbal teas have no caffeine.) **Net Carbs 37 g**

HEALTHY CHOICE

FOOD FACT — **Tea has almost three-quarters less caffeine than coffee. Plus, it is rich in antioxidants that may help keep your blood vessels healthy.**

Jam

1 tbsp (15 mL) pure raspberry jam

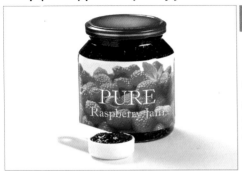

Calories	Carbs	Fiber	Fat	Sodium
55	14 g	0 g	0 g	6 mg

One tablespoon (15 mL) of jam has the same amount of calories and total sugar as a piece of fresh fruit. However, jam does not have the fiber of fresh fruit, so it will raise your blood sugar faster. **Net Carbs 14 g**

1 tbsp (15 mL) "all-fruit" raspberry jam/spread, sweetened only with concentrated fruit juice

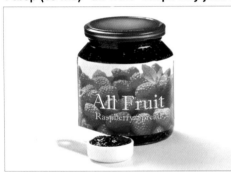

Calories	Carbs	Fiber	Fat	Sodium
50	12 g	0 g	0 g	0 mg

This sugar-free jam has similar amounts of calories and total sugar as regular jam (concentrated grape juice is like adding table sugar). When comparing labels, check the total carbohydrate, which includes the sugar from juice and table sugar. **Net Carbs 12 g**

1 tsp (5 mL) pure raspberry jam

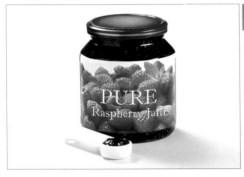

Calories	Carbs	Fiber	Fat	Sodium
18	5 g	0 g	0 g	2 mg

Keep your portion of regular jam to 1 tsp (5 mL) per serving. This is about a thumbtip-size amount of jam. **Net Carbs 5 g**

1 tbsp (15 mL) no-sugar-added jam/spread (10 to 20 calories per tbsp/15 mL)

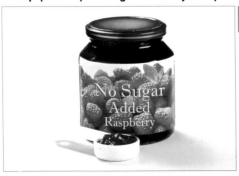

Calories	Carbs	Fiber	Fat	Sodium
10	2 g	0 g	0 g	5 mg

One tablespoon (15 mL) of this jam/spread has 10 to 20 calories. The lowest-calorie variety will be sweetened with a low-calorie sweetener, such as sucralose. **Net Carbs 2 g**

HEALTHY CHOICE

FOOD FACT Some people find that eating 1 to 2 tsp (5 to 10 mL) of jam or honey helps satisfy a sugar craving.

Bagel Breakfast

1 large (4-inch/10 cm or 102 g) bagel (unbuttered) with 3 tbsp (45 mL) cream cheese, 20-oz (600 mL) coffee with 4 creamers (4 tbsp/60 mL) and 4 tsp (20 mL) sugar

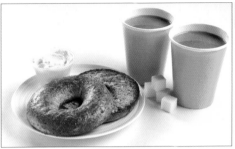

Calories	Carbs	Fiber	Fat	Sodium
640	81 g	3 g	28 g	751 mg

Bagels are a dense type of bread. One 4-inch (10 cm) bagel has the same number of carbs as 4 slices of bread. **Caffeine: 448 mg** (based on filter drip). **Net Carbs 78 g**

1 large (4-inch/10 cm or 102 g) bagel (unbuttered) with 1 tbsp (15 mL) cream cheese, 10-oz (300 mL) coffee with 2 creamers (2 tbsp/25 mL) and 2 tsp (10 mL) sugar

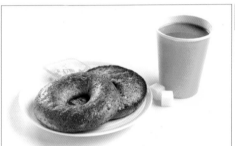

Calories	Carbs	Fiber	Fat	Sodium
445	70 g	3 g	12 g	647 mg

Simply cutting back on the size of your coffee (large to small) makes a big difference in the amount of cream and sugar you'll use. Small changes are easier than big changes. **Caffeine: 224 mg. Net Carbs 67 g**

1 small (3-inch/7.5 cm or 53 g) bagel (unbuttered) with 1 tbsp (15 mL) light cream cheese, 10-oz (300 mL) decaf coffee with 2 tbsp (30 mL) 2% milk

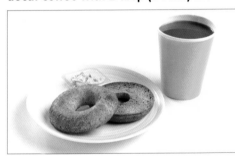

Calories	Carbs	Fiber	Fat	Sodium
206	33 g	1 g	4 g	367 mg

Here's a lighter choice! Not all coffee shops sell small bagels, but you can buy them at the grocery store, toast your bagel at home and spread lightly with cream cheese. **Caffeine: 4 mg. Net Carbs 32 g**

1 small (3-inch/7.5 cm or 53 g) bagel (unbuttered) with 1 tbsp (15 mL) sugar-free jam, 10-oz (300 mL) decaf coffee with 2 tbsp (30 mL) 2% milk

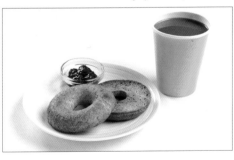

Calories	Carbs	Fiber	Fat	Sodium
192	37 g	1 g	1 g	323 mg

Switching from cream cheese to a sugar-free jam increases your carbs slightly but decreases total calories and fat. Low-calorie sweetener can be added to coffee or tea, if desired. **Caffeine: 4 mg. Net Carbs 36 g**

HEALTHY CHOICE

FOOD FACT Why does a bagel have a hole? Two reasons. The hole provides more even cooking and enabled traditional vendors to carry them on a string or stick.

Deli Sandwich

Rye bread, 2 thin large slices (2 oz/60 g) pastrami, 2 tsp (10 mL) mustard, 2 tsp (10 mL) butter, ¼ cup (60 mL) sauerkraut, 1 medium dill pickle

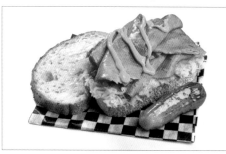

Calories	Carbs	Fiber	Fat	Sodium
330	35 g	6 g	14 g	2,101 mg

Did you notice the sodium? Save this sandwich for a special occasion only or choose one of the options below. **Net Carbs 29 g**

Rye bread, 1 thin slice (1 oz/30 g) pastrami, 2 tsp (10 mL) mustard, 2 tsp (10 mL) butter, 1 medium dill pickle

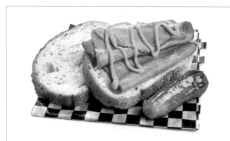

Calories	Carbs	Fiber	Fat	Sodium
286	33 g	5 g	12 g	1,515 mg

If you are buying a pastrami rye sandwich at a restaurant, ask the server to hold the sauerkraut (or the pickle). This helps reduce the sodium. **Net Carbs 28 g**

Rye bread, 1 thin slice (1 oz/30 g) pastrami, 2 tsp (10 mL) mustard, 1 medium dill pickle

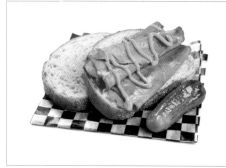

Calories	Carbs	Fiber	Fat	Sodium
218	33 g	5 g	4 g	1,461 mg

To cut calories and sodium further, ask for your bread to be unbuttered. If you use home-cooked sliced roast beef, turkey or chicken, the sodium is even further reduced. **Net Carbs 28 g**

Rye bread, 1 thin slice (1 oz/30 g) pastrami, 1 tsp (5 mL) mustard, lettuce, tomato, ½ medium dill pickle

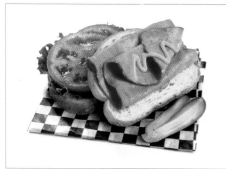

Calories	Carbs	Fiber	Fat	Sodium
215	33 g	5 g	4 g	1,119 mg

This reduced-salt version still contains almost half of the suggested daily intake of sodium. So make sure not to have luncheon meat on a daily basis, or use your own home-cooked sliced roast beef, turkey or chicken. **Net Carbs 28 g**

HEALTHY CHOICE

FOOD FACT

When buying bread, look for thinner or smaller slices that have about 70 to 80 calories per slice.

Cream Soup

Half of a 10-oz (284 mL) can of condensed cream of tomato soup, made with an equal amount of 3.3% (homogenized) milk, 3½-oz (100 g) tea biscuit with 2 tsp (10 mL) butter

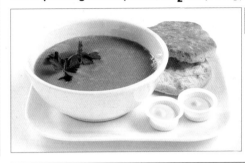

Calories	Carbs	Fiber	Fat	Sodium
617	76 g	3 g	30 g	2,031 mg

The extra fat in this meal comes from the whole milk in the soup and the butter on the biscuit. **Net Carbs 73 g**

Half of a 10-oz (284 mL) can of condensed cream of tomato soup, made with an equal amount of 2% milk, 3½-oz (100 g) tea biscuit with 1 tsp (5 mL) butter

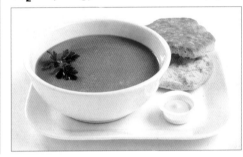

Calories	Carbs	Fiber	Fat	Sodium
568	76 g	3 g	24 g	2,006 mg

The switch to 2% milk cuts some calories and fat.
Net Carbs 73 g

Half of a 10-oz (284 mL) can of condensed reduced-sodium cream of tomato soup, made with an equal amount of skim milk, 3½-oz (100 g) tea biscuit (unbuttered)

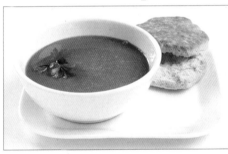

Calories	Carbs	Fiber	Fat	Sodium
523	77 g	2 g	19 g	1,679 mg

When you switch to skim milk, you reduce the calories and fat further. Choosing a reduced-sodium soup can cut salt by 20% to 30%, depending on the brand. Low-sodium varieties reduce the sodium even more, but are more difficult to find. **Net Carbs 75 g**

Half of a 10-oz (284 mL) can of condensed reduced-sodium cream of tomato soup, made with an equal amount of skim milk, 6 unsalted soda crackers, veggies

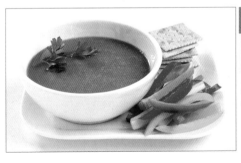

Calories	Carbs	Fiber	Fat	Sodium
262	47 g	3 g	5 g	805 mg

For an even lighter choice, switch to soda crackers and veggies on the side. **Net Carbs 44 g**

HEALTHY CHOICE

FOOD FACT Boil meat or poultry bones for a great soup stock. Add onions and herbs, leftover vegetables and some barley or noodles for a tasty low-salt soup.

Chicken Leg

1 drumstick and thigh, with skin, breaded and deep-fried

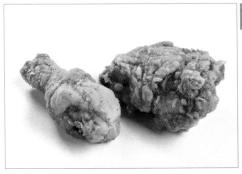

Calories	Carbs	Fiber	Fat	Sodium
360	12 g	0 g	21 g	368 mg

One piece of deep-fried chicken never hurt anyone. But eating fried chicken every day is a health risk. Fried chicken tends to be eaten with other high-fat foods, including fries, gravy and coleslaw laden with high-fat mayonnaise.
Net Carbs 12 g

1 drumstick and thigh, with skin, coated with commercial crumb coating and baked

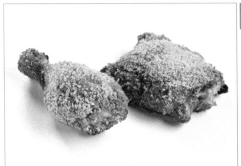

Calories	Carbs	Fiber	Fat	Sodium
286	4 g	0 g	19 g	234 mg

Here's a lower-fat homemade alternative using commercial crumb coating (such as Shake n' Bake™) for the chicken.
Net Carbs 4 g

1 drumstick and thigh, skin removed, coated with commercial crumb coating and baked

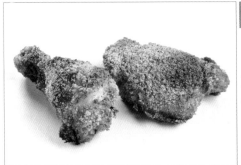

Calories	Carbs	Fiber	Fat	Sodium
173	4 g	0 g	7 g	217 mg

Remove the skin from the chicken and you remove 2½ tsp (12 mL) of fat for this serving. This is still a delicious alternative. **Net Carbs 4 g**

1 drumstick and thigh, skin removed, coated with salt-free spice blend and baked

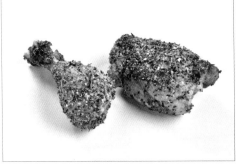

Calories	Carbs	Fiber	Fat	Sodium
148	0 g	0 g	6 g	80 mg

This choice reduces the calories and sodium by using the low-cost homemade Chicken Spice Mix on page 112. You can also use a commercial low-salt spice blend. **Net Carbs 0 g**

HEALTHY CHOICE

FOOD FACT By baking the chicken at home, you're not only making an awesome healthy change, but you're also saving money!

Fish

White fish (5 oz/150 g), battered and deep-fried

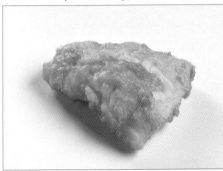

Calories	Carbs	Fiber	Fat	Sodium
329	24 g	1 g	17 g	754 mg

This 5-oz (150 g) choice has 2 oz (60 g) of batter and only 3 oz (90 g) of fish. It is also a poor nutritional choice, as it is high in fat, especially saturated fat. In a restaurant, the fish would typically be served with french fries, further increasing the calories and fat in the meal. **Net Carbs 23 g**

Store-bought frozen "lightly" breaded white fish (5 oz/150 g), baked

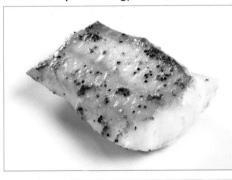

Calories	Carbs	Fiber	Fat	Sodium
244	19 g	0 g	8 g	360 mg

Look for light or lightly breaded fish which is a lighter choice than the standard breaded fish. Have a salad and vegetables and oven-baked fries (see page 156). **Net Carbs 19 g**

White fish (5 oz/150 g), fried, broiled or baked with 1 tsp (5 mL) added fat

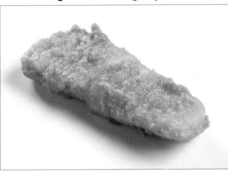

Calories	Carbs	Fiber	Fat	Sodium
193	0 g	0 g	5 g	151 mg

In these next two choices, without batter, you get a 5 oz (150 g) serving of fish. Quickly cook up your fish in 1 tsp (5 mL) of fat (oil, butter or margarine) in a nonstick frying pan. Or bake it in the oven with the small amount of fat. Try Dinner 3 (page 120). **Net Carbs 0 g**

White fish (5 oz/150 g), broiled or steamed with dill or ¼ tsp (1 mL) pesto

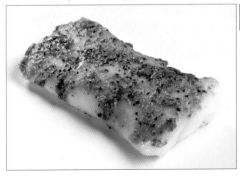

Calories	Carbs	Fiber	Fat	Sodium
159	0 g	0 g	1 g	113 mg

A great way to cook white fish without fat is to wrap it in foil or parchment paper, then bake it. You may want to add chopped vegetables and basil or garlic. Pesto (a combination of basil, garlic and olive oil) can be bought ready-to-use in a squeeze tube. **Net Carbs 0 g**

HEALTHY CHOICE

FOOD FACT Fish is an excellent source of omega-3 fats, which keep your blood vessels healthy. Eating fish twice a week gives you all the omega-3s you need.

Fast-Food Burger with All Toppings

Third-pound beef patty burger (4 oz/112 g cooked weight) with double cheese and bacon (like Angus)

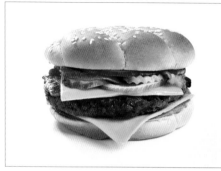

Calories	Carbs	Fiber	Fat	Sodium
770	53 g	2 g	41 g	1,400 mg

Restaurant burgers have layers of tasty ingredients, and that's reflected in the calories, fat and sodium. If you have fries and a drink with this burger, the fat and calories go up even higher. **Net Carbs 51 g**

Two single burgers (each burger = 1 oz/28 g cooked) with cheese and middle bun (like Big Mac)

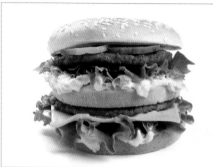

Calories	Carbs	Fiber	Fat	Sodium
520	45 g	3 g	28 g	950 mg

This is a reduction but still pretty loaded. Know what you are eating: check out the calories and nutrients of the fast-food item. This may be listed on the menu, or check it out online before you go out to eat. **Net Carbs 42 g**

Cheeseburger (1 oz/28 g cooked weight burger) with 1 strip of bacon

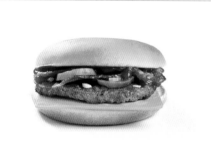

Calories	Carbs	Fiber	Fat	Sodium
360	34 g	2 g	16 g	970 mg

This option has significantly less calories, fat and sodium. It's a good alternative and still tastes great! **Net Carbs 32 g**

Cheeseburger (1 oz/28 g cooked weight burger)

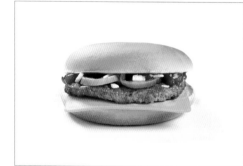

Calories	Carbs	Fiber	Fat	Sodium
290	33 g	2 g	11 g	700 mg

Of the four options here, this is the best choice when you're eating at a fast-food restaurant. Instead of choosing the meal deal, order individual items from the menu. Ask for a small fries or a salad on the side, and have milk instead of a soft drink. Alternatively, try Dinner 27 (page 216). **Net Carbs 31 g**

HEALTHY CHOICE

FOOD FACT It may seem like a waste not to get the meal deal, but remember: all those extra calories go to *your* waist.

Restaurant Pizza

3 pieces of thick-crust 12-inch (30 cm) deluxe pizza (with 6 pieces per pizza)

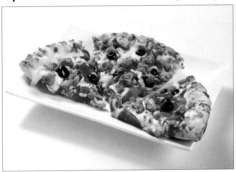

Calories	Carbs	Fiber	Fat	Sodium
1,659	143 g	7 g	87 g	3,474 mg

This option has the same number of calories as a large breakfast, lunch and dinner meal in this book combined — all in just three pieces of pizza! This serving has a whopping $1\frac{1}{2}$ tsp (7 mL) of salt and more than a day's worth of fat. **Net Carbs 136 g**

3 pieces of thin-crust 12-inch (30 cm) deluxe pizza (with 6 pieces per pizza)

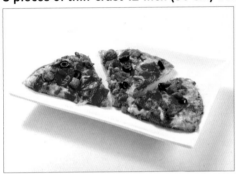

Calories	Carbs	Fiber	Fat	Sodium
1,346	91 g	7 g	81 g	2,757 mg

Cut carbs significantly by switching to thin-crust pizza. To help fill you up, drink water and have a salad or a half plate of your favorite cooked vegetables with your pizza. **Net Carbs 84 g**

2 pieces of thick-crust 12-inch (30 cm) pizza with two toppings, salad with a light dressing

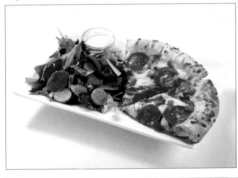

Calories	Carbs	Fiber	Fat	Sodium
944	95 g	4 g	46 g	2,114 mg

To cut calories, fat and sodium, choose a pizza with fewer toppings. For pizza ideas, see Dinner 26 (page 212). **Net Carbs 91 g**

2 pieces of thin-crust 12-inch (30 cm) pizza with two toppings, salad with a light dressing

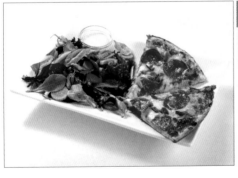

Calories	Carbs	Fiber	Fat	Sodium
782	65 g	4 g	44 g	1,742 mg

Add some extra vegetables to your pizza. Try onions, asparagus, peppers, mushrooms, fresh tomatoes, sun-dried tomatoes and zucchini. Even this choice is salty, so it's best to not choose it every week. **Net Carbs 61 g**

HEALTHY CHOICE

FOOD FACT Slowing down your eating can help you eat less. Eat some vegetables or salad before your pizza, and drink water before and with your meal.

Ready-to-Serve Noodles

Noodles in a bowl, chicken flavor (110 g dry weight)

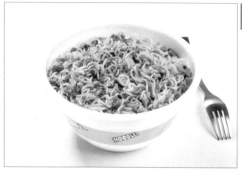

Calories	Carbs	Fiber	Fat	Sodium
481	70 g	3 g	17 g	2,278 mg

This product has a shocking amount of salt. Studies show that people with diabetes are not able to get rid of excess sodium as efficiently as people without diabetes. Eating too much sodium can worsen high blood pressure. **Net Carbs 67 g**

Noodles in a cup, chicken flavor (64 g dry weight)

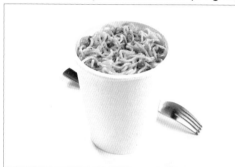

Calories	Carbs	Fiber	Fat	Sodium
280	41 g	2 g	10 g	1,325 mg

The cup serving is smaller than the bowl and so has less sodium. However, this serving is still high in sodium. **Net Carbs 39 g**

Noodles in a cup, chicken flavor (64 g dry weight), made with half the spice mix

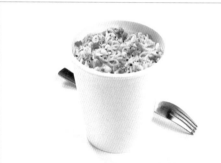

Calories	Carbs	Fiber	Fat	Sodium
274	39 g	1 g	10 g	776 mg

Here's an easy change to cut the salt in half: only add half the package of spice mix! To boost flavor, add some low-salt seasoning, such as Mrs. Dash or McCormick no-salt seasonings. **Net Carbs 38 g**

Noodles in a cup (64 g dry weight) without the chicken flavor mix, made instead with 1 tsp (5 mL) salt-free spice blend (or fresh herbs and/or chili or black pepper)

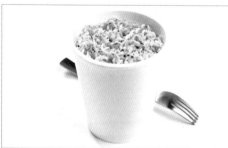

Calories	Carbs	Fiber	Fat	Sodium
268	37 g	1 g	10 g	226 mg

Are you ready to replace the whole package of spice mix with a low-salt seasoning or some tasty fresh herbs? You'll still enjoy the noodles, and you'll no longer have to worry about all that added salt. **Net Carbs 36 g**

HEALTHY CHOICE

FOOD FACT A noodle bowl is the carb equivalent of about **5 slices of bread** and a noodle cup is equivalent to almost **3 slices of bread.**

Potatoes

1 large serving (6 oz/175 g) fast-food french fries

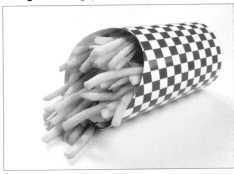

Calories	Carbs	Fiber	Fat	Sodium
560	74 g	6 g	27 g	430 mg

The total fat in a serving of french fries is a concern if they're eaten regularly or daily. Also of concern is that fat heated to a high temperature in a deep-fryer changes into an unhealthy type of fat. **Net Carbs 68 g**

1 large serving (6 oz/175 g) baked frozen french fries, unsalted

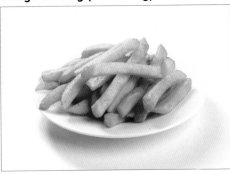

Calories	Carbs	Fiber	Fat	Sodium
350	55 g	6 g	13 g	53 mg

Bake these lower-fat fries at home and serve them as part of a meal. **Net Carbs 49 g**

1 large baked potato with no added fat, with 2 tbsp (30 mL) fat-free sour cream, 1 tsp (5 mL) butter or margarine, and chopped green onion

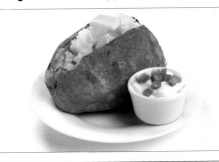

Calories	Carbs	Fiber	Fat	Sodium
298	61 g	5 g	4 g	92 mg

Try a baked potato instead of fries. The life-size photo that accompanies Dinner 1 (page 115) shows the size of 1½ medium potatoes (equivalent to 1 large potato). The carbs are a bit higher in this choice because of the toppings. **Net Carbs 56 g**

1 large potato, cut into sticks, tossed in 1 tsp (5 mL) oil and baked

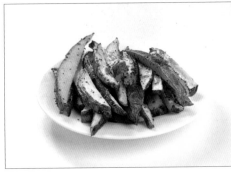

Calories	Carbs	Fiber	Fat	Sodium
276	55 g	5 g	5 g	17 mg

This is a delicious and easy way to make home-baked fries. To spice them up, sprinkle on flavorings such as dried dillweed, chili powder or a commercial salt-free spice blend. **Net Carbs 50 g**

HEALTHY CHOICE

FOOD FACT **Potatoes are an excellent source of vitamin C and potassium.**

Vegetables

Deep-fried onion rings (medium order, 160 g)

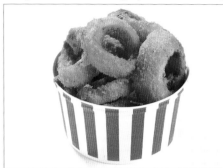

Calories	Carbs	Fiber	Fat	Sodium
501	51 g	4 g	29 g	832 mg

The benefit of the onion (or other vegetable) is lost underneath the battering and frying, so please don't count this deep-fried snack as one of your "vegetables" for the day! The onions are now high in calories, fat and salt. **Net Carbs 47 g**

1½ cups (375 mL) mixed vegetables with ¼ cup (60 mL) cheese sauce, made with skim milk

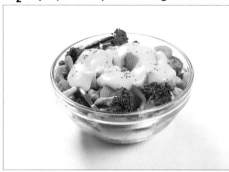

Calories	Carbs	Fiber	Fat	Sodium
155	18 g	4 g	6 g	221 mg

To make cheese sauce for four: In a small saucepan, over medium heat, heat up 1 tbsp (15 mL) fat with 1 tbsp (15 mL) flour until small bubbles form. Add 1 cup (250 mL) skim milk and ½ cup (125 mL) shredded low-fat cheese. Stir with a whisk until smooth and thickened. **Net Carbs 14 g**

1½ cups (375 mL) mixed vegetables with 1 tsp (5 mL) margarine or butter

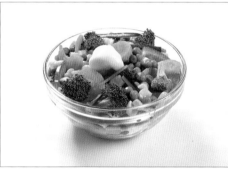

Calories	Carbs	Fiber	Fat	Sodium
95	13 g	4 g	5 g	105 mg

Choose a big serving of vegetables to help fill you up at your meal — you will find that you eat less meat and potatoes. **Net Carbs 9 g**

1½ cups (375 mL) mixed vegetables, lightly steamed, with herbs

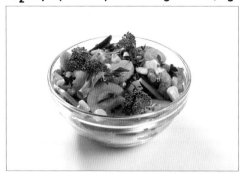

Calories	Carbs	Fiber	Fat	Sodium
63	13 g	4 g	1 g	72 mg

Add black pepper or fresh or dried herbs to your vegetables. This makes them tasty and enjoyable to eat. **Net Carbs 9 g**

HEALTHY CHOICE

FOOD FACT Onions and garlic, eaten raw or cooked, are excellent choices, as they may play a role in reducing blood clots.

Caesar Salad

Restaurant Caesar salad: 4 cups (1 L) romaine lettuce, ¼ cup (60 mL) Caesar salad dressing, ¼ cup (60 mL) croutons and 2 tbsp (30 mL) Parmesan cheese, plus 2 pieces of garlic bread

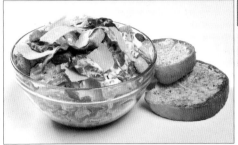

Calories	Carbs	Fiber	Fat	Sodium
798	58 g	8 g	57 g	1,564 mg

Many are surprised that a large Caesar salad from a restaurant has as many calories as a large burger. The reason is that Caesar salad dressing is mostly oil and is high in fat. Topped off with the garlic bread, this salad is not light! **Net Carbs 50 g**

Restaurant Caesar salad: 4 cups (1 L) romaine lettuce, ¼ cup (60 mL) Caesar salad dressing, ¼ cup (60 mL) croutons and 2 tbsp (30 mL) Parmesan cheese

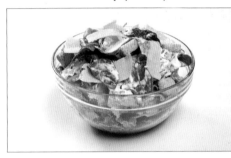

Calories	Carbs	Fiber	Fat	Sodium
442	16 g	5 g	40 g	967 mg

To avoid the extra calories, ask the waiter not to bring out the garlic bread. **Net Carbs 11 g**

Restaurant Caesar salad: 4 cups (1 L) romaine lettuce, 2 tbsp (30 mL) Caesar salad dressing, ¼ cup (60 mL) croutons and 1 tbsp (15 mL) Parmesan cheese

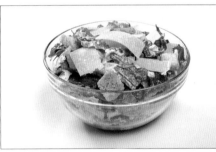

Calories	Carbs	Fiber	Fat	Sodium
263	15 g	5 g	21 g	554 mg

Ask for a small amount of salad dressing on the side and limit your serving of dressing to 2 tbsp (30 mL). Some restaurants have an option for a light salad dressing. **Net Carbs 10 g**

Homemade Caesar salad: 4 cups (1 L) romaine lettuce, 1 tbsp (15 mL) light Caesar salad dressing, ¼ cup (60 mL) croutons and 1 tbsp (15 mL) Parmesan cheese

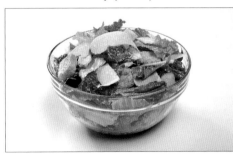

Calories	Carbs	Fiber	Fat	Sodium
125	17 g	5 g	5 g	400 mg

Simple and fast to prepare at home, this light salad choice makes a terrific appetizer or meal accompaniment. Light salad dressing is higher in salt, so you might choose to use regular salad dressing instead. **Net Carbs 12 g**

HEALTHY CHOICE

FOOD FACT Dark green lettuce, such as romaine, is rich in folate, which is helpful for your blood cholesterol.

Yogurt

¾ cup (175 mL) 6% fruit yogurt, sweetened with sugar

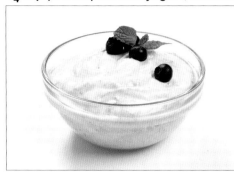

Calories	Carbs	Fiber	Fat	Sodium
240	29 g	0 g	11 g	98 mg

This high-fat yogurt has double the fat of a homogenized milk. Some other yogurts have extra fermenting bacteria added and are labeled as better for you. But look at the label, because they may be made with a higher-fat milk or extra sugar. They may not be the right choice for you. **Net Carbs 29 g**

¾ cup (175 mL) 3% frozen yogurt

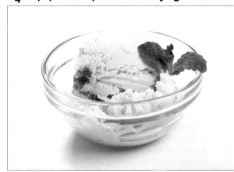

Calories	Carbs	Fiber	Fat	Sodium
150	29 g	0 g	3 g	90 mg

Frozen yogurt is a nice dessert choice and has fewer calories than the high-fat yogurt above. It has similar calories to a 2% sweetened fruit yogurt. **Net Carbs 29 g**

¾ cup (175 mL) fat-free (0% fat) fruit yogurt, sweetened with sugar

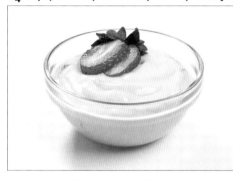

Calories	Carbs	Fiber	Fat	Sodium
173	35 g	0 g	0 g	107 mg

This is a better choice because there's no fat, but there is still added sugar. 0% Greek yogurt is also a great choice. **Net Carbs 35 g**

¾ cup (175 mL) fat-free (0% fat) fruit yogurt, sweetened with a low-calorie sweetener, plus ½ cup (125 mL) blueberries or other fresh or frozen fruit

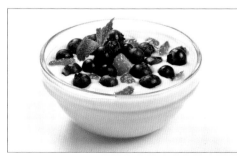

Calories	Carbs	Fiber	Fat	Sodium
128	24 g	2 g	0 g	109 mg

By choosing a fat-free yogurt sweetened with a low-calorie sweetener, you avoid extra fat and added sugar. Like all yogurts, it contains natural sugar (carbohydrate) from the milk. **Net Carbs 22 g**

HEALTHY CHOICE

FOOD FACT

Yogurt is perhaps the oldest fermented milk product. There are records of its use dating back 2,500 years!

Ice Cream

3 scoops (each ½ cup/125 mL) of vanilla ice cream with ¼ cup (60 mL) chocolate sauce and 2 tbsp (30 mL) nuts (strawberry garnish)

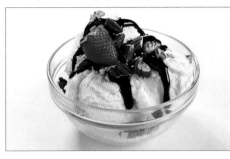

Calories	Carbs	Fiber	Fat	Sodium
728	99 g	3 g	36 g	203 mg

This ice cream with toppings has as much fat and calories as a large fast-food burger (see page 301). This may not be the best choice for you. **Net Carbs 96 g**

3 scoops (each ½ cup/125 mL) of vanilla ice cream (strawberry garnish)

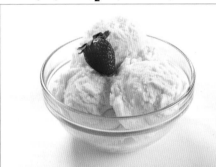

Calories	Carbs	Fiber	Fat	Sodium
442	53 g	2 g	24 g	173 mg

One or two scoops of ice cream in an ice cream cone would have less calories, carbs and fat than the three scoops of regular-fat ice cream. A standard cone has only 20 calories and can make the dessert seem more filling than when the ice cream is served in a bowl. **Net Carbs 51 g**

2 scoops (each ½ cup/125 mL) of vanilla ice cream (strawberry garnish)

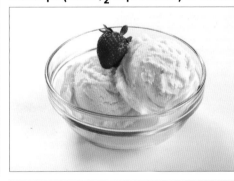

Calories	Carbs	Fiber	Fat	Sodium
293	35 g	1 g	16 g	116 mg

If you put your ice cream in a bowl, remember to use a small bowl, to make it seem like more (see page 253). This may help you cut down to one scoop. **Net Carbs 34 g**

1 scoop (½ cup/125 mL) of vanilla ice cream with 1 cup (250 mL) strawberries or other fresh fruit

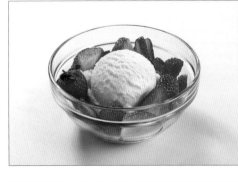

Calories	Carbs	Fiber	Fat	Sodium
198	30 g	4 g	8 g	59 mg

A half cup (125 mL) of ice cream has about the same calories as a ¾-cup (175 mL) serving of yogurt, but has less calcium. Adding fruit helps fill you up. **Net Carbs 26 g**

HEALTHY CHOICE

FOOD FACT   Check labels: not all ice creams are the same. Choose one with less fat, sugar or calories: **125 to 150 calories per ½ cup (125 mL).**

Cookies

Two large (3½-inch/8.5 cm, 114 g) fast-food chocolate chunk cookies

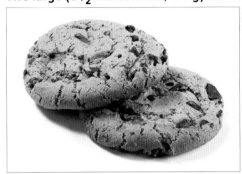

Calories	Carbs	Fiber	Fat	Sodium
460	70 g	2 g	18 g	520 mg

It's probably a good idea to buy only one of these large cookies — but remember, even one has 230 calories, which is more than a large snack (see pages 284–285). **Net Carbs 68 g**

Three 2¼-inch (5.5 cm) commercial chocolate chunk cookies

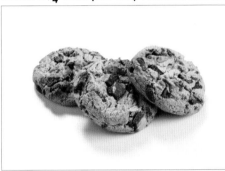

Calories	Carbs	Fiber	Fat	Sodium
255	35 g	2 g	12 g	203 mg

Do you remember the cookies your grandmother used to make? The three of them shown here have fewer carbs and calories than the two supersize cookies above. **Net Carbs 33 g**

Three 2½-inch (6 cm) commercial chocolate chip cookies ("Dad's cookies")

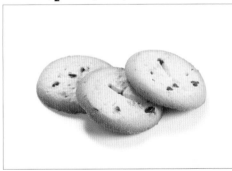

Calories	Carbs	Fiber	Fat	Sodium
195	24 g	0 g	9 g	135 mg

Check the Nutrition Facts table on store-bought cookies. Choose the ones with less saturated fat. **Net Carbs 24 g**

Three 2½-inch (6 cm) thin chocolate cookies

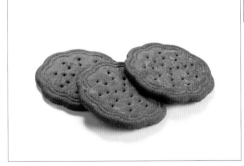

Calories	Carbs	Fiber	Fat	Sodium
98	14 g	1 g	4 g	98 mg

When you buy cookies, look for ones that are thinner and smaller, with less than 100 calories, 20 g of carbohydrates and 5 g of fat per 2 cookies. **Net Carbs 13 g**

HEALTHY CHOICE

FOOD FACT Try not to eat more than two or three small cookies for a dessert or snack. Substitute fruit for cookies more of the time.

Muffin or Donut

Large blueberry bran muffin (128 g)

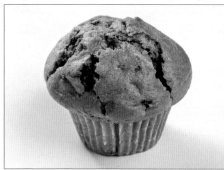

Calories	Carbs	Fiber	Fat	Sodium
380	58 g	5 g	15 g	530 mg

A common misconception is that coffee shop muffins (especially low-fat ones) are healthier than donuts. This is false, because the muffins are made so large, they end up having more sugar and fat than standard-size donuts. **Net Carbs 53 g**

Plain cake donut (60 g)

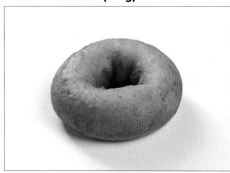

Calories	Carbs	Fiber	Fat	Sodium
253	30 g	1 g	14 g	328 mg

This cake donut has almost 150 calories less than the muffin above. Many coffee shops have the nutrient information of their muffins, donuts and other foods and drinks listed online. If you eat at one regularly, compare the nutrient listings. **Net Carbs 29 g**

3 donut "holes" (50 to 55 g total)

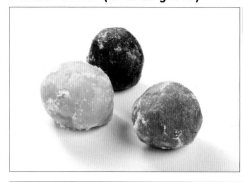

Calories	Carbs	Fiber	Fat	Sodium
219	26 g	1 g	12 g	284 mg

For a lighter donut choice with your coffee or tea, choose two or three donut "holes." **Net Carbs 25 g**

Homemade Bran Muffin (see recipe, page 56)

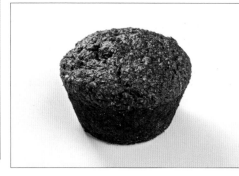

Calories	Carbs	Fiber	Fat	Sodium
163	27 g	3 g	6 g	172 mg

Commercial muffin mixes come in low-fat varieties. Compare the nutrient information to this muffin. Although this choice appears to have more carbs than the 3 donut holes, the available carb is less. It is an excellent source of fiber and is low in fat. **Net Carbs 24 g**

HEALTHY CHOICE

FOOD FACT The size of the muffin determines the total amount of sugar and fat. Bigger muffins can have similar amounts of sugar and fat as donuts.

Apple Dessert

1 piece of homemade double-crust apple pie (¹/₆th of a 9-inch/23 cm pie made with 5 apples)

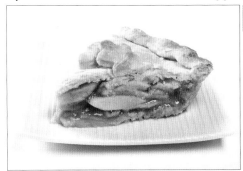

Calories	Carbs	Fiber	Fat	Sodium
556	71 g	3 g	29 g	517 mg

Enjoy apple pie just occasionally. Once you add a double crust to a pie, it's like adding 4 slices of buttered bread to your fruit filling. Ice cream on top of your pie will add more sugar and fat. **Net Carbs 68 g**

³/₄ cup (175 mL) traditional apple crisp (¹/₆th of recipe, see below)

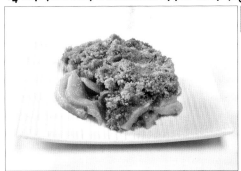

Calories	Carbs	Fiber	Fat	Sodium
314	55 g	2 g	11 g	378 mg

Using a topping rather than a crust cuts the calories and fat. Recipe includes 5 apples, ³/₄ cup (175 mL) flour, 1 cup (250 mL) brown sugar, ³/₄ tsp (3 mL) salt, 1 tsp (5 mL) ground cinnamon and ¹/₃ cup (75 mL) butter or margarine. **Net Carbs 53 g**

³/₄ cup (175 mL) healthier apple crisp (¹/₆th of recipe, see below)

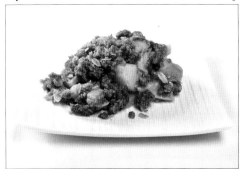

Calories	Carbs	Fiber	Fat	Sodium
224	37 g	3 g	9 g	62 mg

Recipe includes 5 apples, ¹/₄ cup (60 mL) whole wheat flour, ¹/₂ cup (125 mL) rolled oats, ¹/₂ cup (125 mL) brown sugar, 1 tsp (5 mL) ground cinnamon and ¹/₄ cup (60 mL) butter or margarine. If you want, you could replace some of the brown sugar with a low-calorie sweetener. **Net Carbs 34 g**

1 Baked Apple (see recipe, page 165)

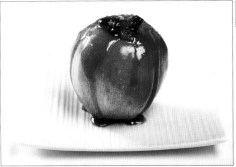

Calories	Carbs	Fiber	Fat	Sodium
150	29 g	3 g	5 g	43 mg

You can still satisfy your sweet tooth with this choice, which has fewer calories and less fat and sugar. **Net Carbs 26 g**

FOOD FACT   Adding cinnamon to desserts and cereals boosts flavor, so you don't need to add as much sugar.

HEALTHY CHOICE

Canned or Fresh Fruit

Two half peaches in syrup

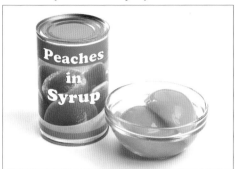

Calories	Carbs	Fiber	Fat	Sodium
145	39 g	3 g	0 g	12 mg

By rinsing the fruit in water, you can remove some of the extra sugar added during the canning process. **Net Carbs 36 g**

Two half peaches in juice

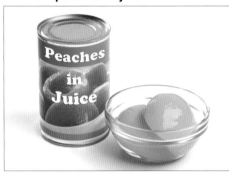

Calories	Carbs	Fiber	Fat	Sodium
86	23 g	3 g	0 g	8 mg

Switching to juice-packed instead of syrup-packed fruit is an easy way to cut calories and carbs. Most stores sell juice-packed fruit for the same price as the syrup-packed fruit. **Net Carbs 20 g**

Two half peaches in water ("no sugar added")

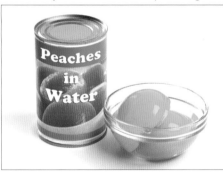

Calories	Carbs	Fiber	Fat	Sodium
47	12 g	3 g	0 g	6 mg

As fresh peaches are seasonal, these canned peaches make an excellent alternative. Unfortunately, peaches canned in water are not always available or may be more expensive. **Net Carbs 9 g**

1 fresh peach (medium-large)

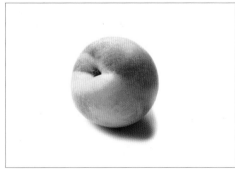

Calories	Carbs	Fiber	Fat	Sodium
50	12 g	3 g	0 g	0 mg

When peaches are in season, go with the fresh fruit. A fresh peach has similar nutrients as peaches canned in water. Calories and carbs vary slightly depending on the size of the peach. **Net Carbs 9 g**

HEALTHY CHOICE

FOOD FACT

Chinese kings and emperors used to consider peaches an exquisite delight — now everyone can eat like a king!

Cheese and Crackers

1½ oz (45 g) regular-fat cheese plus 6 party crackers (20 g)

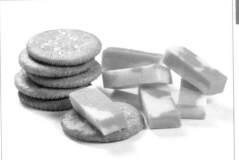

Calories	Carbs	Fiber	Fat	Sodium
271	13 g	0 g	19 g	464 mg

Do party crackers tempt you to overeat? If so, keep them as a "party treat," not an everyday choice. **Net Carbs 13 g**

1½ oz (45 g) regular-fat cheese plus 6 reduced-sodium (61% less sodium) party crackers (20 g)

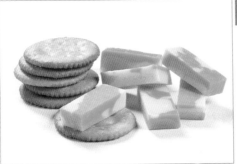

Calories	Carbs	Fiber	Fat	Sodium
271	14 g	1 g	19 g	334 mg

An easy way to reduce salt is to look for low-sodium crackers. Salt is used to preserve cheeses, so low-sodium cheeses don't store as well and are harder to find. **Net Carbs 13 g**

1 oz (30 g) regular-fat cheese plus 4 whole-grain crackers (18 g)

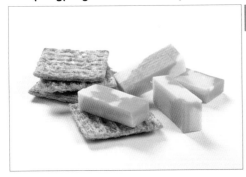

Calories	Carbs	Fiber	Fat	Sodium
194	13 g	2 g	12 g	291 mg

In this choice, four whole-grain crackers replace the six party-type crackers. You can have this option as a snack or incorporate it into your lunch meal (see Lunch 12, page 100.) **Net Carbs 11 g**

1 oz (30 g) regular-fat cheese plus 4 reduced-sodium (61% less sodium) whole-grain crackers (18 g)

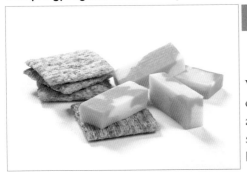

Calories	Carbs	Fiber	Fat	Sodium
194	13 g	2 g	12 g	221 mg

Whole-grain and whole wheat crackers are both good choices. Unfortunately, not all whole wheat crackers are available unsalted. For example, you can buy unsalted plain soda crackers, but whole wheat soda crackers are salted. **Net Carbs 11 g**

HEALTHY CHOICE

FOOD FACT Light Cheddar cheese has less than 20% milk fat (M.F.).

Popcorn

Large buttered movie theater popcorn (20 cups/5 L with 6 pumps of butter, equal to 3 tbsp/45 mL)

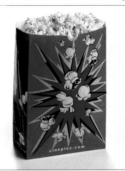

Calories	Carbs	Fiber	Fat	Sodium
1,405	126 g	22 g	96 g	2,190 mg

The amount of fat and salt in this super-sized serving might be enough to scare you or make you cry, if the movie doesn't. **Net Carbs 104 g**

Small buttered movie theater popcorn (7 cups/1.75 L with 3 pumps of butter, equal to 1½ tbsp/22 mL)

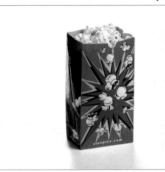

Calories	Carbs	Fiber	Fat	Sodium
538	44 g	8 g	39 g	803 mg

Studies have been done where people were given very stale popcorn at a movie theater, and they still ate it all. If you want to eat less, buy a smaller serving. **Net Carbs 36 g**

4 cups (1 L) home-popped popcorn, made with 1 tsp (5 mL) oil for ¼ cup (60 mL) kernels, plus 3 shakes of salt (¹⁄₁₆ tsp/0.25 mL)

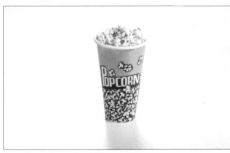

Calories	Carbs	Fiber	Fat	Sodium
164	24 g	4 g	6 g	147 mg

A better choice. It contains about half the fat and sodium of the same amount of movie theater popcorn. Try peanut oil for a great flavor! Electric popcorn makers with motorized stirring rods make yummy popcorn with little oil. **Net Carbs 20 g**

4 cups (1 L) air-popped popcorn

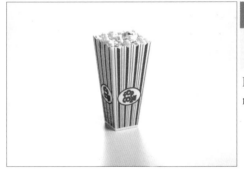

Calories	Carbs	Fiber	Fat	Sodium
122	25 g	4 g	1 g	1 mg

Popcorn can be air-popped with an electric air popper or a microwave popcorn popper. **Net Carbs 21 g**

HEALTHY CHOICE

FOOD FACT Popcorn is believed to have been discovered by Native Americans over 5,000 years ago when corn was being cooked over the open fire.

Juice or Soft Drink

12 oz (355 mL) unsweetened apple juice

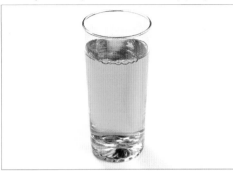

Calories	Carbs	Fiber	Fat	Sodium
168	42 g	0 g	0 g	11 mg

Even unsweetened fruit juice has a lot of natural sugar; in fact, some juices have more total sugar than some soft drinks. It's easy to drink a lot of sugar quickly. Juice has very little fiber, so it does not replace fresh fruit. **Net Carbs 42 g**

12 oz (355 mL) cola

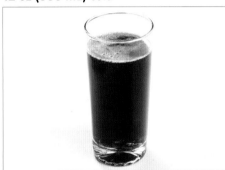

Calories	Carbs	Fiber	Fat	Sodium
155	40 g	0 g	0 g	15 mg

Regular cola is high in added sugar, and has caffeine added. If you drink a 2-quart (2 L) bottle of cola, you get 53 tsp (265 mL) of sugar and 200 to 300 mg of caffeine. Energy drinks can have double or more of this amount of caffeine. **Caffeine: 36–46 mg.** **Net Carbs 40 g**

12 oz (355 mL) diet cola

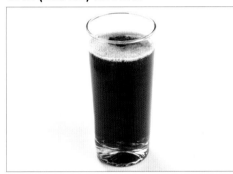

Calories	Carbs	Fiber	Fat	Sodium
4	1 g	0 g	0 g	18 mg

With zero sugar, this is the preferred choice over regular cola. However, diet cola, like regular cola, has added caffeine, and all colas have acids that can damage your teeth. Cola also has phosphates that, when consumed daily, can weaken your bones. **Caffeine: 39–50 mg.** **Net Carbs 1 g**

12 oz (355 mL) water

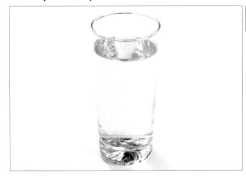

Calories	Carbs	Fiber	Fat	Sodium
0 g	0 g	0 g	0 g	11 mg

Water is the best choice! Fluoridated tap water can help keep your teeth strong. **Net Carbs 0 g**

HEALTHY CHOICE

FOOD FACT All unsweetened juices have a lot of natural sugar, so limit yourself to a ½-cup (125 mL) glass or choose a fresh fruit instead.

Chocolate and Nut Snacks

Super-sized (300 g) milk chocolate and nut bar

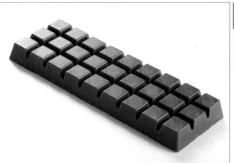

Calories	Carbs	Fiber	Fat	Sodium
1,620	180 g	12 g	96 g	120 mg

Some box stores now carry super-sized chocolate bars. If you are a chocolate fanatic and you buy one of these, you may eat the whole thing in a day or two, or sooner. Avoid the temptation by leaving it on the store shelf. **Net Carbs 168 g**

Large (100 g) milk chocolate and nut bar

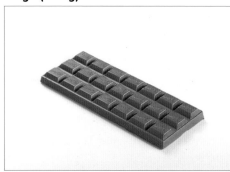

Calories	Carbs	Fiber	Fat	Sodium
522	55 g	2 g	35 g	69 mg

This is a smaller bar than the one above, but still has a whopping 522 calories. It's better to keep large chocolate bars out of sight and out of mind by not buying them in the first place. **Net Carbs 53 g**

Standard-size (43 g) milk chocolate and nut bar

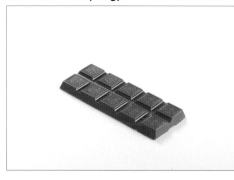

Calories	Carbs	Fiber	Fat	Sodium
240	22 g	1 g	15 g	30 mg

You can fit an "old-fashioned"-sized chocolate bar into your "treat budget." Enjoy one on occasion and don't feel guilty about it. **Net Carbs 21 g**

10 almonds and 2 small pieces (20 g total weight) of dark chocolate (80% cacao)

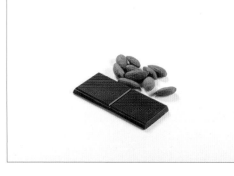

Calories	Carbs	Fiber	Fat	Sodium
176	6 g	3 g	15 g	7 mg

This small serving of almonds, along with a small amount of dark chocolate, would fit into the large snack group (pages 284–285). Chocolate with at least 80% cacao is a good choice, as cacao has healthy antioxidants. **Net Carbs 3 g**

HEALTHY CHOICE

FOOD FACT Chocolate is known for its antioxidants; cocoa is the source of these. Cocoa powder is much lower in fat than chocolate.

Other "Special Treat" Snacks

Large (220 g) bag of potato chips (about 110 chips) with ½ cup (125 mL) commercial chip dip

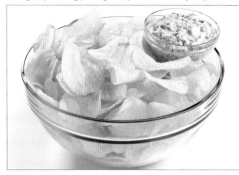

Calories	Carbs	Fiber	Fat	Sodium
1,468	124 g	8 g	103 g	2,283 mg

You are distracted when you watch TV, so you might easily get all the way through this large bag of potato chips. It's shocking to learn that this serving contains the equivalent of about $4\frac{1}{2}$ medium potatoes, 26 tsp (130 mL) of oil and more calories than some people need in an entire day. **Net Carbs 116 g**

Large (220 g) bag of cheese puffs or cheese twists (about 150)

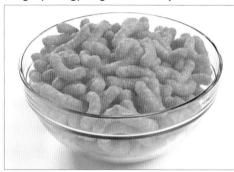

Calories	Carbs	Fiber	Fat	Sodium
1,219	118 g	2 g	76 g	1,940 mg

Don't be fooled into thinking cheese puffs have any cheese in them! Like potato chips, they are mostly starch, fat and salt. **Net Carbs 116 g**

Half of a large (220 g) bag of potato chips (about 55 chips)

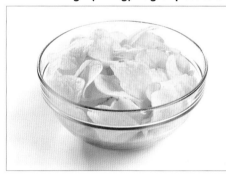

Calories	Carbs	Fiber	Fat	Sodium
614	56 g	4 g	42 g	722 mg

Cutting your portion of chips in half is a good change, as is skipping the dip. However, if you would like a dip with these chips, choose the Vegetable Dip or the low-salt Garlic Vegetable Dip on page 189. **Net Carbs 52 g**

Small (45 g) bag of potato chips (20 to 25 chips)

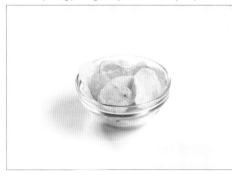

Calories	Carbs	Fiber	Fat	Sodium
241	22 g	2 g	16 g	240 mg

There are 20 to 25 chips in a bag this size, so if you have purchased a larger bag, try putting just that amount in a bowl for your snack. **Net Carbs 20 g**

HEALTHY CHOICE

FOOD FACT One single potato chip has about **1 g of carbohydrate. If you eat 30 chips,** it's like eating **2 slices of bread topped with 5 to 6 tsp (25 to 30 mL) of butter.**

Index